Presented

With the Compliments of

LABAZ: SANOFI UK LTD.

EPILEPTIC SYNDROMES

in INFANCY, CHILDHOOD and ADOLESCENCE

EPILEPTIC SYNDROMES
in INFANCY, CHILDHOOD and ADOLESCENCE

J Roger
(Marseille, France)

C Dravet
(Marseille, France)

M Bureau
(Marseille, France)

F E Dreifuss
(Charlottesville, USA)

P Wolf
(Berlin, FRG)

John Libbey
EUROTEXT
LONDON & PARIS

British Library Cataloguing in Publication Data

Epileptic syndromes in infancy, childhood and adolescence —
   (Current problems in epilepsy; 2)
   I. Epilepsy   II. Youth — Diseases
   I. Roger, J   II. Series
   616.8'53   RC372

ISBN 0-86196-045-9

[Cette edition est réalisée en francais
par John Libbey Eurotext sous le titre *Les syndromes
epileptiques de l'enfant et de l'adolescent*
ISBN 0-86196-046-7]

First English edition
Published by
John Libbey & Company Ltd.
80/84 Bondway, London SW8 1SF, England (01) 582 5266
John Libbey Eurotext Ltd.
6 rue Blanche, 92120 Montrouge, France (1) 657-38-38

Printed in Great Britain by
Whitstable Litho Ltd., Whitstable, Kent.

Preface

It is with pride and emotion that I preface this book devoted to the identification and classification of childhood epilepsies. With pride, because it finally clarifies a previously disordered domain. With emotion, since this work was conceived in the Centre Saint-Paul, the creation of which I proposed following the first meeting of WHO and ILAE experts concerning childhood epilepsies.

During this meeting the recommendation was made that specialized centres should be established with the aim of distinguishing the various epileptic forms hitherto poorly differentiated.

The publication of this work shows that the Centre Saint-Paul has not failed in this task: over a 23-year period it has received representatives of the European Leagues against Epilepsy who proposed, in April 1964, the International Classification of epileptic seizures which was adopted by the ILAE in 1970; and, in July 1983, the description and classification of childhood epilepsies presented in this book.

Acknowledgement from all epileptologists is due to Doctor Joseph Roger, who followed me as Director of the Centre Saint-Paul, and to Doctors Charlotte Dravet and Michelle Bureau who have been responsible for the initiative, organization and success of this major task.

Henri Gastaut

Introduction

The last 20 years have seen substantial advances in knowledge concerning the diagnosis as well as the long-term evolution of epilepsies in infants and children. More accurate observation of seizures, using simultaneous video-recording of the patients and of their EEG tracings, has permitted classification of some epileptic seizures in childhood and their incorporation in the Kyoto International Classification of Epileptic Seizures (1981). However, many gaps must yet be filled and video information concerning many seizure types is lacking.

Above all, there is no general agreement among epileptologists on the framework of the epileptic syndromes. There is little unanimity concerning definitions and what may be included under individual syndromic rubrics. Thus, some authors consider that almost all severe epilepsies in infancy and childhood may be included in the West and Lennox-Gastaut syndromes, using in such cases a variable terminology (for example: 'minor motor epilepsy') while others demand more rigorous criteria. Several syndromes have recently been described, but this information has not been widely disseminated, and these entities remain arcane. This is the case in severe myoclonic epilepsy, benign neo-natal convulsions, myoclonic absences, and epilepsy with continuous spike-waves during slow sleep, for example.

For these reasons a number of specialists working in the field of childhood epilepsy convened in order to review the different types of the childhood epilepsies and to try to more rigorously define a number of epileptic syndromes in infants, children and adolescents. This volume presents the proceedings of the first Workshop on Childhood Epileptology held at the Centre Saint-Paul, Marseille, France in July 1983. To realize the aim of elaborating a uniform terminology, it was felt to be important that such a definition of syndromes must be based on clinical, electroencephalographic, aetiological and evolution data, avoiding, in so far as possible, a consideration of those physiopathological concepts which are often purely hypothetical. It is essential for all researchers working in the field to use the same terminology and to know that if a case is classified as a West syndrome or as a Lennox-Gastaut syndrome by an author, it would not be classified elsewhere by other authors.

However, a classification of syndromes cannot ignore the ultimate place of each syndrome in a classification of the epilepsies, which must take the physiopathological data into account. Thus it is not surprising to see that the reviewers and discussants of the following chapters have used different words pending future classification of epilepsies which is under consideration by the ILAE Committee on Classification and Terminology. Some authors speak of 'primary' epilepsy while others use the word 'idiopathic', and 'secondary' epilepsy when others say 'symptomatic' or 'lesional'.

Because of the interaction between the syndrome classification activity and classification in progress, the members of the ILAE Committee on Classification and Terminology actively participated in the workshop.

As most epileptic syndromes of childhood are age-dependent, the program of the meeting followed a chronological order (neonate, infant, child, adolescent), though some syndromes may cover a larger range of ages.

In order to reduce the number of pages of the book, we have attempted to apportion the length of individual reports and discussions and keep these commensurate with the perceived importance of the topic in the scheme of things.

Implicit in such workshops is the awareness that many problems remain in spite of a few answers. Only the gathering of further data together with the long-term studies of such populations will allow validation of the practical viability of the syndromic classification.

There is no general agreement regarding some problems: what are the nosological limits between benign myoclonic epilepsy, severe myoclonic epilepsy, myoclonic-astatic petit mal and the Lennox-Gastaut syndrome? Is it possible to define an idiopathic West syndrome clearly different from the symptomatic West syndrome and what would be its nosological place? What are the electroclinical forms of symptomatic partial epilepsies in neo-nates and infants? Is it feasible to make a definitive differentiation between simple febrile convulsions and complicated febrile convulsions nosologically? Is there a type of epilepsy with unilateral seizures only?

All these problems will be discussed in further meetings on childhood epilepsy. However we do not pretend that all cases of childhood epilepsy can be subsumed under definite syndromes and recognize that a number of cases will, for the present, remain outside such a syndromic classification even if the elements can be identified and the individual seizures recorded.

The Editors

Acknowledgements

The editors are grateful to all the participants and especially to the chairmen who undertook to summarize the discussion.

They gratefully acknowledge the financial support provided by the Sanofi-Labaz Group, without which the workshop and this book could not have been realized.

They appreciate the technical assistance of the secretaries of the Centre Saint-Paul, the secretary of Sanofi Pharma International and the translators.

Particular thanks are due to Drs A. Perret and D. Brickwood who contributed significantly to the workshop and the publication.

Proceedings of the
International Workshop on Childhood Epileptology
Centre Saint-Paul, Marseille
7-10 July 1983

Participants

AICARDI, J. — France
BEAUMANOIR, A. — Switzerland
BINNIE, C.D. — The Netherlands
BUREAU, M. — France
CAVAZZUTI, G.B. — Italy
DALLA BERNARDINA, B. — Italy
DOOSE, H. — Federal Republic of Germany
DRAVET, C. — France
DREIFUSS, F.E. — USA
DULAC, O. — France
GASTAUT, H. — France
HENRIKSEN, O. — Norway
JEAVONS, P.M. — UK
LERMAN, P. — Israel
LIVET, M.O. — France
LOISEAU, P. — France
MARTINEZ-LAGE, M. — Spain
MONOD, N. — France
MUNARI, C. — France
O'DONOHOE, N.V. — Republic of Ireland
OLLER-DAURELLA, L. — Spain
PINSARD, N. — France
PLOUIN, P. — France
RAVNIK, I. — Yugoslavia
REVOL, M. — France
ROGER, J. — France
SEINO, M. — Japan
SOREL, L. — Belgium
TASSINARI, C.A. — Italy
WOLF, P. — Federal Republic of Germany

Authors

AICARDI, J. — INSERM U 12, Hôpital des Enfants Malades, 149 rue de Sèvres, 75743 Paris Cedex 14, France

AUBOURG, P. — Clinique de Pédiatrie et de Puériculture, Hôpital Saint-Vincent-de-Paul, 74 avenue Denfert-Rochereau, 75674 Paris Cedex 14, France

BANCAUD, J. — INSERM U-97, 2 ter rue d'Alésia, 75014 Paris, France

BEAUMANOIR, A. — Division Neurophysiologie Clinique, Hôpital Cantonal Universitaire, Genève, Switzerland

BUREAU, M. — Centre Saint-Paul, 300 boulevard Sainte-Marguerite, 13009 Marseille, France

CAPOVILLA, G. — Neuropsichiatria Infantile, Università di Verona, Borgo Roma, 37100 Verona, Italy

CAVAZZUTI, G.B. — Istituto di Clinicà Pediatricà, via del Pozzo 7, 41100 Modena, Italy

CHIAMENTI, C. — Neuropsichiatria Infantile, Università di Verona, Borgo Roma, 37100 Verona, Italy

COLAMARIA, V. — Neuropsichiatria Infantile, Università di Verona, Borgo Roma, 37100 Verona, Italy

DALLA BERNARDINA, B. — Neuropsichiatria Infantile, Università di Verona, Borgo Roma, 37100 Verona, Italy

DE MARCO, P. — Divisione di Neuropsichiatria Infantile, Ospedali Riuniti, Trento, Italy

DOOSE, H. — Universitäts Kinderklinik, Schwanenweg 20, 2300 Kiel 1, FRG

DRAVET, C. — Centre Saint-Paul, 300 boulevard Sainte-Marguerite, 13009 Marseille, France

DREIFUSS, F.E. — Department of Neurology, University of Virginia, Charlottesville, VA 22908, USA

DULAC, O. — Clinique de Pédiatrie et de Puériculture, Hôpital Saint-Vincent-de-Paul, 74 avenue Denfert-Rochereau, 75674 Paris Cedex 14, France

GASTAUT, H. — Institut de Recherches Neurologiques (Centre Collaborateur de l'OMS pour l'Enseignement et la Recherche en Neurologie), Faculté de Médecine, 13385 Marseille Cedex 5, France

HENRIKSEN, O. — Statens Senter for Epilepsi, 1301 Sandvika, Norway

JEAVONS, P. — Clinical Neurophysiology Unit, University of Aston in Birmingham, Woodcock Street, Birmingham B47 ET, UK

LERMAN, P. – EEG Department, Beilinson Medical Center, 76100 Petah Tiqva, Israel

LOISEAU, P. – Hôpital Pellegrin/Tripode, Place Amélie-Raba-Léon, 33076 Bordeaux, France

LOUISET, P. – Hôpital Pellegrin/Tripode, Place Amélie-Raba-Léon, 33076 Bordeaux, France

MAGAUDDA, A. – Clinicà Neurologicà, Università di Messina, Messina, Italy

MORIKAWA, T. – National Epilepsy Center, Shizuoka Higashi Hospital, 886 Urushiyama, Shizuoka (MZ 420), Japan

MUNARI, C. – INSERM U-97, 2 ter rue d'Alésia, 75014 Paris, France

O'DONOHOE, N.V. – Department of Paediatrics, National Children's Hospital, Harcourt Street, Dublin 2, Republic of Ireland

OLLER-DAURELLA, L. – Escuelas Pias, 89, Barcelona 17, Spain

OSAWA, T. – National Epilepsy Center, Shizuoka Higashi Hospital, 886 Urushiyama, Shizuoka (MZ 420), Japan

PLOUIN, P. – Laboratoire d'Explorations Fonctionnelles du Système Nerveux, Hôpital Saint-Vincent-de-Paul, 74 avenue Denfert-Rochereau, 75674 Paris Cedex 14, France

RAVNIK, I – Department of Child Neurology and Psychiatry, Laboratory for Functional Neurological Diagnostics, University Children's Hospital, Vrazov trg 1, Ljubljana, Yugoslavia

REVOL, M. – Service d'Explorations Fonctionnelles du Système Nerveux, Centre Hospitalier Lyon Sud, 69310 Pierre-Bénite, France

ROGER, J. – Centre Saint-Paul, 300 boulevard Sainte-Marguerite, 13009 Marseille, France

SEINO, M. – National Epilepsy Center, Shizuoka Higashi Hospital, 886 Urushiyama, Shizuoka (MZ 420), Japan

TASSINARI, C.A. – Clinicà Neurologicà di Bologna, Via Ugo Foscolo 7, Bologna, Italy

TREVISAN, E. – Neuropsichiatria Infantile, Università di Verona, Borgo Roma, 37100 Verona, Italy

WOLF, P. – Abteilung Neurologie, Klinikum Charlottenburg der FU Berlin, Spandauer Damm 130, D-1000 Berlin 19, FRG

YAGI, K. – National Epilepsy Center, Shizuoka Higashi Hospital, 886 Urushiyama, Shizuoka (MZ 420), Japan

Contents

I
Epileptic syndromes
in neonates

Epileptic syndromes in infancy, child-hood and adolescence. J. Roger, C. Dravet, M. Bureau, F.E. Dreifuss and P. Wolf. John Libbey Eurotext Ltd ©1985.

Chapter 1
Benign Neonatal Convulsions (Familial and Non-Familial)

Perrine PLOUIN

Laboratoire d'Explorations Fonctionnelles du Système Nerveux, Hôpital Saint-Vincent-de-Paul, 74 Avenue Denfert-Rochereau, 75014 Paris, France

Summary

Among benign neonatal convulsions, two syndromes may be individualized:
— Benign idiopathic neonatal convulsions (BINNC), occurring around the fifth day of life, at present without known etiology, with a favourable outcome; in most of cases EEG interictal abnormalities are 'théta pointu alternant';
— Benign familial neonatal convulsions (BFNNC), occurring mostly on the second and third days of life, with constant family history of epilepsy; the outcome is favourable but secondary epilepsy may occur (14 per cent); there is no specific EEG pattern.

Introduction

The purpose of this report is, using the results of the literature and our own experience, to decide whether or not two syndromes already described exist: benign idiopathic neonatal convulsions (BINNC) and benign familial neonatal convulsions (BFNNC).

In 1977, Dehan *et al.* focused attention on the existence of neonatal convulsions of unknown etiology and favourable outcome, occurring around the fifth day of life. But in 1980, Gastaut wrote that the electro-clinical characteristics of these convulsions were not precise enough to isolate them as an independent syndrome. In addition, since the first publication of Rett in 1964, several authors have reported new cases of BFNNC: do they represent separate syndromes or do they belong to other benign neonatal convulsions (NNC)?

Benign neonatal convulsions: definition criteria

Benign NNC are defined by their good prognosis, ie, a normal psychomotor development and the absence of secondary epilepsy. The first condition is easy to affirm but the second one is more difficult: a West syndrome occurring in the first months of life can be attributed to the NNC, but if hyperthermic convulsions or benign epilepsy occur, it can be difficult to decide whether or not they are the consequence of NNC. So how long is it necessary to follow these children to confirm that these NNC are benign? (Matsumoto *et al.* 1983).

In the neonatal period, however, several traits indicate a favourable prognosis: infrequent convulsions, normal neurological state between convulsions, normal or moderately altered interictal EEG and electro-clinical correlation of seizures. (Dreyfus-Brisac, 1979).

Neonatal convulsions: review of the literature

We first examined the results of studies published since 1959 about neonatal convulsions and neonatal status epilepticus in order to identify those which could be defined as BINNC. Of course we did not take into account convulsions occurring with metabolic disorders which are known to have a good prognosis as soon as the metabolic disturbances are recognized and treated (Cavazzuti, 1978).

For a diagnosis of BINNC we followed the criteria laid down by Dehan *et al.* (1977) (as far as their data allowed) — infants born after 39 weeks of gestation, APGAR index of 9 or above at the fifth minute of life, presence of a free interval between birth and beginning of convulsions, mean onset around the 104th hour (day 5), duration of the status epilepticus of around 20 hours, clonic and/or apneic seizures, 'théta pointu alternant' on the interictal EEG (75 per cent of the first study of Dehan *et al.* 1977), all other examinations negative, and favourable outcome (see Table 1).

Table 1. *Neonatal convulsions: review of the literature*

Authors	Collection period	Number of cases
Craig	< 1959	374
Harris *et al.*	< 1960	41
Schulte	1961-64	57
Tibbles *et al.*	1955-65	135
Monod *et al.*	1953-68	154
Keen, 1969	1967-69	100
Rose *et al.*	< 1970	137
Keen *et al.* 1973	1967-70	112
Dennis	1970-72	56
Brown	1970-72	142
Gilly *et al.*	< 1973	80
Combes *et al.*	< 1975	174
Eriksson *et al.*	1970-76	77
Watanabe *et al.*	1968-78	282
Dreyfus-Brisac *et al.*	1974-79	121
Total 15	1959-1979	2042

There is a great disparity in the methods of the 15 analysed publications. Most of them do not indicate the results of the EEG; some studies take into account only the convulsions occurring in the first 10 days of life, others all convulsions occurring during the first month. Another problem is that these studies took place between 1959 and 1979, and progress in diagnosis and treatment of NNC has been substantial in these 20 years, so that NNC of unknown etiology in the sixties could have been diagnosed on the basis of etiology in the late seventies.

Among the 2042 cases reported in these 15 studies we found 224 without etiology (mean: 11 per cent, 0 to 37 per cent according to the different authors). The outcome is known in 195 of the 224 cases and is favourable for 120 (mean: 62 per cent, 28 to 93 per cent according to the different authors): it thus appears that NNC of unknown etiology are more likely to have a good outcome than a poor one. Over the 2042 cases the outcome is known for 1807; so NNC of unknown etiology and favourable outcome would seem to represent 6.6 per cent (120 of 1807) of NNC (0 to 28 per cent according to the different authors).

When considering those 120 cases we tried to focus on two important criteria of Dehan *et al.* (1977): the date of onset of convulsions and the interictal aspect of the EEG. The date of onset is only known for 37 infants, 33 of whom began to convulse between d3 and d6. EEG is described in 39 cases: normal in 15 cases, focal or multifocal abnormalities in 13 cases (without precision), with 'théta pointu alternant' pattern found in 11 cases. No traces with a poor prognosis were reported (Monod *et al.* 1972; Plouin *et al.* 1977).

From this, we can conclude that BINNC seem to have already been reported in the literature before they were described in 1977 by Dehan *et al.* Their prevalence can be evaluated around 7 per cent, perhaps only 2 per cent if we only take into account the cases for which the date of occurrence and the interictal EEG patterns are known.

Benign idiopathic neonatal convulsions described in the literature as 'fifth day fits'

Since the first report of Dehan *et al.* (1977), several workers have reported such convulsions, either in France(André *et al.* 1978; Dreyfus-Brisac *et al.*, 1981; Navelet *et al.*, 1981; Plouin *et al.*, 1981) or in Australia (Pryor *et al.* 1981). Table 2 records the 182 cases that have been reported.

Table 2. Benign idiopathic neonatal convulsions

Authors	Collection period	Number of cases
Dehan *et al.*	1973-76	20
Andre *et al.*	1972-76	4
Pryor *et al.*	1973-77	90
Dreyfus-Brisac *et al*	1974-79	11
Plouin *et al.*	1966-80	39
Navelet *et al.*	1976-80	18
Total *n* = 6	1966-1980	182

The prevalence of BINNC is extremely variable from study to study and probably depends on the way patients are recruited by the different authors: it varies from 4 to 20 per cent of NNC. Twenty per cent is certainly excessive; the 4 per cent figure is in better agreement with the 2-6 per cent range estimated above.

The sex ratio is known for 139 infants and shows a majority of boys (*n* = 86; 62 per cent).

In all cases the convulsions occurred between d 1 and d 7, 80 per cent between d 4 and d 6, and 95 per cent between d 3 and d 7.

When described, the convulsions are always of a clonic type, mostly partial, and/or apneic, never tonic. Convulsions are often lateralized, changing side, and rarely generalized. They last from one to three minutes. They are repeated frequently, leading to a status epilepticus. The mean duration of status epilepticus is about 20 h, but can be shorter (2 h) or longer (up to 3 days).

The neurological state of the infants is usually normal between the convulsions at the beginning of the status epilepticus. Then, infants become drowsy, hypotonic, but the various antiepileptic drugs given to stop the convulsions may be responsible for this. Drowsiness and hypotonia may last several days after the end of the status epilepticus. Then, the infants return to a normal neurological state.

Interictal EEG patterns are described in 101 cases among the 182 published. The interictal EEG was normal in 10 infants, discontinuous in 6, and showed 'focal or multifocal' abnormalities in 25 cases. In the other 60 infants the 'théta pointu alternant' pattern was present (Fig. 1). This pattern was first described by Dehan *et al.* (1977) as a dominant théta activity, which is alternating or discontinuous, unreactive, with sharp waves and frequent interhemispheric asynergy. The maturational age cannot be precisely defined. The pattern can be present when the patient is awake as well as during active or quiet sleep: it is then difficult to differentiate between the two stages of sleep. When the convulsions have stopped, the 'théta pointu alternant' pattern can be recorded up to the 12th day and it is possible to contemplate diagnosis of BINNC even if the EEG is performed after the end of the status epilepticus. The 'théta pointu alternant' pattern can be seen in other neonatal status epilepticus (hypocalcemia, neonatal meningitis, subarachnoid hemorrhage) and cannot be considered as specific to BINNC (Navelet *et al.*, 1981; Poulin, unpublished data). Nevertheless it is associated with a good prognosis.

Seizures have been recorded in most of the 101 cases (Fig. 2). They last from 1 to 3 minutes and have no remarkable features. They can be localized in any area but are found on the rolandic area in the majority of cases. They can be strictly unilateral, immediately generalized, or first localized and then generalized. Electro-clinical seizures or sub-clinical discharges can be seen, as well as clinical seizures without EEG

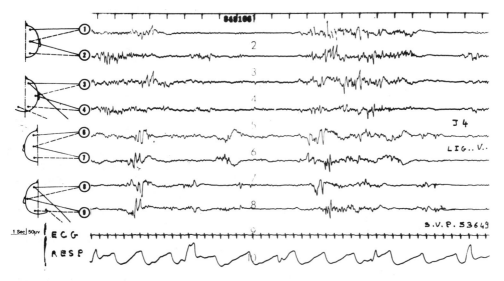

Fig. 1. Interictal EEG in a 4-day-old infant with BINNC; 'théta pointu alternant' pattern: bursts of théta rhythms mostly on rolandic areas, often asynchronous, record speed: 15mm/s.

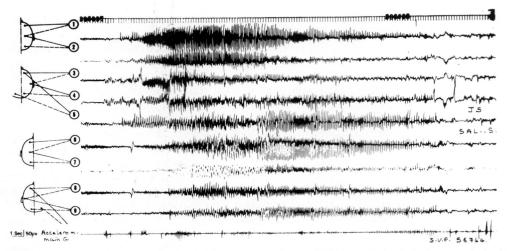

Fig. 2. Recorded seizures in a 5-day-old infant with BINNC; left hand clonic jerks recorded with an accelerometer (last channel); record speed: 2.5mm/s.

discharges. At the beginning of the status epilepticus seizures are clinical and/or electro-clinical, and at the end sub-clinical discharges may persist up to several hours. The EEG patterns during seizures are essentially rhythmic spikes or rhythmic slow waves. No alpha-like ictal activity has been recorded.

Many anti-epileptic drugs have been used for these BINNC, often in association: phenobarbitone, phenytoin, diazepam, paraldehyde, chloral hydrate, clomethiazole, clonazepam. Treatments have not had a consistent effect on the duration of seizures. Most often the convulsions stopped without treatment, but occasionally the end seemed to be related to administration of diazepam or phenytoin. Now Dehan proposes not to treat these infants if alternative diagnoses have been eliminated.

The differential diagnosis is of major importance. BINNC remains a diagnosis of exclusion and any other etiology must be sought, such as metabolic disturbances, neonatal meningitis and viral infections.

Only one etiologic hypothesis is proposed by Goldberg and Sheehy (1983) who, after a three-year prospective study, found that there was an acute zinc deficiency in the CSF of infants suffering from BINNC when compared with a group of infants in whom a cause of convulsions had been identified, and with another group of infants without convulsions but with other health problems. No other hypothesis, viral, toxic or metabolic has been confirmed.

This syndrome must be isolated with regard to all the clinical and paraclinical elements which compose it. Its recognition allows one to forecast a favourable neurological outcome. However the 'théta pointu alternant' EEG pattern is present in only 60 per cent of cases and is not specific. Finally, the long-term favourable outcome must be confirmed by more numerous and more extensive studies. The 90 cases recorded by Pryor *et al.* (1981) have not been followed up beyond the neonatal period. Other infants (92) were followed from 3 months to 6 years: in five cases a transitory psychomotor retardation was noted until the age of one year, one child had a hyperthermic convulsion and another one a convulsion without fever at the age of 3 (Dehan *et al.* (1982). In six other children, between the age of $2^{1}/_{2}$ and 6, foci of spikes appeared on the EEG with no clinical seizures.

Benign familial neonatal convulsions

Eighty-three observations of BFNNC have been reported in the literature since the first paper by Rett *et al.* (1964). We have added two families seen at Saint Vincent de Paul's hospital, which gives us 87 individuals, belonging to 14 families. The number of generations affected varies from 1 to 5. (Table 3).

It is not possible to define the prevalence of these BFNNC as they are not compared with other NNC in any study.

The date of occurrence of the convulsions is precisely known in only 49 cases: 80 per cent of them start on the 2nd and the 3rd days of life. But one infant began to convulse on the 21st day, another at one month of age and three at 3 months of age.

In documented cases (49) birth was at full-term with normal birthweight. There was always a free interval between birth and occurrence of convulsions. The sex-ratio, based upon 77 cases, shows a majority of boys (43) against 34 girls.

No etiology was found except one case with a transitory hypomagnesemia.

When described, seizures are of a clonic type, sometimes with apneic spells. One case of tonic seizures is reported. These seizures are short (lasting from 1 to 3 minutes), repeated frequently up to the 7th day, and some isolated seizures can occur during the following weeks.

The EEG is described in only 14 cases. In three cases seizures have been recorded: they do not seem to have any particular character. The interictal EEG is normal in four cases, discontinuous in three cases, with focal or multifocal abnormalities in six cases and with 'théta pointu alternant' pattern in one case. Patterns suggesting a poor prognosis such as a paroxysmal or an inactive EEG have never been reported.

The outcome of these BFNNC is favourable with regard to the psychomotor development. But in 11 cases (14 per cent) epilepsy developed in infancy (five cases), in childhood (three cases) and in adulthood (three cases). Different authors give only few details about the symptomatology of these seizures; usually they are rare and easily controlled by medication. No case with severe epilepsy has been reported. In five other cases febrile convulsions took place.

Table 3. Benign familial neonatal convulsions

Authors	Date of publication	Cases in each family (No. of generations)	
Rett *et al.*	1964	8	(3)
Bjerre *et al.*	1968	14	(5)
Steejohnsen	<1968	8	(?)
Rose *et al.*	1975	3	(3)
Goutieres	1977	8	(3)
		2	(1)
Carton	1978	9	(4)
Quattelbaum	1979	15	(4)
Pettit *et al.*	1980	5	(3)
Tibbles	1980	2	(2)
		6	(2)
		3	(2)
Plouin (in this report)	1983	2	(2)
		2	(1)

Total, 1964–1983: 87 cases, 14 families

Studies of families with several affected generations and with a sufficient number of siblings, show an equal sex-ratio and a probability around 1/2, confirming the dominant autosomal character of the transmission.

BFNNC are different from BINNC on several counts:
— the family history, (neonatal epilepsy or later epilepsy) is constant in BFNNC, but is rare in BINNC (2 per cent),
— age of occurrence is earlier in BFNNC (d 2, d 3,) than in BINNC (d 4, d 5),
— persistence of convulsions is longer in BFNNC,
— occurrence of secondary epilepsy is more frequent in BFNNC (14 per cent) compared to 0.5 per cent in BINNC.

These two syndromes must be considered as different. They must be identified and recognized because they allow to forecast a favourable neurological outcome from the neonatal period.

References

André, M., Vert, P., Bouchez, T. (1978): A propos des convulsions du cinquième jour. *Archs Franc. Péd.* **35**, 922-923.

Bjerre, I., Corelius, E. (1968): Benign familial neonatal convulsions. *Acta Paediatr. Scand.* **57**, 557-561.

Brown, J.K. (1973): Convulsions in the newborn period. *Develop. Med. Child Neurol.* **15**, 823-846.

Carton, D. (1978): Benign familial neonatal convulsions. *Neuropädiatrie* **9**, 167-171.

Cavazzuti, G.B. (1978): Nosologia ed etiologia delle convulsioni del neonato. *Boll. Lega It. Epil.* **22-23**, 95-98.

Combes, J.C., Rufo, M., Vallade, M.J., Pinsard, N., Bernard, R. (1975): Les convulsions néonatales. Circonstances d'apparition et critères de pronostic. *Pédiatrie* **30**, 477-492.

Craig, W.S. (1960): Convulsive movements occurring in the first ten days of life. *Archs Dis. Child.* **35**, 336-344.

Dehan, M., Quilleron, D., Navelet, Y., D'Allest, A.M., Vial, M., Retbi, J.M., Lelong-Tisier, M.C., Gabilan, J.C. (1977): Les convulsions du 5e jour de vie: un nouveau syndrome? *Archs Franc. Péd.* **34**, 730-742.

Dehan, M., Navelet, Y., D'Allest, A.M., Vial, M., Ropert, J.C., Boulley, A.M., Gabilan, J.C. (1982): Quelques précisions sur le syndrome des convulsions du 5ème jour de vie. *Archs Franc. Péd.* **39**, 405-407.

Dennis, J. (1978): Neonatal convulsions: aetiology, late neonatal status and long term outcome. *Develop. Med. Child Neurol.* **20**, 143-158.

Dreyfus-Brisac, C. (1979): Neonatal electroencephalography. In *Reviews in perinatal medicine,* vol. 3, ed E.M. Scarpelli, E.V. Cosmi, pp 397-412. Raven Press: New York.

Dreyfus-Brisac, C., Peschanski, N., Radvanyi, M.F., Cukier-Hemeury, F., Monod, N. (1981): Convulsions du nouveau-né. Aspects clinique, électroencéphalographique, étiopathogénique et pronostique. *Rev. EEG Neurophysiol.* **11**, 367-378.

Eriksson, M., Zetterstom, R. (1979): Neonatal convulsions. *Acta Paediatr. Scand.* **68**, 807-811.

Gastaut, H. (1981): Individualisation des épilepsies dites bénignes ou fonctionnelles aux différents âges de la vie. Appréciation des variations correspondantes de la prédisposition épileptique à ces âges. *Rev. EEG Neurophysiol.* **11**, 346-366.

Gilly, R., Revol, M., Dutruge, J., Mamelle, J.C., Challamel, M.J. (1973): Convulsions et états de mal du nouveau-né. *Lyon Médical* **229**, 357-366.

Goldberg, H.J., Sheehy, E.M. (1983): Fifth day fits: an acute zinc deficiency syndrome? *Archs Dis. Child.* **57**, 633-635.

Goutières, F. (1977): Convulsions néonatales familiales bénignes. In *Congrès de la Société de Neurologie Infantile,* pp 281-286. Diffusion Générale de Librairie: Marseille.

Harris, R., Tizard, J.P.M. (1960): The electroencephalogram in neonatal convulsions. *J. Pediatr.* **57**, 501-520.

Keen, J.H. (1969): Significance of hypocalcaemia in neonatal convulsions. *Archs Dis. Child.* **44,** 356-361.

Keen, J.H., Lee, D. (1973): Sequelae of neonatal convulsions: study of 112 infants. *Archs Dis. Child.* **48,** 542-546.

Matsumoto, A., Watanabe, K., Sugiura, M., Negoro, T., Takaesu, E., Iwase, K. (1983): Long term prognosis of convulsive disorders in the first year of life: mental and physical development and seizures persistance. *Epilepsia* **24,** 321-329.

Monod, N., Dreyfus-Brisac, C., Sfaello, Z. (1969): Dépistage et pronostic de l'Etat de Mal néonatal. *Archs Franc. Péd.* **26,** 1085-1102.

Monod, N., Pajot, N., Giudasci, S. (1972): The neonatal EEG: statistical studies and prognostic value in full-term and pre-term babies. *Electroenceph. Clin. Neurophysiol.* **32,** 529-544.

Navelet, Y., D'Allest, A.M., Dehan, M., Gabilan, J.C. (1981): A propos du syndrome des convulsions néonatales du cinquième jour. *Rev. EEG Neurophysiol.* **11,** 390-396

Pettit, R.E., Fenichel, G.M. (1980): Benign familial neonatal seizures. *Archs Neurol.* **37,** 47-48.

Plouin, P., Moussali, F., Lerique, A., Mises, J., Lavoisy, P., Navelet, Y. (1977): Evolution clinique après un tracé néonatal considéré comme grave. *Rev. EEG Neurophysiol.* **7,** 410-415.

Plouin, P., Sternberg, B., Bour, F., Lerique, A. (1981): Etats de mal néonataux d'étiologie indéterminée. *Rev. EEG Neurophysiol.* **11,** 385-389.

Pryor, D.S., Don, N., Macourt, D.C. (1981): Fifth day fits: a syndrome of neonatal convulsions. *Archs Dis. Child.* **56,** 753-758.

Quattlebaum, T.G. (1979): Benign familial convulsions in the neonatal period and early infancy. *J. Pediatr.* **95,** 257-259.

Rett, A., Teubel, R. (1964): Neugeborenen Krampfe im Rahmen einer epileptisch belasten Familie. *Wien. Klin. Wschr.* **76,** 609-613.

Rose, A.L., Lombroso, C.T. (1970): Neonatal seizure states. A study of clinical pathology and EEG features in 137 full-term babies with a long term follow-up. *Pediatrics* **45,** 405-425.

Schulte, F.J. (1966): Neonatal convulsions and their relation to epilepsy in early childhood. *Develop. Med. Child Neurol.* **8,** 381-392.

Tibbles, J.A.R., Prichard, J.S. (1965): The prognostic value of the electroencephalogram in neonatal convulsions. *Pediatrics* **35,** 778-786.

Tibbles, J.A.R. (1980): Dominant benign neonatal seizures. *Develop. Med. Child Neurol.* **22,** 664-667.

Watanabe, K., Kuroyanagi, M., Hara, K., Miyazaki, S. (1982): Neonatal seizures and subsequent epilepsy. *Brain & Development* **4,** 341-346.

*　　　　　*　　　　　*

Discussion
Summarized by Perrine PLOUIN

Dr *Monod* opened the discussion.

Aicardi: a risk exists of a closed loop thought process since the exposed population is ill-defined: the percentage of cases of benign outcome is difficult to calculate when they are not compared with cases with similar initial signs but with an unfavourable outcome. This criticism holds for all the epileptic syndromes presently discussed.

Martinez-Lage: what are the immediate and long-term treatments used in BINNC and BFNNC?

Plouin: the most widely used treatments for status epilepticus have been diazepam and phenytoin. As a rule treatment is discontinued at the end of the status epilepticus, but in some studies it has been prolonged up to the third month. Concerning the first question, the definition of benign NNC does not exclude symptomatic convulsions with benign outcome. The evaluation of the percentage of BINNC among NNC is given in three studies: *Dehan* (20 percent), *Plouin* (16 per cent of recorded status epilepticus) and *Dreyfus-Brisac* (7 per cent).

Sorel: to define an epileptic syndrome, is it necessary to rely on strict electro-clinical associations, or, taking into account mostly the clinical outcome, must we describe atypical or incomplete forms? The Gaussian distribution of the date of onset of seizures must be emphasized. The familial component is not necessarily a criterion of a benign epilepsy.

Plouin: long term outcome is reported in 50 per cent only of BINNC. Until what age is it necessary to follow these children to rule out a secondary epilepsy?

Munari: what is the prognosis in the case of seizures with an electro-clinical correlation?

Plouin: Port Royal's team has shown a better outcome when an electro-clinical correlation is present.

Beaumanoir: what is the percentage of children followed up to the age of 6 among the 2042 cases of NNC?

Plouin: 1807 have been followed from the age of 3 months to 6 years, but few of them up to 6 years.

Revol: can the 'théta pointu alternant' EEG pattern be differentiated from the physiological 'tracé alternant' during quiet sleep in full-term newborns?

Plouin: this pattern can be seen during quiet sleep and in some records devoid of the physiological lability; such records can be connected with the effect of drugs.

Dalla Bernardina: what is the percentage of favourable outcome in status epilepticus with unknown aetiology?

Plouin: 80 per cent in my own material; 62 per cent in all 15 studies I have reported; this leaves 20 to 38 per cent of cases with poor outcome.

Wolf: the common clinical characteristics of this syndrome are clonic or apneic seizures. Are both types present in the same infant?

Plouin: in one given infant, seizures may be clonic, apneic, or clonic and apneic.

Dreifuss: apneic and clonic (but not multifocal) neonatal convulsions have a good outcome in 60 to 70 per cent of cases, mostly when the interictal EEG is normal.

Plouin: when tonic seizures are present, prognosis is indeed worse.

Ravnik: emphasizes that many works concerning NNC do not refer to EEG although the prognostic usefulness of EEG has been documented for over 30 years.

Cavazzuti: presented his film on the semiological differences between convulsions which are secondary to anoxic or ischaemic encephalopathy, and benign convulsions.

In the first situation (anoxic or ischaemic encephalopathy), the infants are in a state of coma. The seizures are polymorphous: violent, symmetrical or non-symmetrical myoclonic jerks involving all four limbs. With these are associated clonus of the eyelids, jerking of the eyeballs, jerking of the diaphragm and axial tonic spasm. This polymorphism, combined with a dissociation between clinical signs and EEG tracings, indicates a poor prognosis.

A case of benign convulsions of undetermined etiology beginning on 9th day of life is then presented: the seizures are mainly clonic, of varying localizations, and correlated with EEG discharges localized on the opposite hemisphere. The clonic nature of the seizures, associated with a correlation of clinical signs with EEG tracings, indicates a good prognosis.

The final case shown is of ante-natal encephalopathy with cerebral atrophy found at autopsy. The child is extremely hypertonic. The seizures are characterized by bouts of polypnea, abnormal eye movements and massive myoclonus.

The characteristics of the seizures may enable differentiation, in a certain number of cases, between seizures with benign evolution and those with unfavourable outcome.

Epileptic syndromes in infancy, childhood and adolescence. J. Roger, C. Dravet, M. Bureau, F.E. Dreifuss and P. Wolf. John Libbey Eurotext Ltd ©1985.

Chapter 2
Early Myoclonic Encephalopathy

Jean AICARDI

INSERM U12, Hôpital des Enfants Malades, 149 rue de Sèvres, 75743 Paris Cedex 14, France

Summary

Twenty-five cases of early myoclonic encephalopathy including 7 unpublished cases are reviewed. The onset is almost always in the neonatal period, and the ictal manifestations include: (1) fragmentary or partial erratic myoclonus; (2) massive myoclonias; (3) partial motor seizures; (4) tonic infantile spasms. The EEG manifestations include complex bursts of spikes, sharp waves and slow waves, separated by episodes of flattening of the tracing and localized discharges resembling usual neonatal seizure discharges. The EEG later evolves into atypical hypsarrhythmia. All infants are severely abnormal neurologically and more than half of them die before one year of age. Early myoclonic encephalopathy is a syndrome with several causes, one of the most important being non-ketotic hyperglycinaemia. The relationship between early myoclonic encephalopathy and early infantile epileptic encephalopathy, as described by Ohtahara, is discussed.

Introduction

A syndrome characterized clinically by the occurrence of erratic, fragmentary myoclonus of early onset, in association with other types of seizures (especially partial motor seizures and massive myoclonias or infantile spasms), and electroencephalographically by the so-called suppression-burst pattern was first described in five patients by Aicardi and Goutières (1978). Thirteen additional cases have since been reported under various names: neonatal myoclonic encephalopathy (Vigevano *et al.* 1981); myoclonic encephalopathy with neonatal onset (Cavazzuti *et al.* 1978); neonatal epileptic encephalopathy with periodic EEG bursts (Martin *et al.*, 1981); early myoclonic epileptic encephalopathy (Dalla Bernardina *et al.*, 1982, 1983). These 18 reported cases, together with 7 new personal patients, observed since 1978, form the basis of this study. Analysis of these 25 cases has permitted a more precise delineation of the syndrome but its etiology remains unknown. A few atypical cases (Cansiani *et al.*, 1982; Menegati *et al.*, 1982; Turcker and Solitare, 1963) have not been included, although they were reported as early myoclonic encephalopathy or shared several features with the typical cases.

Table. Early myoclonic encephalopathy-reported cases

Authors		Sex	Age of onset (days)	Familial involvement	Course	Remarks
Aicardi and Goutières (1978)	Case 1	F	1	One affected brother	Died 2 mnth	
	Case 2	M	5		Died 4 yr. 1 mnth	
	Case 3	M	4		Living at 11 mnth (vegetative)	
	Case 4	M		One affected brother died at 2.5 mnth	Died 2 mnth	Poliodystrophy at post-mortem
	Case 5	M			Died 3 mnth	Minor cortical malformations
Cavazzuti *et al.* (1978)		F	1/2		Died 9 mnth	
Martin *et al.*(1981)		F	4		Died 13 mnth	
Dalla Bernardina *et al.* (1982, 1983)	Case 1	M	28	Brother of case 2	Died 23 mnth	
	Case 2	M	15	Brother of case 1	Died 6.5 mnth	
	Case 3	F	2		Died 26 mnth	X-linked disease (Menkes) in same family
	Case 4	F	70		Alive at 37 mnth	
	Case 5	M	4		Alive at 20 mnth	
	Case 6	F	7		Alive at 20 mnth	
	Case 7	F	2	One brother died 8 mo. from epileptic encephalopathy	Alive at 23 mnth	
	Case 8	F	8		Died 2 mnth	
	Case 9	F	4		Died 2 mnth	
Vigevano *et al.* (1981)		M	7		Died 4 mnth	
Vigevano *et al.* (1982)		M	4		Died 2 mnth 20 days	High levels of propionic acid in blood
Alcardi (1983)	Case 6	F	1		Died 37 mnth	
	Case 7	M	2	Brother of case 8	Died 17 mnth	
	Case 8	M	1	Brother of case 7	Living at 22 mnth (vegetative state)	
	Case 9	M	45		Living at 23 mnths (vegetative state)	Progressive cerebral atrophy
	Case 10	F	10		Died 13 mnth	
	Case 11	F	2	Sister of case 12	Living 4 yr 11 mnth (severely retarded)	
	Case 12	F	30	Sister of case 11	Living 3 yr 7 mnth	

13

Clinical and EEG manifestations

The main data on these patients are shown in the table. The onset of the syndrome is either neonatal, i.e. during the first 28 days of life (23 cases) or early infantile, before the age of three months (2 cases).

The ictal manifestations include: (1) fragmentary or partial erratic myoclonus; (2) massive myoclonias; (3) simple partial seizures; (4) infantile spasms of a tonic type. Erratic, partial myoclonus usually constitutes the first ictal manifestation and may appear as early as a few hours of life (case 3). The jerks may involve the face or limbs. They may be restricted to a very limited territory, e.g. one finger or eyebrow, or they may affect a whole limb. In most patients, the jerks are frequently repeated or almost continuous. They may persist during sleep (Dalla Bernardina *et al.,* 1982, 1983) and shift incessantly from one part of the body to another in an anarchic and asynchronous manner. Occasionally the jerks are few and are seen only with prolonged observation. Massive (bilateral) myoclonias are not mentioned in all reports. They may appear early in the course and alternate with the erratic jerks. The occurrence of partial seizures has been especially emphasized by Dalla Bernardina *et al.* (1982, 1983). Their clinical expression may be very limited, for example to a deviation of the eyes with or without clonias, or to autonomic phenomena (apnea, flushing of the face). These partial seizures usually follow rapidly the appearance of erratic myoclonus. Infantile spasms

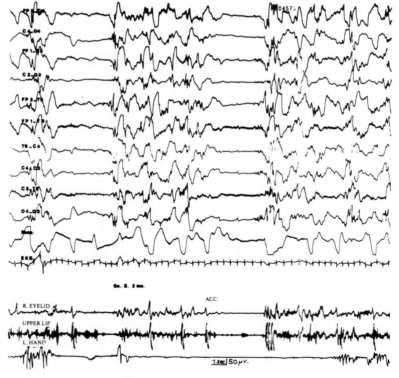

Fig. 1. Case 8 — Suppression-burst pattern with asynchronous erratic myoclonias of the face and arms: (Acc: Accelerometer).

of a tonic type almost always appear later than the other types of seizures, usually around 3-4 months of age. They occur in wakefulness and occasionally in sleep, in a repetitive manner.

The *EEG manifestations* of early myoclonic encephalopathy are distinctive. There is no normal background activity and the tracings, both in the waking and sleeping states, consist only of complex bursts of spikes, sharp waves and slow waves irregularly intermingled, lasting 1 to 5 seconds, and separated by episodes of flattening of the tracing which becomes almost inactive (Fig. 1) and last from 3 to 10 seconds. The paroxysmal bursts may occur synchronously or asynchronously over both hemispheres. They tend to be shorter in the initial phase of the disorder. Their individual components (spikes or sharp waves) are never bilaterally synchronous. The paroxysmal bursts of this suppression-burst pattern are not synchronous with the jerks of the erratic myoclonus (Fig. 1). They may occur synchronously with massive myoclonus (Martin *et al.*, 1981 and Fig. 2). The partial seizures have the usual EEG features of neonatal fits. The spike discharges remain localized to part of one hemisphere. During these seizures, the suppression burst pattern may persist unchanged (Fig. 3). The suppression-burst pattern tends to be replaced by atypical hypsarrhythmia or by a tracing of multifocal paroxysms after the first 3-5 months of life. Infantile spasms which also occur at this time may not have EEG concomitants.

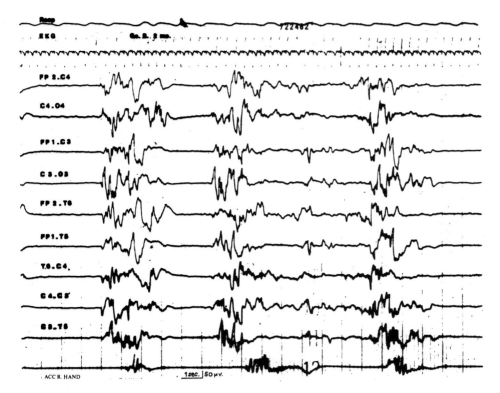

Fig. 2. Case 8 — Suppression-burst EEG pattern with myoclonias of the right hand roughly synchronous with the paroxysmal bursts. Myoclonias always follow the EEG burst with a slightly variable latency (Acc: Accelerometer).

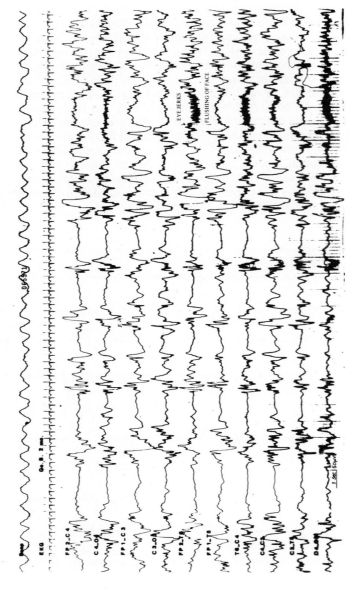

Fig. 3. (A) Case 8 – Onset of a *right* temporo-frontal discharge at 10 c/s. Note the persistence of the suppression-burst pattern.

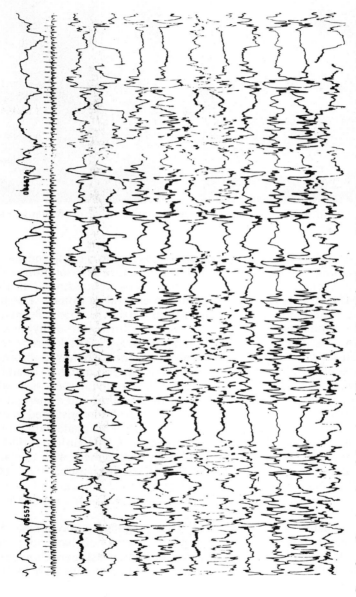

Fig. 3. (B) Case 8 — Continuation of the seizure (20 seconds after 3A). Note eyelid jerks, irregular respiration and high voltage spikes and spike-wave complexes more marked over posterior part of the *left* hemisphere.

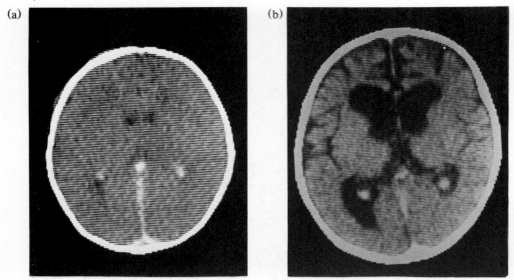

Fig. 4. Case 9 — (a) Normal CT scan image at age 2 months; (b) Gross dilatation of ventricles and sulci at age 12 months.

The *neurological status* of affected infants is always severely compromised from birth or from the beginning of seizures in cases of later onset. A deterioration or an arrest of developmental performances has been reported (Dalla Bernardina *et al.* 1982, 1983) but is indeed difficult to appreciate owing to the early age of onset. The progressive character of the symptomatology which is emphasized by Dalla Bernardina *et al.* (1983) is, for the same reason, almost impossible to affirm. Marked hypotonia of truncal muscles is the rule, but hypertonia of the limbs and at times decerebrate posturing may develop. Head circumference was normal at birth whenever information was available, but moderate microcephaly developed in several patients. Bilateral pyramidal tract signs were constantly present. Mental development was essentially nil. Involvement of peripheral nerves, with signs of denervation and a marked slowing of both motor and sensory nerve conduction velocities, was demonstrated in one familial case (case 8). Neuroradiological examination (pneumoencephalography or CT scan) was initially normal in most studied patients. In one case (Martin *et al.*, 1981), CT scan showed an asymmetrical enlargement of the right hemisphere with dilatation of the corresponding lateral ventricle. In five patients (Dalla Bernardina *et al.*, 1982, 1983; Aicardi, case 9), repeated scanning showed progressive cortical and periventricular atrophy (Fig. 4). In several patients, however, repeated CT scan examination was consistently normal.

The course in all patients studied so far, has been regularly unfavourable. Several patients have died before one or two years of age. Most survivors have not been followed up for long periods but all were in a vegetative state when last seen. Conventional antiepileptic drugs as well as ACTH or cortico-steroids and pyridoxine were ineffective.

Etiological data.

The incidence of early myoclonic encephalopathy is unknown. The condition is certainly rare. The syndrome has been observed in both sexes (11 boys and 14 girls). The most remarkable fact is the frequent occurrence of familial cases. In 4 of our 10 families, two siblings were affected and this was also the case in 2 of the 8 families of Dalla Benardina *et al.* (1983). The parents of affected siblings have always been healthy and no case of parental consanguinity is on record. Thus, although an autosomal recessive inheritance appears likely, at least in some of the cases, it has not been proved so far. In no case were obstetrical complications or perinatal abnormalities present. Neuropathological examination in one of our familial cases (case 1) showed a drop out of cortical neurones and an astrocytic proliferation consistent with a diagnosis of non-specific poliodystrophy. Familial cases of non-specific poliodystrophy have been reported (Alpers, 1960; Christensen and Hojgaard, 1964; Greenhouse and Neuburger, 1964; Jellinger and Seitelberger, 1970) so the pathological data in this patient are consistent with the hypothesis of a genetic disorder recessively transmitted. In the first patient of Vigevano *et al.* (1982), severe multifocal spongy changes in the white matter and PAS-positive perivascular concentric bodies were noted. These changes also seem consistent with a metabolic, possibly familial, disorder, although this was an isolated case. In the second patient of the same worker (1982), there was a marked poverty of myelin without spongiosis in the cerebral hemispheres but not in the spinal cord. In other patients, however, the neuropathological appearance was that of a malformation. Thus in our patient 3, minor disturbances of neuronal migration (imperfect lamination of the deeper cortical layers with occasional small heterotopias) were noted. In the patient of Martin *et al.* (1981) hemimegalencephaly with astrocytic proliferation, but without disturbance of the cortical architectonics, was present. In 2 patients of Dalla Bernardina *et al.* (1983) no striking abnormality was evident at post-mortem examination.

Laboratory investigations, including amino-acid and organic acid studies, lysosomal enzyme studies, very long chain fatty acid determinations, detailed study of CSF with electrophoresis, have been negative in all patients investigated, except that of Vigevano *et al.* (1982) in whom a high level of propionic acid in the serum was demonstrated. Skin biopsy performed in 6 patients never demonstrated any storage material.

Present evidence from neuroradiological, biological and neuropathological data seems to favour a syndrome of diverse causes rather than a single disorder. It can be argued, however, that some of the reported cases, especially familial cases, may represent a distinct subgroup with a progressive course and a probable metabolic origin. Such an interpretation is supported by the occurrence of a similar, if not identical, syndrome in glycine encephalopathy and in D-glyceric acidemia, two conditions of proven metabolic causation (Brandt *et al.*, 1974; Dalla Bernardina *et al.*, 1979; Grandgeorge *et al.*, 1980) and by the case of Vigevano *et al.* in which propionic acidemia was found. A case of early myoclonic encephalopathy with excretion of an unusual oligosaccharide has been recently presented (Michalski *et al.*, 1984). Whether such a subgroup, if it exists, could be separated from cases with other causes, especially non-familial ones, remains to be seen.

Diagnostic and nosological problems

Three conditions share several characteristics with early myoclonic encephalopathy: non-ketotic hyperglycinaemia and D-glyceric acidemias on the one hand, and the early infantile epileptic encephalopathy (EIEE) reported by Ohtahara *et al.* (1976) and Ohtahara, (1978). The clinical and EEG picture of non-ketotic hyperglycinaemia is virtually indistinguishable from that of early myoclonic encephalopathy and, indeed, glycine encephalopathy should be regarded as one of its major causes, rather than a differential diagnosis. The same applies to D-glyceric acidemia which is indistinguishable from non-ketotic hyperglycinaemia clinically and by EEG. The syndrome, as produced by disturbances of the metabolism of glycine however, has an even more severe course with a mortality of about 50 per cent before the age of one month.

EIEE, according to Ohtahara (1976, 1978) is characterized by tonic spasms occurring before the age of 20 days and associated with an EEG tracing of 'suppression-burst' activity. Erratic myoclonus and partial seizures were not mentioned in Ohtahara's description. EIEE undoubtedly has several causes and major brain abnormalities, especially of a malformative nature, are usually responsible for the syndrome. Ohtahara includes among them Aicardi's syndrome and various other encephalopathies, in which early infantile spasms are commonly associated with partial seizures, an association which is indeed the rule rather than the exception. Therefore, erratic myoclonus is probably the main distinctive feature between early myoclonic encephalopathy and EIEE, unless the latter differs from most other early infantile spasms by the absence of associated partial seizures. Whether the occurrence of erratic myoclonus is sufficient to separate the two syndromes remains unsettled. In some patients with non-ketotic hyperglycinaemia, the erratic myoclonus may be absent altogether, or may occur only for brief periods or may be quite inconspicuous, and the same can conceivably apply to myoclonic encephalopathies of other causes. The progressive course, emphasized by Dalla Bernardina *et al.,* is difficult to evaluate and was not evident on repeated clinical and neuroradiological examination in several of my patients, even in familial cases.

It seems likely that there is some overlap between early myoclonic encephalopathy and EIEE and that some cases (e.g. the case of Martin *et al.,* 1981) may be considered either as myoclonic encephalopathy, with mainly massive rather than erratic myoclonias, or as EIEE with occasional partial seizures and massive myoclonus. Whether the presence of erratic myoclonus is sufficient to separate the two syndromes cannot be established until more is known about their etiology, biochemistry and neuropathology. Meanwhile, the prominence of erratic myoclonus justifies, on a purely clinical basis, the provisional separation of EMIE.

References

Aicardi, J., Goutières, F. (1978): Encéphalopathie myoclonique néonatale. *Rev. EEG Neurophysiol.* **8**, 99-101.

Alpers, B.J. (1960): Progressive cerebral degeneration of infancy. *J. Nerv. Ment. Dis.* **130**, 442-448.

Brandt, N.V., Rassmussen, K., Brandt, S., Schonheyder, F. (1974): D-glyceric acidemia with hyperglycinemia. A new inborn error of metabolism. *Br. Med. J.* **4**, 334.

Cansiani, F., Mangano, S., Stranci, G. (1982): Encefalopatia mioclonica precoce con epilessia. *Boll. Lega It. Epil.* **39**, 199-200.

Cavazzuti, G.B., Nalin, A., Ferrari, F., Grandori, L., Beghini, G. (1978): Encefalopatia epilettica ad insorgenza neonatale. *Clinica Pediatrica* **60**, 239-246.

Christensen, E., Hojgaard, K. (1964): Poliodystrophia cerebri progressiva infantilis. *Acta Neurol. Scand.* **40**, 21-40.

Dalla Bernardina, B., Aicardi, J., Goutières, F., Plouin, P. (1979): Glycine encephalopathy. *Neuropädiatrie* **10**, 209-225.

Dalla Bernardina, B., Dulac, O., Bureau, M., Dravet, C., del Zotti, F., Roger, J. (1982): Encéphalopathie myoclonique précoce avec épilepsie. *Rev. EEG Neurophysiol.* **12**, 8-14.

Dalla Bernardina, B., Dulac, O., Fejerman, N., Dravet, C., Capovilla, G., Bondavalli, S., Colamaria, V., Roger, J. (1983): Early myoclonic epileptic encephalopathy (E.M.E.E.). *Eur. J. Pediatr.* **140**, 248-252.

Grandgeorge, D., Favier, A., Bost, M., Frappat, P., Bonjet, C., Garrel, S., Stoebner, P. (1980): L'acidémie D-glycérique. A propos d'une nouvelle observation anatomo-clinique. *Archs Franc. Pédiatr.* **37**, 577-584.

Greenhouse, A.H., Neueburger, K.T. (1964): The syndrome of progressive cerebral poliodystrophy. *Archs Neurol.* **10**, 46-57.

Jellinger, K., Seitelberger, F. (1970): Spongy glio-neuronal dystrophy in infancy and childhood. *Acta Neuropathol.* **16**, 125-140.

Menegati, E., Perini, A., Tiberti, A. (1982): Encefalopatia mioclonica precoce nella sindrome de Menkes. *Boll. Lega It. Epil.* **39**, 186-187.

Martin, H.J., Deroubaix-Tella, P., Thelliez, P. (1981): Encéphalopathie épileptique néonatale à bouffées périodiques. *Rev. EEG. Neurophysiol.* **11**, 397-403.

Michalski, J.C., Bouquelet, S., Montreuil, J., Strecker, G., Dulac, O., Munnich, A. (1984): Abnormal galactosid excretion in urine of a patient with early myoclonic epileptic encephalopathy. *Clin. Chim. Acta* **137**, 43-51.

Ohtahara, S., Ishida, T., Oka, E., Yamatogi, Y., Inique, H., Ohtsuka, Y., Kanda, S. (1976): On the age-dependent epileptic syndromes: the early infantile encephalopathy with suppression-burst. *Brain and Development* **8**, 270-288.

Ohtahara, S. (1978): Clinico-electrical delineation of epileptic encephalopathies in childhood. *Asian Med. J.* **21**, 7-17.

Turcker, J.S., Solitare, G.B. (1963): Infantile myoclonic spasms. Clinical, electrographic and neuropathologic observations. *Epilepsia* **4**, 45-59.

Vigevano, F., Bosman, C., Giscondi, A., Maccagnani, F., Sevanti, G., Sergo, M. (1981): Neonatal myoclonic encephalopathy without hyperglycinemia. *Electroenceph. Clin. Neurophysiol.* **52**, 52P-53P.

Vigevano, F., Maccagnani, F., Bertini, E., Sabetta, G., Parisella, G., Bosman, C., Bachman, C. (1982): Encefalopatia mioclonica precoce associata ad alti livelli di acido propionico nel siero. *Boll. Lega It. Epil.* **39**, 181-182.

*   *   *

Discussion
Summarized by Jean AICARDI

Dreifuss remarks that there is little difference between waking and sleep EEGs in this syndrome.

Beaumanoir enquires about the mortality rate during the 1st year of life. Aicardi gives a figure of 60 per cent.

Dulac presents slides and films of 3 infants who all died before age 2 months. One of them excreted urinary oligosaccharides so far undetected in any human disorder. Dulac emphasizes the hypertonus with opisthotonus which may suggest a diagnosis of tetanus. Aicardi indicates that hypotonia may exist in the syndrome, even outside non-ketotic hyperglycinaemia.

Lerman has seen 4 or 5 similar cases and favours a dysmetabolic origin.

Dalla Bernardina believes that the early infantile encephalopathy of Ohtahara is distinct from the myoclonic encephalopathy. In the former, no partial seizures or myoclonias were described, and the only common feature was the suppression-burst tracing. Dalla Bernardina thinks that all cases of early myoclonic encephalopathy of known cause are due to inborn errors of metabolism. The onset is in the neonatal period, the course is progressive and the EEG tracings show initial periodic abnormalities followed by multifocal paroxysms. The outcome is death in all patients after variable duration.

Aicardi thinks that EIEE and early myoclonic encephalopathy share several features (except for the erratic myoclonus). An inborn error of metabolism has never been proved (outside hyperglycinaemia) and other causes, especially brain malformation, cannot be excluded.

Seino indicates that Ohtahara's description mentions tonic spasms, not myoclonias.

Jeavons indicates that EIEE features tonic spasms, as in West's syndrome, but the spasms are often isolated. He agrees that the suppression-burst EEG is unspecific.

Dreifuss asks for a precise definition of tonic spasms and underlines the necessity of videoscopic and polygraphic data.

Cavazzuti describes a case in which ultrasonic examination evidenced hydrocephalus and a porencephaly. He wonders whether there are 2 main causes: (1) inborn error of metabolism; (2) brain malformations.

Aicardi indicates that the frequency of familial cases suggests dysmetabolic causes in the broadest meaning of the term. Two of 3 pathological examinations in his series displayed images of non-specific poliodystrophy. In a third case, minor abnormalities of brain gyration were present.

Epileptic syndromes in infancy, child-
hood and adolescence. J. Roger,
C. Dravet, M. Bureau, F.E.
Dreifuss and P. Wolf. John Libbey
Eurotext Ltd ©1985.

Chapter 3
Other Epileptic Syndromes
in Neonates

Olivier DULAC, Patrick AUBOURG and Perrine PLOUIN

*Service de Neurologie Infantile, Clinique de Pédiatrie et de Puériculture, Hôpital Saint-Vincent-de-Paul,
74 Avenue Denfert-Rochereau, 75674 Paris, Cedex 14, France*

Summary

Three specific neonatal epileptic syndromes are reviewed. They are characterized by severe idiopathic status epilepticus starting within the first 5 days of life, mostly before 3 days, with frequent
generalized tonic seizures and abnormal interictal neurological status lasting several weeks
before progressive improvement. Focal status epilepticus appears between 8 and 72 hours of age
with frequent clonic seizures all localized in the same muscle groups, usually resulting from
hemispheric infarct or haematoma. Early infantile epileptic encephalopathy with suppression-
burst is characterized by the progressive appearance of frequent seizures described as flexion, extension or asymmetrical spasms associated with various other types of seizures and a
suppression-burst EEG pattern, resulting in most cases from malformation or diffuse prenatal
brain lesion.

Introduction

Most neonatal convulsions result from acute brain insult and persist repeatedly for a
few hours or days before remitting spontaneously (Dreyfus-Brisac and Monod, 1972;
Lombroso, 1983). Although the pathophysiology can be controversial in some cases
(Kellaway and Hrachovy, 1983), the etiological diagnosis is usually rapidly reached.
Indeed, neurological, digestive, cardiorespiratory or other manifestations precede
onset of seizures, and the cause of the brain lesion is often evident before they appear.
This is the case after trauma and anoxia, in infection and in various inherited metabolic
diseases including aminoacidopathies (Kohlschütter, 1983), nonketotic hyperglycinemia (Dalla Bernardina *et al.,* 1979) and D-glyceric acidemia (Brandt *et al.,* 1976;
Grandgeorge *et al.,* 1980). It is also the case in several brain malformations such as
holoprosencephaly with facial dysmorphia (De Myer, 1977).

   In some cases, however, the anamnesis gives no clue as to the precise etiology, and
the seizures are the main clinical manifestation. Benign neonatal convulsions (see
Plouin, chapter 1) and early myoclonic encephalopathy (see Aicardi, chapter 2)
belong to this group and are described elsewhere. In addition, three other clinical con-

ditions deserve attention: severe idiopathic status epilepticus, focal status epilepticus, and early infantile epileptic encephalopathy with suppression-bursts.

I — Severe idiopathic status epilepticus

Several authors have reported that some of the cases of neonatal status epilepticus of unknown cause evolve unfavourably.

Indeed, among 2042 patients with idiopathic neonatal convulsions, reported from 1959 to 1979, 75 (ie 38 per cent) of the cases with status epilepticus had a poor outcome (see chapter 1). In fact, the proportion is probably overestimated, since several cases were observed at a time when neither CT scan nor detailed metabolic investigations were available. Since 1975, we had the opportunity to observe 12 such patients in the Hôpital Saint Vincent de Paul. After a normal delivery and an apparently normal status during the first hours or days of life, an acute neurological distress with frequent seizures and abnormal interictal consciousness appeared.

Indeed, the first seizures appeared early, within the first 5 days of life, and before day 3 in two-thirds of the cases. They lasted no longer than 1 or 2 minutes. They consisted of a tonic phase in all cases, and in some patients this was the only clinical ictal manifestation. In most cases, however, the seizures also included generalized (three cases), unilateral (two cases) or partial (three cases) clonic jerks; upward (two cases) or lateral (one case) deviation of the eyes, and vegetative manifestations. Among the latter, apnea (two cases), cyanosis (four cases), erythrosis (two cases) and chewing movements (one case) were the most frequent.

Interictal neurological abnormalities were observed from onset in all cases. They consisted of hypotonia, disorders of consciousness and abnormal movements, including pedalling (four cases), chewing (two cases) and frequent very pronounced jittering (seven cases).

The seizures were repeated, very frequently in some cases. In nine patients, they persisted whatever the drugs administered, for a period of 3 to 6 weeks with a mean of 5 weeks. One patient died on the 10th day of life. In only two patients, the status was interrupted during the second week of life.

The interictal EEG tracings lacked sleep organization. They were characterized by diffuse bursts of slow waves, sharp waves and spikes of very high amplitude lasting a few seconds and alternating with periods of low activity (Fig. 1). However, the tracing was never inactive and was therefore different from the suppression burst pattern. Ictal discharges consisted of a suddenly reduced amplitude; an 'alpha' activity was often observed either at the onset or at the end of the discharge (Fig. 2a, b).

The various radiological, CSF and blood biological studies remained negative.

The patients' psychomotor development had been slow, although most of the eldest walked before three years of age, and pronounced a few words before five years. During the first two years of life, all the patients suffered from further generalized or partial motor seizures of variable frequency and four developed West syndrome.

The clinical pattern is therefore quite marked, including acute onset of frequent seizures with interictal neurological distress, and spontaneous remission after several weeks. The progressive long-term improvement and the EEG ictal and interictal trac-

see page opposite

Fig. 1. Severe idiopathic status epilepticus. Interictal tracing characterized by diffuse bursts of slow waves, sharp waves and spikes of very high amplitude alternating with periods of low activity.

Fig. 2. Ictal discharge characterized by sudden reduction of amplitude and appearance of an 'alpha' activity.

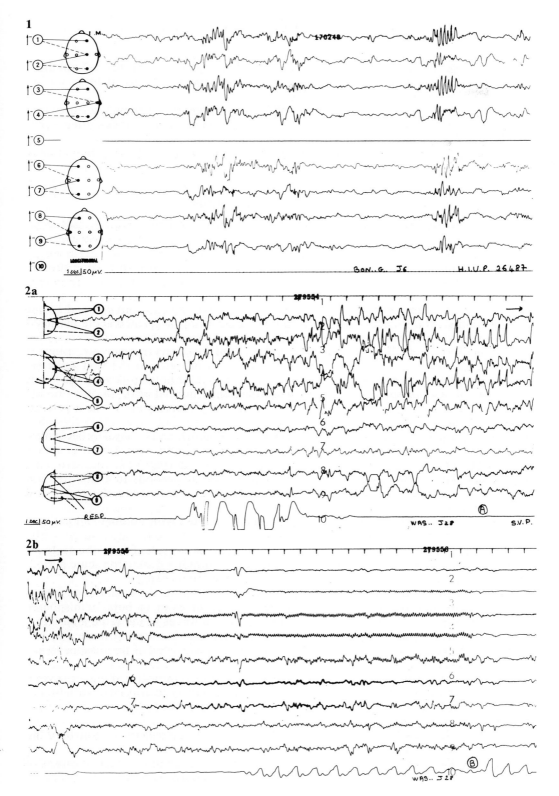

ings also suggest some kind of acute brain insult. Although careful prepartum monitoring of fetal heart frequency had been performed in several patients, damage during parturition cannot be completely ruled out.

This pattern may easily be distinguished from pyridoxine-dependency seizures that usually appear during the first hours of life, or even prenatally. Jitteriness, cries, agitation and myoclonias occur. The seizures last several hours and eventually respond transiently to conventional antiepileptic drugs; between the seizures, the child initially appears normal (Banker *et al.*, 1983).

II — Focal status epilepticus

Neonatal seizures are often partial motor and this characteristic is usually said to be devoid of any significance as to the existence and localization of an eventual brain lesion. However, Billard *et al.* (1982) and Bour *et al.* (1983) reported patients in whom acute onset of frequently repeated partial seizures, all localized in the same muscle groups, resulted from a localized brain lesion. Although the seizures were frequent, they remitted spontaneously within two or three days.

An obvious predominance of boys was recorded in both series: 6 out of 8 and 15 out of 21 patients. Abnormal parturition with low Apgar scores suggested acute perinatal foetal distress in five cases; eight patients developed status epilepticus after surgery for cardiac malformation (Bour *et al.*, 1983); and in 8 and 7 patients respectively, minimal or no abnormalities were noticed in the perinatal period prior to the first seizures. Status epilepticus appeared after a delay ranging from 8 to 72 hours following the insult — abnormal birth or surgery — or following apparently normal birth. In only one patient was the delay of 6 days. The seizures were very stereotyped in each patient. Rhythmic jerks of mean amplitude of 1 or 2 limbs or the face, with vegetative phenomena — ie apnea, tachycardia — or chewing movements, and eventually secondary generalization were the main ictal manifestations. Four patients were drowsy or comatose after surgery and had no clinical manifestations during EEG-recorded ictal discharges. The seizures were very brief, lasting from 30 seconds to 1 minute, and were very frequent in most cases. They resisted to intravenous diazepam and phenobarbital.

Interictal neurological status was variable and correlated with etiology: all patients whose delivery had been abnormal were comatose and hypotonic; after surgery, the patients were either normal or drowsy, probably in part as a result of anaesthesia. In no patient was it possible to detect the slightest motor asymmetry during the acute period. Axial hypotonia was a frequent finding and persisted for 10 to 20 days.

Ictal EEG recordings consisted of rhythmic slow spikes on the rolandic or frontal areas, eventually diffusing to the whole hemisphere or even to both hemispheres asymmetrically (Fig. 3). Interictal EEG disclosed sharp waves in the same areas (Fig. 4) and poor sleep organization; alterations on the opposite hemisphere were only observed in the cases following abnormal parturition and consisted of the disappearance of physiological activity.

CT scan in patients with apparently normal parturition demonstrated one or several triangular hypodense areas suggesting brain infarct secondary to arterial obstruction in 8 and 3 patients respectively. An intracerebral haematoma was observed in 3 other patients (Bour *et al.*, 1983).

Evolution demonstrated appearance of mild to frank hemiplegia in one fourth of the cases, and epilepsy in respectively one of 8 and 2 of 20 patients.

Although localized infarcts and haematomas seem to be the most frequent causes of such localized or unilateral status epilepticus of the newborn, various acute and local-

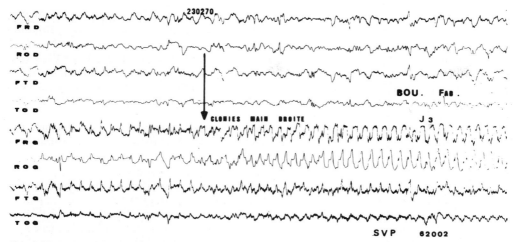

Fig. 3. Unilateral status epilepticus. Seizure characterized by unilateral rhythmic slow spikes.

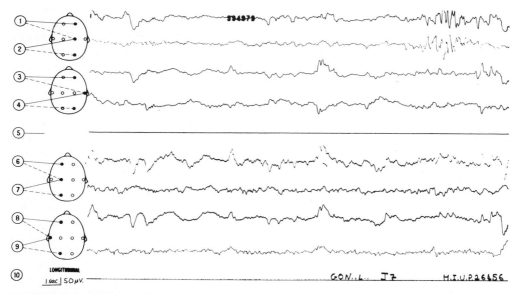

Fig. 4. Unilateral status epilepticus. Interictal tracing. Burst of spikes and sharp waves localized on the same area as the ictal discharges.

ized brain lesions may give rise to such manifestations, including bacterial meningitis, and exceptionally Sturge-Weber disease and Incontinentia Pigmenti.

III — Early infantile epileptic encephalopathy with suppression-bursts

Over the last decade, several authors have called attention to a group of patients who develop severe epileptic encephalopathy earlier than 3 months of age (Maheshwari and Jeavons 1975; Ohtahara *et al.,* 1976; Ohtahara 1978, Martin *et al.,* 1981), mostly during the first weeks: 7 of 9 before 20 days in Ohtahara's series (1978). Contrary to the 2 precedent groups, this syndrome appears as a subacute clinical condition worsening progressively over a period of several days or weeks, and not remitting spontaneously. After normal delivery and apparently normal early days, seizures appear with a progressively increasing frequency. They are generalized and most often described as flexor, extensor or asymmetrical spasms, eventually associated with tonic-clonic or unilateral seizures. Although interictal neurological status is normal at onset, severe mental retardation progressively becomes evident and various neurological abnormalities — spastic diplegia, hemiplegia or quadriplegia, ataxia or dystonia — are observed in half the cases.

EEG demonstrates no basal activity, but a suppression-burst pattern. A nearly flat tracing lasting several seconds alternates with $150\text{-}300\mu$V diffuse high amplitude slow wave and spike bursts (Fig. 5). The latter is sometimes unilateral or asynchronous on both hemispheres. This pattern is poorly modified by sleep-wake stages.

Prognosis is very poor since there is poor response to treatment, half the patients dying in infancy or childhood and most of the remainder being severely handicapped.

Etiology is variable and predominantly includes brain malformations and diffuse prenatal lesions, the precise nature of which remains unknown in over half the cases.

Thus, as opposed to early myoclonic encephalopathy, this group lacks severe myoclonic activity.

The clinical and EEG characteristics of neonatal seizures appear therefore to be the most helpful features of etiological diagnosis. Acute onset of frequent seizures suggest

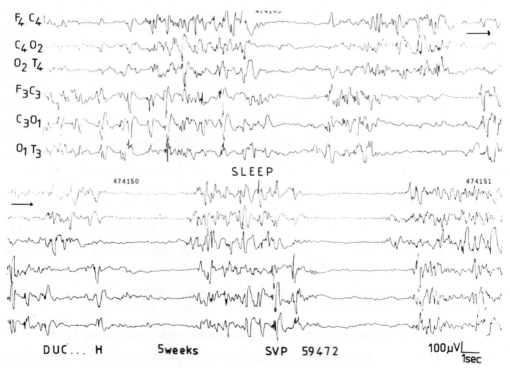

Fig. 5. Early infantile epileptic encephalopathy with supression-bursts. Interictal tracing demonstrating diffuse bursts of spikes and slow waves alternating with periods of inactivity. Notice that the latter are slightly asymmetrical. This infant had severe congenital malformations of the cerebellum and brain stem.

benign neonatal seizures if they are clonic and erratic with no severe clinical or EEG interictal abnormalities; they suggest an acute focal brain lesion if they are clonic and localized repeatedly in the same muscle groups; tonic seizures and interictal neurological distress results from severe idiopathic status. Progressive increase in seizure frequency with myoclonias most likely expresses an inborn metabolic disease. On the contrary, progressive increase in seizure frequency with suppression-burst, but without myoclonias, suggest a brain malformation or a severe prenatal brain lesion. However, the latter group does not include all types of chronic epilepsy appearing in the first weeks of life. Indeed, several malformations such as agyria, focal cerebral dysplasia or Aicardi's syndrome may result in various types of epilepsy with onset in infancy, and sometimes even in the first weeks of life.

Furthermore, some chronic partial epilepsies appear in the first weeks of life.

References

Banker, A., Turner, M., Hopkins, I.J. (1983): Pyridoxine dependent seizures — a wider clinical spectrum. *Archs Dis. Child.* **58**, 415-418.

Billard, C., Dulac, O., Diebler, C. (1982): Ramollissement cérébral ischémique du nouveau-né. *Archs Fr. Pédiatr.* **39**, 677-683.

Bour, F., Plouin, P., Jalin, C., Frenkel, A., Dulac, O., Bonifas, P. (1983): Les états de mal unilatéraux au cours de la période néo-natale. *Rev. EEG Neurophysiol.* **13**, 162-167.

Brandt, N.J., Rassmussen, K., Brandt, S., Kolvraa, S., Schonheyder, F. (1976): D-glyceric acidemia and non-ketotic hyperglycinemia. *Acta Paediatr. Scand.* **65**, 17-22.

Dalla Bernardina, D., Aicardi, J., Goutières, F., Plouin, P. (1979): Glycine encephalopathy. *Neuropädiatrie* **10**, 209-225.

De Myer, W. (1977): Holoprosencephaly (cyclopia-arhinencephaly). In *Handbook of clinical neurology,* vol. 30. *Congenital malformations of the brain,* Part I, ed P.J. Vinken, G.W. Bruyn. Amsterdam: North Holland .

Dreyfus-Brisac, C., Monod, N. (1972): Neonatal status epilepticus. *Electroencephalogr. Clin. Neurophysiol.* **15**, 38-52.

Grandgeorge, D., Favier, A., Bost, M., Frappat, P., Bouget, C., Garrel, S., Stoebner, P. (1980): L'acidémie D-glycérique. *Archs Fr. Pédiatr.* **37**, 577-584.

Kellaway, P., Hrachovy, R.A. (1983): Status epilepticus in newborns: a perspective on neonatal seizures. In *Status epilepticus,* ed Delgado-Escueta *et al.,* pp 93-99. Raven Press: New York.

Kohlschütter, A. (1983): The clinical presentation of organo acidopathies: when to investigate. *Neuropediatrics* **14**, 191-196.

Lombroso, C.T. (1983): Prognosis in neonatal seizures. In *Status epilepticus,* ed Delgado-Escueta *et al.,* pp 101-113. Raven Press: New York.

Maheshwari, M.C., Jeavons, P.M. (1975): The prognostic implications of suppression-burst activity in the EEG in infancy. *Epilepsia* **16**, 127-131.

Martin, H.J., Deroubaix-Tella, P., Thelliez, P. (1981): Encéphalopathie épileptique néo-natale à bouffées périodiques. *Rev. EEG Neurophysiol.* **11**, 397-403.

Ohtahara, S., Yamatogi, Y., Ohtsuka, Y. (1976): Prognosis of the Lennox syndrome. Long-term clinical and electroencephalographic follow-up study, especially with special reference to relationship with the West syndrome. *Folia Psychiat. Neurol. Jap.* **30**, 275-287.

Ohtahara, S. (1978): Clinico-electrical delineation of epileptic encephalopathies in childhood. *Asian Med. J.* **21**, 7-17.

Discussion
Summarized by Giovanni Battista CAVAZZUTI

Cavazzuti: It seems to me to be more correct to speak of epilepsies of infants and children which may begin in the neonate, rather than of neonatal epilepsies as such. Epilepsies beginning in the neonate — although this indeed occurs rarely — are no different from the epilepsies which begin a few months later. Their symptomatology has nothing specific about it: as in infantile epilepsies, we find erratic myoclonus, tonic seizures and partial seizures. Their outcome is particularly severe.

Monod: Neonatal epilepsy is very rare. Convulsions in the neonate, on the other hand, are frequent, benign or secondary to various lesions which often leave serious encephalopathic sequelae, sometimes associated with epilepsy. Evolution of neonatal convulsions towards delayed isolated epilepsy is exceptional. We personally have seen no more than 10 cases in 30 years.

Dulac: Some subjects have a fixed antenatal lesion (malformation or ischaemic lesion) and an epilepsy which begins during the first days of life and continues for a long time, with stereotyped partial seizures.

Wolf: It is interesting to see that this type of epilepsy, which may also have its onset later in life, may begin during the neonatal period. This is true for both malformations and ischaemic lesions.

Revol: I agree with Dulac that there is a neonatal epilepsy which later evolves towards partial epilepsy originating from the same hemisphere.

Aicardi: There is no doubt as to the existence of a syndrome of repeated neonatal seizures with fixed localization. After a period of popularizing the idea that partial seizures had no focal value, we are now re-discovering that they may also have the value of a focal lesion. But is there continuity between neonatal seizures and subsequent epilepsy? I myself am not sure.

Pinsard: I speak as a paediatrician. Epilepsy is a chronic disease: for the paediatrician, there is no such thing as chronic pathology in the neonate.

Cavazzuti: Dulac has shown that there are some epilepsies which begin during the neonatal period and continue afterwards. However, the vast majority of infants who suffer from seizures during the neonatal period do not continue to do so in later life, and we cannot refer to them as epileptics. Are we in future to consider all paroxysmal events of limited duration as epilepsies?

Monod: I agree with Cavazzuti — otherwise we have to call everything epilepsy, including effects of ischaemia, anoxia, etc.

Roger: The name is of little importance. What is important is to know whether neonatal convulsions of unknown etiology occurring in normal infants, and having specific clinical and EEG characteristics, are sufficiently recognizable and stereotyped to constitute a syndrome. This could be called benign epilepsy, or, equally well, benign convulsions in the neonate.

Dravet: The value of determining syndromes is to be able to give a prognosis.

Jeavons: The idea behind the meeting is not to classify epilepsies or seizures, but rather to identify syndromes which can be given international recognition.

Roger: Because we are trying to identify syndromes, the following questions come to mind:
- Syndrome of benign neonatal convulsions with no known etiology, with or without genetic substratum
- Syndrome of early myoclonic encephalopathy, with two subgroups: metabolic errors, and unknown etiology
- Partial epilepsy symptomatic of a non-evolutive focal lesion.

II
Epileptic syndromes in infancy and childhood

Epileptic syndromes in infancy, child-
hood and adolescence. J. Roger,
C. Dravet, M. Bureau, F.E.
Dreifuss and P. Wolf. John Libbey
Eurotext Ltd ©1985.

Chapter 4
Febrile Convulsions

Niall V. O'DONOHOE

Department of Paediatrics, National Children's Hospital, Harcourt Street, Dublin 2, Republic of Ireland

Summary

Febrile convulsions are an age-related disorder characterized by almost always generalized seizures occurring during an acute febrile illness. The majority of febrile convulsions are brief and
uncomplicated but a minority may be more prolonged and followed by transient or permanent
neurological sequelae. There is a tendency to recurrence of febrile convulsions in about one-
third of those affected. Controversy about the risks of developing later epilepsy have largely
been resolved by some recent large studies and it seems that the overall risk is not greater than 4
per cent. The indications for prolonged drug prophylaxis against recurrence of febrile convulsions are more clearly defined now and the majority do not require it. Essentially, this condition
is a relatively benign disorder of early childhood.

General

Febrile convulsions are characteristically generalized seizures which occur during an
acute febrile illness. Convulsions which occur in association with infections of the nervous system should be considered separately since the central nervous system infection modifies the typical course of the illness. Febrile convulsions are an age-related
and usually benign disorder in the majority of patients. Febrile convulsions should be
distinguished from epilepsy which is usually characterized by recurrent non-febrile
seizures. However, any child who already has clinical epilepsy or who has a predisposition to primary generalized epilepsy may suffer a generalized seizure during the course
of a febrile illness and this can occur at any age, although it is more frequent in the
young. Febrile convulsions occur in about 3 per cent of the population at risk, that is
children from the age of 6 months to 5 years of age. Although usually generalized and
brief and terminating spontaneously, a small proportion show lateralizing or focal features even in attacks of short duration, and a proportion, perhaps a quarter or more,
may be prolonged for 30 minutes or longer. The cause of the febrile illness is a disseminated virus infection of the upper respiratory tract in nearly 90 per cent of cases
(Lewis *et al.* 1979). The percentage of patients with febrile convulsions whose family
history shows the occurrence of either epilepsy or febrile convulsions is at least 10 per

cent (Newmark and Penry, 1980). An autosomal dominant pattern with incomplete penetrance has been suggested as the most common mode of inheritance but poly-genetic mechanisms may also be involved and the pattern of inheritance may vary from family to family. There are genetic links with primary generalized epilepsy of the petit mal type and with benign partial epilepsy of childhood.

The level of fever inducing a febrile convulsion is usually in excess of 39°C. Febrile convulsions represent a response on the part of the child to pyrexia and to an invasion of the body by a micro-organism, which is usually a virus occurring in an individual who is predisposed genetically and at a period in childhood when the convulsive threshold of the immature brain is lowered. Experiments in animals suggest that this age-related susceptibility to febrile seizures may be related to neuro-chemical and neuro-transmitter alterations associated with genetically-determined enzyme deficits in the brain with resultant ionic and metabolic changes contributing to seizure sus-ceptibility (Glaser, 1982). A further factor of importance may be the sex of the child, girls of 18 months or less being more likely to suffer more frequent and more severe febrile seizures (Taylor and Ounsted, 1971).

Clinical data

It is customary nowadays to categorize febrile convulsions into (1) those which are simple and uncomplicated, that is generalized tonic-clonic seizures occurring in child-ren of normal development where the seizures are short in duration, do not occur in series on the same day and where there are no focal or transient neurological sequelae, and (2) those which are complicated, that is seizures which are long in duration, may occur in series on the same day, are often focal or lateralized and which may be fol-lowed by transient or permanent neurological sequelae. The incidence of complicated febrile convulsions is difficult to assess but may be as high as 30 per cent in infants of 1 year or younger. Over 75 per cent of complicated febrile convulsions are first convul-sions and the children are usually not recognized as being febrile before the convulsion occurs.

The recurrence rate of febrile convulsions varies from 25 to 50 per cent with 33 per cent as an average estimate. About 9 per cent of affected children have three or more convulsions. The younger the child at the time of the first convulsion the greater the risk of recurrence, especially in females, and a family history of febrile convulsions in first degree relatives can double the risk of recurrence (Lennox-Buchthal, 1973). Fifty per cent of second febrile convulsions occur within six months of the first seizure, 75 per cent occur within a year and 90 per cent within two years (Nelson and Ellenberg, 1978). There is no evidence that severe initial convulsions are more likely to be fol-lowed by a recurrence but the overall risk of having a severe convulsion increases as the number of convulsions increases, particularly with third and subsequent attacks.

A correct diagnosis of a febrile convulsion is of considerable importance. Rigors, drug intoxications, and syncopal episodes need to be distinguished from febrile sei-zures and the important work of Stephenson (1983) in distinguishing and defining reflex anoxic seizures from febrile seizures should be recognized. Serious conditions such as meningitis, encephalitis and Reye's syndrome should be considered and ruled out.

EEG examination is of limited value in the diagnosis and assessment of the child with a febrile seizure. Marked generalized slowing usually occurs after the attack and may persist for some days. Focal or asymmetrical slowing in the EEG soon after the seizure may identify the focal or lateralized nature of the attack. Doose et al. (1972) claimed that persistent posterior theta rhythms at 4-7 c/s indicated an increased risk of recurrence, especially if there were associated spike-wave discharges. Spike-wave paroxysms are an expression of a genetic predisposition to epilepsy but do not necessarily indicate that later epilepsy will evolve in an individual patient.

There is considerable evidence that febrile seizures which last for more than 15-30 minutes or are repeated within 24 hours may cause cerebral damage, particularly in the vulnerable temporal lobe areas of the brain where the H1 or Sommer sector of the hippocampus is likely to show pathological changes, usually termed mesial temporal sclerosis. It has been suggested by Wallace (1976) and others that hereditary and minor alterations in brain structure are inseparable predisposing factors to febrile seizures, especially prolonged and potentially damaging seizures. There is evidence that children who have prolonged febrile seizures have an increased incidence of factors associated with suboptimal neurological development, and it is suggested that a convulsion of this type is drawing attention to a developmental defect which may be a consequence of pre or perinatal adverse events. It can be argued, therefore, that this is a distinct epileptic syndrome, which is different from the simple or complicated febrile seizure occurring in a normal child with a genetic predisposition to convulse with high fever. The latter group, it should be emphasized, comprises the great majority of children who suffer febrile seizures.

Long-term evaluation

There has been controversy about the risks of developing later epilepsy following febrile seizures. Controversy has arisen because of differing definitions of a febrile seizure, because of differing methods of selecting cases for follow-up and because of variations in the duration of follow-up of the cohort chosen. Definitions of what constitutes later epilepsy have also varied. Some studies require two or more afebrile seizures for a diagnosis of epilepsy while others have accepted a single afebrile seizure as evidence of epilepsy. Several large studies in the past decade have made it possible to reach a consensus about prognosis. They have indicated that the incidence of subsequent epilepsy in those who have experienced febrile seizures is of the order of 2 to 4 per cent. The incidence of epilepsy in the general population is 0.5 per cent. The features associated with the likely development of later epilepsy include prolonged febrile seizures, lateralized seizures, repeated seizures, onset of seizures in the first year of life, antecedent cerebral injury, associated mental handicap, female sex, and a family history of epilepsy.

In their prospective study in the United States, Nelson and Ellenberg (1978) identified three important risk factors for the development of later epilepsy, namely, a family history of epilepsy in a parent or sibling, complicated initial febrile seizures, and the presence of neuro-developmental abnormalities prior to the occurrence of the first febrile convulsion. In 60 per cent of their cohort, no risk factors were present and the risk of later epilepsy developing by the age of seven years was only marginally increased compared with those children who had not suffered febrile seizures at all (1 per cent compared with 0.5 per cent). Of those children with one risk factor, comprising 34 per cent of the cohort, 2 per cent of the patients developed later epilepsy, that is four times the rate in normal controls. Children who had two or more risk factors, constituting 6 per cent of the cohort, had a 10 per cent chance of developing later epilepsy. When they considered the risk factors individually they were unable to demonstrate that prolonged duration of febrile convulsions was a major determinant of later epilepsy, although children whose initial febrile convulsion was prolonged or repeated or associated with focal features were three times more likely to have epilepsy by the age of 7 years of age than those children whose initial febrile convulsion was not complicated. However, more than 90 per cent of the children who developed later epilepsy after febrile seizures had never had a febrile seizure which lasted as long as 30 minutes.

Annegers *et al.* (1979) in their 20-year follow-up Rochester Study showed that a combination of atypical features in the first febrile convulsion and prior neuro-developmental disorder was associated with a 17 per cent chance of developing epilepsy by the age of 20 years, compared with a 2.5 per cent chance in their low risk patients with neither of these factors. They also found that a family history of febrile convulsions or epilepsy in a parent or sibling was associated with an increased risk of epilepsy. Wallace (1977), in her hospital-based study of 112 children aged between 2 months and 7 years at the time of their initial seizure, of whom 55 were aged less than 19 months at the time of the first seizure and 75 had a complicated initial seizure, found that 12 per cent of the patients developed later epilepsy and that prolonged unilateral seizures were more likely to be followed by the development of complex partial seizures related to temporal lobe damage.

The overall risk of later epilepsy for all children developing febrile seizures is now considered to be of the order of 4 per cent at most.

Apart from the development of later epilepsy the child with febrile seizures may have a neurological deficit such as mental retardation. It is generally believed that these central nervous system deficits, when present, have usually antedated the febrile seizures. There is no convincing evidence that these deficits reflect neurological injury occurring at the time of the febrile seizure in the vast majority of cases. Wallace (1976) however, has suggested that approximately 5 per cent of normal children who sustain febrile seizures acquire neurological abnormalities as a result. There is no convincing evidence available that there is a long-term risk of impaired cognitive development following febrile seizures.

Prophylaxis and treatment

Prophylaxis to prevent further febrile seizures has also been a controversial matter in recent years. There is no doubt that prophylaxis will prevent the recurrence of febrile seizures but there is no certain evidence that prophylaxis will prevent the development of later epilepsy.

Furthermore, there is no ideal drug available for prophylaxis. Anticonvulsant prophylaxis is recommended to-day (Consensus Development Panel, 1980) following a complicated febrile seizure, in the presence of neurodevelopmental abnormality, where there is a history of epilepsy of genetic origin in a parent or sibling, where there is marked parental anxiety about the possibility of recurrences, and possibly where the first febrile seizure has occurred in a child under the age of one year especially if female. Using this regimen of selective medication almost two thirds of children with febrile convulsions will be excluded from prophylactic drug treatment. Parents should be taught how to control fever and how to manage possible further convulsions. The use of tepid sponging, antipyretic drugs and the administration of rectal diazepam should be taught to parents. The initial febrile convulsion warrants admission to hospital especially if meningitis is suspected and a lumbar puncture indicated, but subsequent febrile convulsions may safely be managed at home. Parents need, above all, an adequate explanation of the condition and an optimistic outlook in order to allay their reasonable anxiety.

References

Annegers, J.F., Hauser, W.A., Elveback, L.R., Kurland, L.T., (1979): The risk of epilepsy following febrile convulsions. *Neurology* 29, 277-303.

Consensus Development Panel (1980): Febrile seizures: long term management of children with fever-associated seizures. *Pediatrics* **66,** 1009-1012.

Doose, H., Gerken, H., Völzke, E. (1972): On the genetics of EEG-Anomalies in childhood. I. Abnormal theta rhythms. *Neuropädiatrie* 3, 386-401.

Glaser, G. (1982): Critical periods in brain development related to behaviour: the developing neurophysiology of self. In *One child* ed J. Apley, C. Ounsted, pp 54-74. Clinics in Developmental Medicine, No. 80. Spastics International Medical Publications. William Heinemann Medical Books: London.

Lennox-Buchthal, M.A., (1973): *Febrile convulsions: a reappraisal.* Elsevier: Amsterdam.

Lewis, H.M., Parry, J.V., Parry, R.P., Davies, H.A., Sanderson, P.J., Tyrrell, D.A.J., Valman, H.B. (1979): Role of viruses in febrile convulsions. *Archs Dis. Child.* **54,** 869-876.

Nelson, K.B., Ellenberg, J.H. (1978): Prognosis in children with febrile convulsions. *Pediatrics* **61,** 720-727.

Newmark, M.E., Penry, J.K. (1980): *Genetics of epilepsy: a review,* pp 54-58. Raven Press: New York.

Stephenson, J.B.P. (1983): Febrile convulsions and reflex anoxic seizures. *Research progress in epilepsy,* ed F.C. Rose, pp 244-252. Pitman: London.

Taylor, D.C., Ounsted, C. (1971): Biological mechanisms influencing the outcome of seizures in response to fever. *Epilepsia* 12, 33-45.

Wallace, S.J. (1976): Neurological and intellectual deficits; convulsions with fever viewed as acute indicators of life-long developmental defects. In *Brain dysfunction in infantile febrile convulsions,* ed M.A.B. Brazier, F. Coceani: pp 259-277. International Brain Research Organization Monograph. Raven Press: New York.

Wallace, S.J. (1977): Spontaneous fits after convulsions with fever. *Archs Dis. Child.* **52,** 192-196.

*   *   *

Discussion
Summarized by Niall V.O'DONOHOE

Aicardi opened the discussion remarking that, in recent years, the pendulum of opinion about febrile convulsions (FC) had swung back in favour of their being a benign syndrome in general and one which was not followed by later epilepsy in 97 per cent of cases. He was still concerned, however, about FCs in the very young, below 13 or even 18 months of age, and whether the risk of a damaging seizure in that epoch was related to the neurological status of the child prior to the convulsions or to the duration of the convulsion. He had been surprised by the data from Nelson and Ellenberg's prospective study which indicated that 22 per cent of children who had a prolonged FC had had an abnormal neurodevelopmental status beforehand. He referred to his study with Chevrie (1975)* which showed that the proportion of genetic antecedents in children with prolonged FC was only half that in children with the usual simple type of FC (18 per cent compared with 35 per cent).

He speculated that perhaps half of the cases of prolonged FCs did not conform to the classic pattern of the condition, that is convulsions solely due to the effect of high fever on a genetically predisposed individual, but were examples of prolonged seizures occurring as a result of factors operating in the pre or perinatal stages. The argument for defining two separate groups of children with prolonged FCs was, he considered, a valid one.

*Chevrie, J.J., Aicardi, J. (1975): Duration and lateralization of febrile convulsions. Etiological factors. *Epilepsia* **16,** 781-789.

Lerman emphasized that the duration of the seizure was all-important. If the seizure lasted 2-6 hours then the child was invariably brain-damaged. He wondered if the HHE syndrome (hemiconvulsions, hemiplegia and later epilepsy) should be excluded from the rubric of FCs. He thought that a rapid rise of temperature (over 10-15 minutes) was all-important in triggering a FC.

Martinez-Lage asked about the role of sodium valproate in prophylaxis and noted that there had not been any cases of hepatotoxicity in Spain after 15 years' use of the drug. *O'Donohoe,* replying to this comment, argued that it was difficult to justify the use of a potentially toxic agent for the prophylaxis of what was essentially a benign condition in the vast majority of cases.

Jeavons referred to his analysis of reported cases of hepatotoxicity following valproate therapy and said that most of the cases had occurred in brain-damaged children who were on multiple anti-epileptic agents. There had, however, been one case reported in the USA in a child with recurrent FCs. He agreed that it was preferable to instruct the parents how to deal with the seizure when it occurred and he hardly ever resorted to continuous prophylaxis nowadays. He disliked phenobarbitone as a drug for young children and favoured the use of rectal diazepam.

He pointed out, however, that some parents, for various reasons, are unable to handle this preparation at home and continuous prophylaxis may be necessary to protect the child.

Jeavons, O'Donohoe and *Aicardi* agreed that focal features were not important in a brief FC and that duration was the important factor. It was agreed that duration was the most important factor in influencing long-term outcome and that an attack lasting more than 15 minutes might be dangerous. Unilateral features were common in prolonged seizures. *Aicardi* pointed out that it was difficult to collect a group of brief focal FCs but that the long-prognosis for these was the same as for brief generalized FCs. He also emphasized that the differentiation between simple and complicated FCs was very much a *post hoc* exercise and that the distinction was not apparent during the first minutes of the seizure. It was therefore important to instruct parents how to cope with the next FC.

Dreifuss compared the two varieties of FCs with the division into primary and secondary epilepsies, the former with a strong hereditary background and a good prognosis, and the latter usually a lesional epilepsy with a less certain outcome. He preferred the terms uncomplicated and complicated to the use of simple and complex. He emphasized the unique nature of Nelson and Ellenberg's prospective study of 54,000 pregnant women, pointing out that it was unlikely to be replicated and that the results obtained would stand scrutiny as definitive.

Wolf asked if there were any hard data on duration of FCs and the potential for brain damage. He objected to the word 'focal' to describe features of the actual seizure since a focal seizure should start focally to be so categorized. In discussion, *Aicardi* and others suggested the term 'lateralized features' as preferable.

Dreifuss added that certain localized features in FCs had no localizing significance, eg versive turning of head and eyes. He advised caution, however, where unilateral or partial features of the seizure had been observed.

Doose wondered if FCs should be labelled as an epileptic syndrome. There was a broad overlap between FCs and other epileptic syndromes with a good prognosis, for example, the primary myoclonic epilepsies of early childhood where one may find a high prevalence of FCs in the families.

His data showed that, if children with FCs are followed to puberty with serial EEGs, inconstant signs of a genetic predisposition to epilepsy will be detected in 81 per cent, consisting of spike-wave discharges (sometimes only in sleep), photosensitivity, and 4-7 c/s rhythms or a combination of these findings. There were no correlations between these findings and any clinical criteria, however. He compared these findings with similar findings in patients with primary generalized epilepsies.

He suggested that those children who go on to develop a primary epilepsy after FCs are indicating clinically a high expressivity of the genetic predisposition. In a reply to *Dulac* he stated that the frequency of EEG abnormalities was the same in those with simple and complicated FCs and that there was no correlation between EEG abnormalities and the type of FC which occurred.

There was also no correlation between the rate of recurrences of FCs and EEG findings with one exception, namely, that if spike-wave discharges were constantly seen in every record then the rate of recurrences was high.

Sorel emphasized the importance of making an exact diagnosis of the type of FC in order to give precise prognostic information to the parents. He excluded lateralized convulsions and atonic seizures from his description of a FC, confining the diagnostic label to short tonic-clonic seizures without post-ictal paralysis of any kind and with a normal EEG between attacks. He considered that FCs during sleep did not indicate a good prognosis and emphasized again the overriding importance of duration of the seizure. He referred also to the need to exclude anoxic seizures after breath-holding, or after syncope, from the diagnostic category of FCs.

Oller-Daurella suggested that simple FCs often had a tonic or atonic component only and that such seizures were more benign than tonic-clonic FCs. He commented on the value of the EEG in identifying a lateralized FC through the presence of post-ictal focal slowing and on the desirability of giving prophylactic treatment to those patients with post-ictal spike-wave discharges.

Dalla Bernardina referred to the important relationships between the age and sex of the child, the occurrence of simple or complicated FCs, and the incidence of later epilepsy. His studies had shown a close correlation between FCs in the first year of life and later epilepsy. Duration and lateralization were partially age-dependent and a long lateralized FC was more likely to occur under 18 months. The incidence of later epilepsy was higher for girls who had FCs before 1 year but this difference compared with boys disappeared progressively after that age.

Cavazzuti presented data from a study of 95 infants who developed FCs in the first year. The incidence of prolonged or repeated convulsions in the same illness was high. 23 children went on to develop afebrile seizures, 18 after a few years and 5 at a later stage. 10 of the cases were mentally handicapped to a varying extent. The recurrence rate for FCs was 50 per cent and frequent recurrences were common, even before the first birthday. He commented on the very bad prognosis attached to FCs appearing before the age of 6 months. Familial factors were less common in FCs occurring in the first year. He stressed that the prognosis for FCs occurring in this epoch of life was completely different from that obtaining for older children with FCs.

Beaumanoir commented that these early FCs may represent an entirely different epileptic syndrome.

Pinsard and *Roger* noted the marked decline in the incidence of the HHE syndrome in recent years and ascribed this to the better general health of children and to the availability of more effective anti-epileptic agents for terminating prolonged seizures.

Epileptic syndromes in infancy, child-hood and adolescence. J. Roger, C. Dravet, M. Bureau, F.E. Dreifuss and P. Wolf. John Libbey Eurotext Ltd ©1985.

Chapter 5
West Syndrome: Infantile Spasms

Peter M. JEAVONS

Clinical Neurophysiology Unit, Department of Ophthalmic Optics, University of Aston in Birmingham, Woodcock Street, Birmingham BA 7ET, United Kingdom

Summary

Typical West Syndrome consists of infantile spasms, mental retardation and hypsarrhythmia. Spasms may be flexor, extensor, lightning or nods but most commonly are mixed. Mental retardation is almost invariable. Hypsarrhythmia is present in at least two thirds. There is a characteristic ictal EEG pattern. Onset peaks between 4 and 7 months, and is nearly always before 1 year. Males are more affected. There are two aetiological groups. In the primary group development is normal prior to onset; in the secondary group development is abnormal and there is known aetiology. Half the cases show neurological abnormality. The prognosis depends on early therapy with ACTH or oral steroids, and on a number of other factors, the most important being early normal development. Complete recovery is confined to the primary group. Atypical forms are those with early or late onset, and those in whom one element of the triad is missing.

Introduction

West syndrome (infantile spasms), so called because the first clinical account was given by Dr W. J. West in 1841, consists of a triad (first described by Vazquez and Turner, 1951) of infantile spasms, psychomotor retardation or deterioration and a characteristic EEG pattern, called hypsarrhythmia by Gibbs and Gibbs (1952). In 1958, Sorel and Dusaucy-Bauloye reported the first successful treatment, using ACTH.

Detailed accounts of West's syndrome, including reviews of the early literature, were given by Jeavons and Bower (1964), Gastaut *et al.* (1964), Lacy and Penry (1976) and a more recent comprehensive account was given by Aicardi and Chevrie (1978).

West's syndrome is rare, and it has been estimated that the incidence is 1 in 4000-6000 (Lacy and Penry, 1976; Riikonen and Donner, 1979).

The onset is usually between 3 and 7 months, and onset before the age of one year occurs in 80-95 per cent, with a peak at 5 months. If onset is after the age of 1 year it is probable that the diagnosis is Lennox syndrome.

Boys are more often affected than girls, and although the ratio varies according to different authors, in 1245 patients reported in the literature, the male/female ratio was 1.5: 1. Lombroso (1983) found the male preponderance was mainly in the symptomatic group.

A family history of infantile spasms is rare and is from 3-6 per cent (Lacy and Penry, 1976; Lombroso, 1983). Infantile spasms may occur in a wide variety of disorders some of which are genetically determined.

Clinical aspects

The various descriptions of spasms depend broadly on the musculature involved and the duration of the spasms. Spasms are usually divided into flexor, extensor, and mixed spasms, whilst some authors separate head nods and lightning spasms.

Flexor spasms may involve the neck, trunk and limbs with abduction or adduction of the arms. Flexor spasms have been described as 'jack-knife' when flexion is very marked and the legs are drawn up. In salaam spasms, the arms are flung outwards. The arms may appear to hug the head, or adopt a posture similar to warding off a blow to the head, or resemble the Moro reflex. In extensor spasms ('cheer-leader') the neck and trunk are extended with limbs in extension, abduction or adduction. Head nods are brief flexor spasms confined to the muscles of the neck. Lightning spasms are distinguished by their brevity, being only observed if one is looking at the infant at the time of their occurrence. Asymmetrical or unilateral spasms are rare and almost always are a reflection of some cerebral pathology. The duration of the spasm is usually between 1 and 15 s.

Most authors state that flexor spasms are the most common, mixed spasms the next most common and extensor spasms the rarest. Jeavons and Bower (1964) reported flexor spasms in 68 per cent, mixed spasms in 22 per cent, extensor in 6 per cent, nods in 2 per cent and lightning in 2 per cent. However, in a detailed study of 5042 spasms in 24 infants Kellaway *et al.* (1979) found mixed spasms to be present in 42 per cent, flexor in 34 per cent and extensor in 22.5 per cent. Lombroso (1983) reported mixed spasms in 50 per cent, flexor in 42 per cent and extensor in 19 per cent.

It is characteristic of infantile spasms to occur in series (present in 50-66 per cent) and up to 30 attacks may occur in quick succession. Spasms are present during waking and during sleep, and have been reported as being more common prior to going to sleep and immediately after waking.

There is no consensus of opinion as to whether there is any disturbance of consciousness. However, smiling and increased alertness (psychic awakening: Launay *et al.,* 1959), have been noted during the period of EEG attenuation associated with a spasm. A variety of events have been noted to occur in association with spasms, the most common of these being a scream or a cry which may lead to the misdiagnosis of colic.

Mental retardation
Mental retardation or psychomotor regression is present at the onset in about 95 per cent of cases and is usually severe (88 per cent). Normal mentality is found in 5 per cent (Jeavons and Bower, 1964; Sorel, 1973).

Neurological abnormalities
Neurological abnormalities may be found in nearly half the patients, the most common being spastic diplegia or quadriplegia or hemiparesis, quite often with associated microcephaly. Neurological abnormalities are of course commoner in symptomatic cases.

Other seizures
Seizures of types other than spasms may precede, accompany, or follow the acute period of spasms. Such seizures may be generalized or partial, and are most likely to

occur in the symptomatic group. Seizures preceding or accompanying spasms occur in 20-30 per cent, whilst at least half the patients will have seizures after the spasms have ceased, the most common being generalized tonic-clonic fits.

EEG

Hypsarrhythmia is defined as a grossly chaotic mixture of very high amplitude (exceeding 200 μV) slow waves at frequencies of 1-7 c/s. with sharp waves and spikes which vary in amplitude, morphology, duration and site (Fig. 1). Modified hypsarrhythmia has a more organized appearance with some bilaterally synchronous discharges. Jeavons and Bower (1964) reported hypsarrhythmia or modified hypsarrhythmia in 66 per cent (a similar figure to that of Lombroso, 1983) whilst in 32 per cent the EEG was not hypsarrhythmic but showed paroxysmal discharges of slow waves and spikes. Unilateral hypsarrhythmia or marked asymmetry of hypsarrhythmia is usually associated with cerebral pathology. In some patients hypsarrhythmia may only appear during sleep whilst in others it becomes less marked during sleep. Suppression-burst activity is seen mainly in the younger infant, before the age of four months, and may occur during waking or during sleep.

The most common ictal pattern is an initial high amplitude slow wave with or without a spike followed by a period of flattening of the trace for several seconds (Fig. 2). This pattern was found in 38 per cent of ictal patterns reported by Kellaway et al. (1979). During the period of attenuation there may be fast activity, or some rhythms which are normal for the age of the patient. The next most common pattern of ictal discharge consists of high amplitude sharp wave, slow wave, or spike and slow wave without attenuation. In some instances periods of EEG attenuation occur without any preceding discharge and without any apparent spasms though the child may be staring. These would appear to be tonic attacks of early Lennox syndrome.

The EEG during a series of attacks may show high amplitude spike and slow waves associated with each spasm without attenuation.

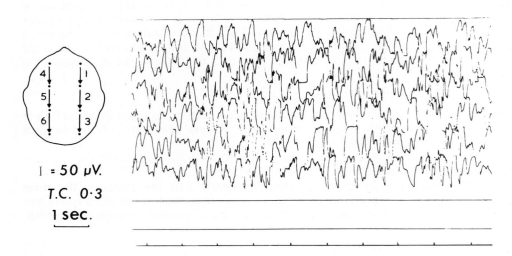

I = 50 μV.
T.C. 0·3
1 sec.

Fig. 1. Hypsarrhythmia, gain 50 μV. Time constant 0.3. Paper speed 3 cm/s (from Jeavons & Bower, 1964. Heinemann: London).

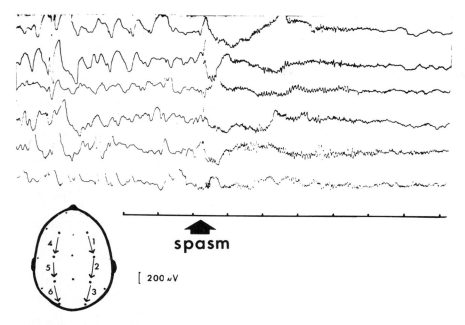

Fig. 2. Typical ictal EEG pattern of spasm, showing attenuation and fast activity (from Jeavons & Bower, 1964. Heinemann: London).

Aetiology

West syndrome can be divided into two groups, cryptogenic or primary, and symptomatic or secondary. In the cryptogenic group psychomotor development of the infant is normal up to the onset of spasms and there is no evidence of any cerebral disorder. In the symptomatic group there is evidence of early abnormal development with psychomotor retardation or neurological abnormality prior to the onset. With increasing sophistication of investigatory techniques the proportion of symptomatic cases has increased and it is probable that 70 per cent are symptomatic.

There are innumerable causes of West syndrome including pre and perinatal damage, neuro-cutaneous syndromes (especially tuberose sclerosis), cerebral malformations, metabolic disorders, and cerebral infections (Lacy and Penry, 1976; Aicardi and Chevrie, 1978).

Neuroradiology

Investigation using computerised tomography has shown abnormality in 81 per cent of 37 patients in one study (Gastaut *et al.,* 1978) and in 66 per cent of 30 patients (Singer *et al.,* 1982). The most common abnormalities are cerebral atrophy and congenital malformations.

Response to therapy

There is general agreement that ACTH or oral steroids remain the therapy of choice especially in cryptogenic cases, though some improvement has occurred with benzodiazepines and sodium valproate. Recent publications have confirmed previous theories that early and intensive treatment is important in achieving a complete cure (Pinsard, 1980; Lerman and Kivity, 1982; Lombroso, 1983).

Complete recovery (cessation of all seizures and a normal or near normal intellectual level) is confined to the cryptogenic or primary group. The mean figure, based on 12 reports (Snyder, 1967; Pache and Troger, 1967; Chevrie *et al.*, 1968; Cavazzuti, 1973; Jeavons *et al.*, 1973; Sorel, 1973; Bachet and Gallet, 1978; Pinsard, 1980; Singer *et al.*, 1980; Matsumoto *et al.*, 1981; Lerman and Kivity, 1982; Lombroso, 1983), is 41 per cent but when there is early and intensive treatment, better results, between 59 and 85 per cent, have been achieved (Pinsard, 1980; Lerman and Kivity, 1982; Lombroso, 1983).

Prognosis

Spasms usually disappear by the age of 5 years whether or not treatment has been given.

Achievement of the normal or near normal mentality is rare in untreated patients, but may occur in cryptogenic cases if psychomotor retardation was only mild, or absent, at the onset of the spasms and if spasms occurred over a period of a few months (Jeavons *et al.*, 1973; Sorel, 1973).

Complete recovery is confined to the primary or cryptogenic group and depends in part on the therapy, though other factors are very important and these are shown in Table 1.

Figures for mortality vary between 6 and 24 per cent, the mean figure in eight large studies being 16 per cent (Gibbs *et al.*, 1954; Trojaborg and Plum, 1960; Mizutani, 1969; Friedman and Pampiglione, 1971; Cavazzuti, 1973; Jeavons *et al.*, 1973; Pinsard, 1980; Matsumoto *et al.*, 1981).

Differential diagnosis

Some other syndromes occurring at the same age must be well differentiated.

(1) The first is benign myoclonus of early infancy, described by Lombroso and Fejerman in 1977. In this the ictal symptomatology consists of typical spasms, there is never any associated psychomotor retardation, the EEG is normal, even during spasms, and remission occurs in a short time without therapy.

(2) The other epileptic syndromes in infancy described in this book: benign myoclonic epilepsy, myoclonic-astatic epilepsy, early myoclonic encephalopathy.

Table 1. Factors in prognosis

Good	*Poor*
1 Primary group	1 Secondary group
2 Normal development prior to onset	2 Abnormal development prior to onset
3 Normal mentality or only mild retardation at onset	3 Severe initial mental retardation
4 No other seizures	4 Other seizures
5 No neurological abnormality	5 Neurological abnormality
6 Early therapy in primary group	6 Onset before 3 months
7 Short acute phase of spasms	

Atypical forms and nosological limits

Atypical forms of West syndrome are those in which the age of onset is atypical and those in which one element of the triad is missing.

Atypical age of onset

I think that the cases with onset before the age of 3 months can be included in West syndrome provided all three elements of the triad are present. If the onset is after the age of 1 year, on the contrary, the case should be excluded from West syndrome and is most likely to be Lennox syndrome.

One element of the triad is missing

If there is no evidence of typical spasms the case should be excluded. If the infant has staring attacks, occurring in association with typical EEG attenuation of the type usually seen with spasms, these should be regarded as tonic attacks and excluded. Yamatogi and Ohtahara (1981) have described a syndrome of neonatal epileptic encephalopathy with suppression burst, the onset being within the first 3 months of life. The associated attack is a tonic spasm and this syndrome should be separated from typical West syndrome, as it is probably a form of early Lennox syndrome.

The absence of psychomotor retardation does not exclude the diagnosis of West syndrome though it is rare for this to occur.

On the contrary, the absence of EEG abnormality must lead to exclusion of this diagnosis.

If at least two EEGs are normal, including sleep recording, in infants in whom the onset of spasms was later than 3 months West syndrome is excluded.

But the absence of hypsarrhythmia or modified hypsarrhythmia is not an exclusion criterion. Children should be included if this EEG shows asymmetrical or unilateral hypsarrhythmia. In the same way cases should be included if their EEG shows non-specific paroxysmal abnormalities, provided they have infantile spasms and development retardation. For this reason we include the Aicardi syndrome (Aicardi et al., 1969) as it is clearly defined, characterized by female sex, spasms, a particular EEG (often asymmetric suppression bursts), absence of the corpus callosum, retinal lacunae and vertebral abnormalities.

References

Aicardi, J., Chevrie, J-J. (1978): Les spasmes infantiles. *Archs Franc. Pédiatr.* **35**, 1015-1023.
Aicardi, J., Chevrie, J-J., Rousselie, F. (1969): Le syndrome spasmes en flexion, agénésie calleuse, anomalies choriorétiniennes. *Archs Franc. Pédiatr.* **26**, 1103-1120.
Bachet, J., Gallet, J.P. (1978): Spasmes infantiles ou syndrome de West. *Rev. Pédiatr.* **14**, 76-82.
Cavazzuti, G.B. (1973): Infantile spasms with hypsarrhythmia. In *Evolution and prognosis of epilepsies*, ed E. Lugaresi, P. Pazzaglia, C.A. Tassinari, pp 109-117. Aulo Gaggi: Bologna.
Chevrie, J-J., Aicardi, J., Thieffry, St. (1968): Traitement hormonal de 58 cas de spasmes infantiles. Résultats et pronostic psychique à long terme. *Archs Franc. Pédiatr.* **25**, 263-276.
Friedman, E., Pampiglione, G. (1971): Prognostic implications of electro-encephalographic findings of hypsarrhythmia in first year of life. *Br. Med. J.* **2**, 323-325.
Gastaut, H., Roger, J., Soulayrol, R., Pinsard, N. (1964): *Encéphalopathie myoclonique infantile avec hypsarythmie (syndrome de West)*. Masson: Paris.
Gastaut, H., Gastaut, J.L., Régis, H., Bernard, R., Pinsard, N., Saint-Jean, M., Roger, J., Dravet, C. (1978): Computerized tomography in the study of West's syndrome. *Develop. Med. Child Neurol.* **20**, 21-27.

Gibbs, F.A., Gibbs, E.L. (1952): *Atlas of electroencephalography, vol. II, Epilepsy*. Addison-Wesley: Cambridge, Mass.

Gibbs, F.A., Gibbs, E.L., Fleming, M.M. (1954): Diagnosis and prognosis of hypsarrhythmia and infantile spasms. *Pediatrics* **13**, 66-73.

Jeavons, P.M., Bower, B.D. (1964): *Infantile spasms. A review of the literature and a study of 112 cases*. Heinemann: London.

Jeavons, P.M., Bower, B.D., Dimitrakoudi, M. (1973): Long term prognosis of 150 cases of "West Syndrome". *Epilepsia* **14**, 153-164.

Kellaway, P., Hrachovy, R.A., Frost, J.D., Zion, T. (1979): Precise characterization and quantification of infantile spasms. *Ann. Neurol.* **6**, 214-218.

Lacy, J.R., Penry, J.K. (1976): *Infantile spasms*. Raven Press: New York.

Launay, C., Blanc, C., Rebufat-Deschamps, M. (1959): Spasmes en flexion et hypsarythmie. Mise au point à propos de dix observations personnelles. *Presse Méd.* **67**, 887-890.

Lerman, P., Kivity, S. (1982): The efficacy of corticotropin in primary infantile spasms. *J. Pediatr.* **101**, 294-296.

Lombroso, C.T. (1983): A prospective study of infantile spasms: clinical and therapeutic correlations. *Epilepsia* **24**, 135-158.

Lombroso, C.T., Fejerman, N. (1977): Benign myoclonus of early infancy. *Ann. Neurol.* **1**, 138-143.

Matsumoto, A., Watanabe, K., Negoro, T., Sugiura, M., Inase, K., Miyazaki, S. (1981): Long-term prognosis after infantile spasms: a statistical study of prognostic factors in 200 cases. *Develop. Med. Child Neurol.* **23**, 51-65.

Mizutani, I. (1969): Clinical study of infantile spasms. *Acta Paediatr. Jap.* **73**, 110-130.

Pache, H.D., Troger, H. (1967): Das West-Syndrom und seine Behandlung mit ACTH. *Münch. Med. Wschr.* **109**, 2408-2413.

Pinsard, N. (1980): Evolution à long terme du syndrome de West (à propos de 100 cas). *Gaslini.* **12**, (Suppl 1), 24-27.

Riikonen, R., Donner, M. (1979): Incidence and aetiology of infantile spasms from 1960 to 1976. A population study in Finland. *Develop. Med. Child. Neurol.* **21**, 333-343.

Singer, W.D., Rabe, E.F., Haller, J.S. (1980): The effect of ACTH therapy upon infantile spasms. *J. Pediatr.* **96**, 485-498.

Singer, W.D., Haller, J.S., Sullivan, L.R., Wolpert, S., Mills, C., Rabe, E.F. (1982): The value of neuroradiology in infantile spasms. *J. Pediatr.* **100**, 47-50.

Snyder, C.H. (1967): Infantile spasms: favourable responses to steroid therapy. *J.Am.Med.Ass.* **201**, 198-200.

Sorel, L. (1973): A propos de 187 observations de la maladie des spasmes en flexion de la première enfance à symptomatologie typique et atypique et son traitement; évolution thérapeutique à long terme. In *Evolution and prognosis of epilepsies*, ed E. Lugaresi, P. Pazzaglia, C.A. Tassinari, pp 85-99. Aulo Gaggi: Bologna.

Sorel, L., Dusaucy-Bauloye, A. (1958): A propos de 21 cas d'hypsarythmie de Gibbs. Son traitement spectaculaire par l'ACTH. *Acta Neurol. Belg.* **58**, 130-141.

Trojaborg, W., Plum, P. (1960): Treatment of hypsarrhythmia with ACTH. *Acta Paediatr.* **49**, 572-582.

Vasquez, H.J., Turner, M. (1951): Epilepsia en flexion generalizada. *Archs Argent. Pediatr.* **35**, 111-141.

West, W.J. (1841): On a peculiar form of infantile convulsions. *Lancet* **1**, 724-725.

Yamatogi, Y., Ohtahara, S. (1981): Age-dependent epileptic encephalopathy: a longitudinal study. *Folia Psychiatr. Neurol. Jpn.* **35**, 321-332.

Discussion
Summarized by P.M. JEAVONS

Dulac presented a number of slides illustrating the EEG aspects of West syndrome, stressing the heterogeneity of its aetiology, and he illustrated Leigh's disease, agyria, Aicardi syndrome, tuberose sclerosis and Von Recklinghausen disease. He did not feel that the type of spasm was important, but it was important to know whether the epilepsy was primary or secondary. He then stressed the heterogeneity of EEG patterns and suggested that further individual patterns, such as those of Aicardi syndrome, needed to be identified. His patients who recovered fully were all of the primary group and were neurologically normal apart from hypotonia and mental regression, and none had shown focal EEG abnormality following the administration of diazepam. Finally, he felt it important to identify further clinical and EEG characteristics of a homogenous group who make a complete recovery, since there may be factors other than normal development and early therapy.

Pinsard stressed the importance of using strict criteria in defining the primary or cryptogenic group in order to evaluate therapies and prognosis. The main criteria were onset after the age of 3 months but before 1 year, lack of antecedent disease or seizures prior to the spasms, no neurological signs, normal psychomotor development, and a characteristic symmetrical hypsarrhythmia, and normal CT scan.

The secondary or symptomatic types may be atypical or partial but still belong to West syndrome.

Sorel commented that one describes a syndrome as consisting of many symptoms. He felt that it was important to add the age of onset, the evolution, and possibly the age at which the syndrome ceased. He preferred the term epileptic entity, which was defined as a syndrome with particular clinical and EEG features, a typical evolution, and probably a common physiopathology, though aetiology was variable.

Gastaut felt it necessary to distinguish primary and secondary forms but thought primary were rare because in most cases there must often be slight brain damage. Many cases of tuberose sclerosis presented as primary cases, the diagnosis being made by CT scan.

Lerman mentioned that some patients may have focal partial seizures prior to the onset of spasms, indicating secondary generalisation.

Beaumanoir did not think it essential to differentiate primary and secondary forms, and said that it was important to say what the syndrome was symptomatic 'of ', or secondary 'to'. On the other hand, *Pinsard* felt it was necessary to differentiate the two forms because of the prognosis, which was worse in the secondary form. Evolution, prognosis and results of therapy were better evaluated in primary cases.

Loiseau indicated the need for participants to define entities or syndromes, and discussion of the criteria for inclusion or exclusion followed. It was generally agreed that onset before the age of 3 months could be included and onset after 1 year be excluded. For *Sorel, Jeavons and Gastaut* hypsarrhythmia was not an essential element for diagnosis, which had to be made early, possibly before the appearance of hypsarrhythmia.

However, the EEG must be abnormal. For *Sorel* it was possible to have West syndrome without spasms, but for *Jeavons, Aicardi and Doose* spasms were essential. *Tassinari* indicated that spasms might not be present initially, but agreed that their occurrence at some time was essential. *Doose* had never seen hypsarrhythmia without spasms. *Sorel* said it was important to treat any child with hypsarrhythmia as soon as possible, whether or not there were spasms. *Munari* considered the presence of spasms to be fundamental in defining West Syndrome.

Dreifuss indicated the danger of rigid definitions which could exclude something very pertinent, but stressed that one must avoid the 'forme fruste', and he felt that hypsarrhythmia without spasms should be excluded.

Dalla Bernardina spoke about the difference between scientific discussions concerning classification and practical clinical problems. It was important to retain typical and atypical syndromes.

Throughout the discussion there had been agreement that decisions on therapy were independent of decisions on classification and the criteria involved in defining the syndrome.

Finally *Dreifuss* stressed the importance of full polygraphic recording in the differential diagnosis of the 'staring' attacks which were associated with an ictal pattern typical of an infantile spasm, since he felt that clinical signs could be very slight in some spasms. *Jeavons* agreed, but thought that many of the children who showed these 'staring' attacks were cases of early Lennox-Gastaut syndrome, and not West syndrome.

Epileptic syndromes in infancy, childhood and adolescence. J. Roger, C. Dravet, M. Bureau, F.E. Dreifuss and P. Wolf. John Libbey Eurotext Ltd ©1985.

Chapter 6
Benign Myoclonic Epilepsy in Infants

Charlotte DRAVET, Michelle BUREAU and Joseph ROGER

Centre Saint-Paul, 300 Boulevard Sainte-Marguerite, 13009 Marseille, France

Summary

Benign infantile myoclonic epilepsy is certainly rare, since reports of only 17 such cases have been published to date. It is characterized by brief bouts of generalized myoclonus which occur during the first or second year of life in normal children who often have a family history of convulsions or epilepsy. EEG recordings show generalized spike-waves occurring in brief bursts during the early stages of sleep. These attacks are easily controlled by suitable treatment. They are not accompanied by any other types of seizure, although generalized tonic-clonic seizures may occur later, during adolescence. If treatment is not begun sufficiently early, the epilepsy may be accompanied by a relative slowing down of intellectual development and minor personality disorders.

It seems as if this type of epilepsy could be the earliest expression of primary generalized epilepsy.

General

We have found no description of a syndrome of this kind in data published before 1981, although many authors have studied the subject of myoclonic epilepsy in infants. We observed the syndrome in 1981 in seven infants (Dravet and Bureau, 1981) and Dalla Bernardina *et al.,* reported 10 such cases in 1983.

Prevalence
This condition is most probably a rare one, since the cases we observed represented only 7 per cent of a total of 142 subjects with different types of myoclonic epilepsy and the cases observed by Dalla Bernardina represented only 2 per cent of 504 children whose epilepsy had begun during the first three years of life.

Sex
Boys out-numbered girls amongst the children studied (five versus two).

Genetic factors
The number of cases observed so far is too small for us to draw any definite conclusions.

Two of the seven children in our patient series had a family history of epilepsy: one girl had a second degree cousin who suffered from absence seizures, and one boy had a maternal uncle who died 10 months following febrile convulsions. Dalla Bernardina *et al.,* mention 33 per cent of cases with a positive family history.

Age of onset
Age of onset was between 6 months and 2 years for our patients, and between 4 months and 2 years 8 months for those of Dalla Bernardina.

Electroclinical semiology

The seizures are brief, generalized *myoclonic attacks,* varying in intensity and occurring in normal children. These attacks may be barely noticeable initially. For this reason, parents sometimes have difficulty in determining the exact age of onset and frequency. They often speak of the seizures as 'spasms' or as 'head nodding'. Later, these attacks occur several times a day, and when the children learn to stand, they cause loss of balance possibly leading to falls.

Observation on video and polygraphic recordings have enabled us to make a precise analysis of these attacks. They are more or less massive myoclonic seizures involving the axis of the body and the limbs, causing the head to drop suddenly onto the trunk,

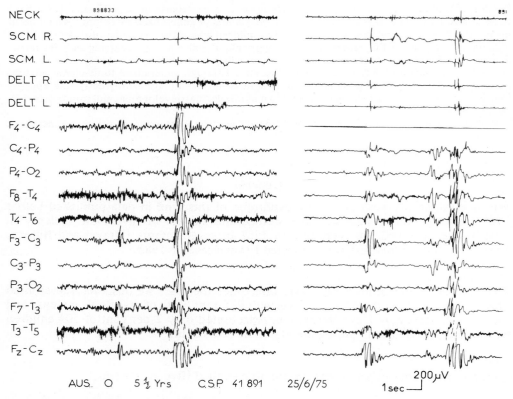

Fig. 1. Myoclonic fits in a 5.5 years old boy before VPA treatment. Top: EMG of neck, right and left sterno-cleido-mastoids and deltoids. Each very brief fit is accompanied by a generalized spike-wave discharge.

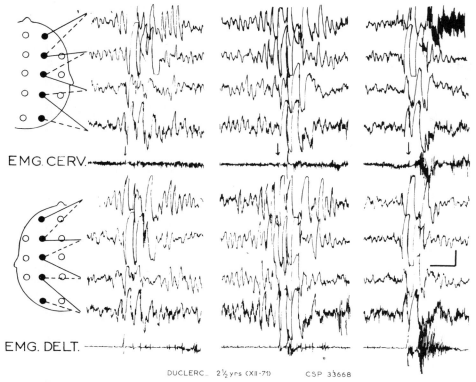

EMG. CERV.

EMG. DELT.

DUCLERC.. 2½ yrs (XII-71)   CSP 33668

Fig. 2. Three short myoclonic fits, polygraphically recorded. Each fit is accompanied by a very high generalized spike-wave discharge. On the recorded muscles myoclonias (deltoid) are sometimes followed by an atonia (cervical muscle).

and an upwards-outwards movement of the upper limbs, with flexion of the lower limbs. They may also provoke a rolling up of the eyeballs. The intensity of the seizures varies greatly from one child to another, and sometimes from one attack to another in the same child. The most severe forms cause the child to fail suddenly and to involuntarily project any objects he may be holding in his hand; the mildest forms provoke only a brief forwards movement of the head, or even a simple closing of the eyes.

As a rule, the attacks are very brief (1-3s), although they may be longer (5-10s), especially in older children, consisting of pseudorhythmically repeated jerks (Figs 1 and 2). In these cases, alertness may be reduced, but the children never lose consciousness and continue their activity during the seizure. These myoclonic attacks do not occur in series and there is no known triggering factor. They may occur at any time of day, and disappear during deep sleep.

On EEG recordings (Figs 1 and 2), myoclonic seizures are always accompanied by a discharge of generalized spike-waves (SW) or polyspike-waves (PSW) occurring in rapid succession (3 c/s) and lasting the same length of time as the seizure (1-3s).

Polygraphic recordings reveal myoclonus in the muscles. In two of the cases we observed, the seizures appeared to be favoured by IPS.

No other types of seizure were observed in the children affected: in particular, no absence seizures and no tonic seizures. However, two of the children had suffered from simple febrile convulsions prior to onset of the seizures (at the age of 20 months in one case, and at the age of 10 months and 15 months in the second case).

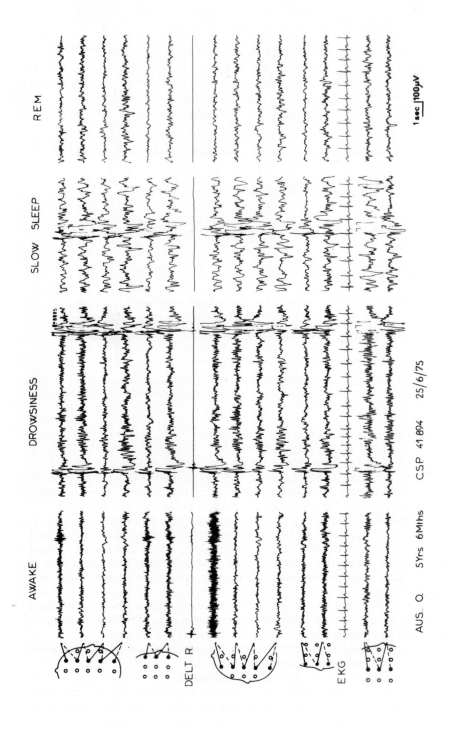

Fig. 3. In the same child as in Fig. 1, from the left to the right: normal interictal awake EEG; EEG during drowsiness showing generalized spike-waves and multiple spike-waves associated with small myoclonias on the right deltoid; slow sleep EEG showing subclinical generalized spike-waves; REM sleep EEG without abnormality.

Interictal EEG recordings (Fig. 3) are normal for the children's age. During waking hours, there are few interictal abnormalitites. Almost all spike-wave or polyspike-wave discharges have some form of clinical expression. In cases where SW or PSW are provoked by photic stimulation, they are accompanied by myoclonus. Drowsiness and the early stages of sleep activate generalized SW. During light sleep, they are almost always accompanied by myoclonus. The discharges then tend to become less frequent during slow wave sleep, and myoclonus disappear. Similarly, during REM sleep, we observe neither SW nor myoclonus.

Clinical examination is normal, and there is no interictal myoclonus. Neurological examination and X-rays (one pneumoencephalography, two CT scans) were conducted in three cases and showed|no abnormalities.

Evolution

If left untreated, the myoclonic seizures tend to persist (up to the age of 8.5 years in one of our patients). They are easily controlled by sodium valproate (Na VPA) alone in therapeutic doses. Generalized tonic-clonic seizures may occur subsequently in later childhood or at puberty (two cases). but they disappear when treatment is re-introduced.

EEG disturbances improve at the same time as the clinical signs, although rare, isolated, generalized SW may persist for several years. It should also be born in mind that prescription of unsuitable drugs (barbiturates or benzodiazepines in high doses) may aggravate both clinical and EEG disturbances, causing in particular a slowing down of background rhythm.

Our seven patients are now aged between 6 and 17 years. The seizures have disappeared in all cases during a follow-up period ranging from 4 to 11 years. Two patients are no longer receiving treatment and the follow-up period is 5 years and 11 years respectively. The psychological evolution of the patients is less favourable than the clinical evolution of the seizures. Although psychomotor development was normal in all cases, the children who did not receive adequate treatment at a sufficiently early stage presented behavioural disturbances and learning difficulties when they started school (four cases out of seven). These difficulties remained slight, and the children were able to continue their education in specialized schools. This disturbance in development is probably related to the early stage of onset of the seizures and to their frequency. All authors, Aicardi and Chevrie (1970) in particular, have insisted on the possibility of unfavourable psychological prognosis in children suffering from epilepsy of any type at an early stage.

Diagnosis

It may be difficult initially to determine the epileptic nature of the bouts of myoclonus, unless one of them occurs during an EEG recording. They could be confused with benign, non-epileptic myoclonus, as described by Fejerman and Medina (1977) and Lombroso and Fejerman (1977), which are never accompanied by EEG disturbances. However, this type of myoclonus begins earlier (4-8 months) and disappears spontaneously during the child's second year.

It is easy, on the other hand, to distinguish benign myoclonic epilepsy from most types of secondary generalized epilepsy occurring at this age: West syndrome (Gastaut et al., 1964) (no serial spasms, no hypsarrhythmia, no psychomotor regression, occurring at a later age), Lennox-Gastaut syndrome (Gastaut et al., 1966) (no atypical absence seizures, no tonic seizures, no diffuse slow SW, no immediate psychological repercussions, earlier onset).

Severe myoclonic epilepsy (Dravet *et al.,* 1982) is also different: the bouts of myoclonus are preceded by severe, repeated convulsive seizures, with or without fever. Most treatment is ineffective. Generalized SW appear later on the recordings and are associated with focal abnormalities. Partial seizures may occur. Development is seriously disturbed after the child's second year, and abnormal neurological signs and interictal myoclonus appear.

Nosological place

We have found very few descriptions amongst published studies which correspond to the cases we report here. The cases described by Harper in 1968 under the name of 'true myoclonic epilepsy' have been reviewed by Jeavons and do not constitute a homogeneous group.

Kruse (1973) refers to similar cases, but his description is extremely brief. Jeavons, in 1977, gave the name of 'infantile myoclonic epilepsy' to a type of epilepsy similar to that which we describe, but beginnning at a later age (3 years) in children with no mental retardation.

All the other authors who have studied what they call 'infantile myoclonic epilepsy' report series which no doubt included cases similar to ours but which were not given individual characterization.

In a group of 51 patients with centrencephalic myoclonic-astatic petit mal, Doose *et al.,* (1970) mention five subjects who suffered from myoclonic seizures only, but give no details as to the age of onset, EEG patterns or outcome.

Aicardi and Chevrie's series in 1971 included a group with infantile cryptogenic myoclonic epilepsy, which was recognized as being non-homogeneous by the authors. It should have included a sub-group of cases with benign evolution, corresponding to the cases we describe. This sub-group was better defined by Aicardi in 1980.

In their taxonomic classification in 1974, Loiseau *et al.,* identify a 'Group C' corresponding to Aicardi's cryptogenic myoclonic epilepsy, specifying that there is no myoclonic status epilepticus in this group.

The Italian authors Pazzaglia *et al.,* (1979) and Giovanardi-Rossi *et al.,* (1979) make no distinction in their group of 'true myoclonic epilepsies' between cases with favourable outcome and those with unfavourable outcome.

It would appear, however, that out of all the different forms of myoclonic epilepsy, we can distinguish one which appears early in life and has a favourable prognosis, which belongs to the group of primary generalized epilepsy, and which we propose calling 'benign infantile myoclonic epilepsy'. It probably is the infantile equivalent of juvenile myoclonic epilepsy, both being an expression of primary generalized epilepsy at different moments of the brain maturation (Gastaut, 1981). It would be necessary to get a larger number of cases to study myoclonias more accurately by comparing them to those in juvenile myoclonic epilepsy.

We have observed too few cases to be able to determine incidence or genetic characteristics. Similarly, the number of cases we have seen beginning at the same age and in the same way but progressing unfavourably, is too small for us to make a comparative study.

References

Aicardi, J. (1980): Course and prognosis of certain childhood epilepsies with predominantly myoclonic seizures. In *Advances in Epileptology:* the Xth Epilepsy International Symposium, pp 159 - 163, ed J.A. Wada, J.K. Penry. Raven Press: New York.
Aicardi, J., Chevrie, J.J. (1971): Myoclonic epilepsies of childhood. *Neuropädiatrie* 3, 177 - 190.

Aicardi, J., Chevrie, J.J. (1978): Convulsive disorders in the first year of life: neurological and mental outcome and mortality. *Epilepsia* **19**, 67 - 74.

Dalla Bernardina, B., Colamaria, V., Capovilla G., Bondavalli, S. (1983): Nosological classification of epilepsies in the first three years of life. In *Epilepsy: an update on Research and Therapy*, pp 165-183, ed G. Nisticó, R. Di Perri, H. Meinardi. Alan Liss: New York.

Doose,H., Gerken, H., Leonardt, R., Völzke, E., Völz, C. (1970): Centrencephalic myoclonic-astatic petit mal. *Neuropädiatrie* **2**, 59 - 78.

Dravet, C., Bureau, M. (1981): L'épilepsie myoclonique bénigne du nourrisson. *Rev. EEG Neurophysiol.* **11**, 438-444.

Dravet, C., Roger, J., Bureau, M., Dalla Bernardina, B. (1982): Myoclonic epilepsies in childhood. In *Advances in Epileptology*: XIIIth Epilepsy International Symposium, pp 135 - 140, ed H. Akimoto, H. Kazamatsuri, M. Seino, A. Ward. Raven Press: New York.

Fejerman, N., Medina, C.S. (1977): *Convulsion en la Infancia*. Ergon: Buenos Aires.

Gastaut, H. (1981): Individualisation des épilepsies dites "bénignes" ou "fonctionnelles" aux différents âges de la vie. *Rev. EEG Neurophysiol.* **11**, 346 - 366.

Gastaut, H., Roger, J., Soulayrol, R., Pinsard, N. (1964): *L'Encéphalopathie myoclonique infantile avec hypsarythmie (syndrome de West)*. Masson: Paris.

Gastaut, H., Roger, J., Soulayrol, R., Tassinari, C.A., Régis, H., Dravet, C., Bernard, R., Pinsard,N., Saint-Jean, M. (1966): Childhood epileptic encephalopathy with diffuse slow spike-waves (otherwise known as 'petit mal variant') or Lennox syndrome. *Epilepsia* **7**, 139 - 179.

Giovanardi Rossi, P., Pazzaglia, P., Cirignotta, F., Moschen, R., Lugaresi, E. (1979): Le epilessie miocloniche nell'infanzia. *Riv. ital. Elettroencef. Neurofisiol. clin.*, **2**, 321 - 328.

Harper, J.R. (1968): True myoclonic epilepsy in childhood. *Archs Dis. Chiid.* **43**, 28-35.

Jeavons, P.M. (1977): Nosological problems of myoclonic epilepsies in childhood and adolescence. *Develop. Med. Child Neurol.* **19**, 3 - 8.

Kruse, R. (1973): Epilepsien des Kindesalters. In *Neuropädiatrie*, pp 354 - 425, ed A. Matthes, R. Kruse. George Thieme Verlag: Stuttgart.

Loiseau, P., Legroux, M., Grimond, P., du Pasquier, P., Henry, P. (1974): Taxometric classification of myoclonic epilepsies. *Epilepsia* **15**, 1 -11.

Lombroso, C., Fejerman, N. (1977): Benign myoclonus of early infancy. *Ann. Neurol.* **1**, 138-143.

Pazzaglia, P., Giovanardi Rossi, P., Cirignotta, F., Moschen, R., Lugaresi, E. (1979): Nosografia delle epilessie miocloniche. *Riv. ital. Elettroencef. Neurofisiol. Clin.*, **2**, 245 - 252.

* * *

Discussion pages 100-104

Epileptic syndromes in infancy, childhood and adolescence. J. Roger, C. Dravet, M. Bureau, F.E. Dreifuss and P. Wolf. John Libbey Eurotext Ltd ©1985.

Chapter 7
Severe Myoclonic Epilepsy in Infants

Charlotte DRAVET, Michelle BUREAU and Joseph ROGER

Centre Saint-Paul, 300 Boulevard Sainte Marguerite, 13009 Marseille, France

Summary

Severe myoclonic epilepsy (SME) in infants is a recently-defined syndrome, and only 82 case studies have been published. Their characteristics are homogeneous: family history of epilepsy or febrile convulsions, no previous personal history of disease, seizures beginning during the first year of life in the form of generalized or unilateral febrile clonic seizures, secondary appearance of myoclonic jerks and often partial seizures. EEG recordings show generalized spike-waves and polyspike-waves, early photosensitivity and focal abnormalities. Psychomotor development is retarded from the second year of life onwards, and ataxia, pyramidal signs and interictal myoclonus appear. This type of epilepsy is very resistant to all forms of treatment and all the children affected suffer from intellectual deficiency and personality disorders.

General

As with benign myoclonic epilepsy in infants, we found no syndrome of this type in data published before 1978. In 1978, our attention was drawn to several very severe cases of epilepsy beginning early in life which, despite certain similarities, could not be categorized as Lennox-Gastaut syndrome for several reasons, especially their stereotyped mode of onset and the absence of axial tonic seizures (Dravet, 1978). At the 13th International Epilepsy Symposium in 1981, we reported 42 cases of what we then termed severe myoclonic epilepsy (SME) (Dravet *et al.*, 1982). In 1982, Dalla Bernardina *et al.* reported 20 such cases. Dulac and Arthuis also reported 20 cases in the same year.

Prevalence
The incidence is unknown.

Our 42 cases represented 29.5 per cent of a group of 142 children with various types of myoclonic epilepsy. In a study on 504 subjects whose epilepsy had begun in the first three years of life, Dalla Bernardina *et al.* (1983) found that SME accounted for 7 per cent of the cases.

Sex

Of the 82 cases published, the number of boys (47) is slightly higher than the number of girls, (35) although the difference is not statistically significant.

Genetic factors

We found a high percentage of family history of epilepsy or convulsions (26 per cent). Six children had a family history of epilepsy, four of convulsions, and one of both epilepsy and convulsions. In only one case could we be certain that a brother and a sister both suffered from SME.

Among 20 cases, Dalla Bernardina *et al.* (1982) noted five cases with a family history of epilepsy (25 per cent) and three cases with a family history of febrile convulsions (15 per cent). Dulac and Arthuis (1982) found that five of their 20 subjects had a family history of epilepsy or convulsions.

Age of onset

Epilepsy began during the first year of life in all cases: the average age of onset was 5 months 9 days in our series (with a range from 2 months to 10 months), 6 months in the series of Dalla Bernardina *et al.* (1982) and 5 months 7 days in the series of Dulac and Arthuis (extremes of 3 months and 8 months).

Clinical and EEG characteristics

The children were all apparently normal before onset of the seizures, and only three of the 42 children in our study had suffered from neonatal anoxia. None of the children in the other two series had a history of previous illness.

The first seizure took the form of a *clonic seizure* in all cases, either generalized (37 cases) or unilateral (five cases). In some cases (14), it was of short duration, but was more often long (more than 15 minutes in 21 cases). We were unable to ascertain the precise duration of the first seizure in seven children. In most cases (30 out of 42), the first seizure was associated with fever. In all cases, the seizures recurred after short intervals (2 months on average for Dalla Bernardina *et al.* (1982) and 6 weeks for Dulac and Arthuis between the first two seizures), and were accompanied by a rise in temperature, suggesting febrile convulsions. However, the seizures later recurred with only slight rises in temperature and even in the absence of any fever. The febrile seizure tended to be long and to produce status epilepticus.

Between the ages of 1 and 4 years (with an average of 1 year 6 months in our series and 1 year 9 months in the series of Dalla Bernardina), a second type of seizure appeared, in the form of *generalized myoclonic attacks.* They were devoid of any specific characteristics. They occurred several times a day, did not appear in sudden bouts, but were very frequent and sometimes continuous (particularly during the period preceding a convulsive seizure). When they were particularly intense, they could cause the children to fall and sometimes to injure themselves. The less intense seizures were sometimes difficult to discern in very young children. They could be demonstrated by giving the child a precise activity to accomplish (drinking, holding a spoon, piling up cubes . . .). The children did not appear to suffer any disturbance in consciousness, unless the seizures occurred at very close intervals (of a few seconds). They could be initiated by variations in light intensity. We are not entirely in agreement with the term 'atypical absences' used by Dalla Bernardina *et al.* (1982) to describe these seizures of short duration with no detectable disturbance in consciousness.

A third type of seizure sometimes appeared at the same time as the myoclonic jerks, namely *partial seizures* evocative of complex partial seizures, with either autonomic (pallor, cyanosis of the lips,) or atonic phenomena and automatisms (14 of the 42

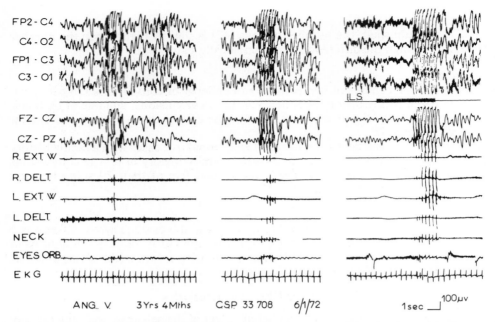

FP2 - C4
C4 - O2
FP1 - C3
C3 - O1
FZ - CZ
CZ - PZ
R. EXT. W
R. DELT.
L. EXT. W
L. DELT.
NECK
EYES ORB.
E K G

ANG. V.   3 Yrs 4 Mths   CSP 33 708   6/1/72   1 sec   100 μv

Fig. 1. Girl, 3 years 4 months old. Three generalized myoclonic fits are polygraphically recorded, corresponding to generalized fast spike-waves and polyspike-waves. The last one is provoked by IPS.

cases in our series). In certain cases, the partial seizure later became generalized, in the form of clonic or hemiclonic seizures.

Finally, some of the children presented in obtunded states accompanied by myoclonus, with varying degrees of diminished alertness.

EEG recordings were generally normal at the beginning of the disease, even during sleep. During the second year, paroxysmal abnormalities appeared (Fig. 1) in the form of rapid, generalized spike-waves or polyspike-waves, occurring either in isolation or in brief bursts, with an eventual predominance on one or other side. They were influenced by intermittent photic stimulation (30 out of 42 cases) and increased by drowsiness or slow-wave sleep (32 cases) (Figs 1 and 2). Photosensitivity appeared very early: during the first year of life in one case and between the ages of 1 and 2 years in six cases in the study of Dalla Bernardina *et al.* (1982). The polyspike-waves recorded ed during sleep were never characterized by repeated bursts of polyspikes observed during sleep in children with Lennox-Gastaut syndrome. Localized paroxysmal abnormalities were also very frequent (36 out of 42 cases) and mostly multifocal (21 cases), appearing as spikes and spike-waves. Background activity was normal to begin with, although Dalla Bernardina *et al.* (1982) insist on the presence of theta rhythms at 4 to 5 c/s during waking hours, in the fronto-central regions and the vertex (Fig. 3).

The recorded seizures were hemiclonic, myoclonic (Fig. 1) or partial (Fig. 4) seizures and obtunded states. In the last case, there were no continuous spike-waves on the EEG, but only a slowing in rhythm and sporadic discharges of spikes and spike-waves with no relationship to the myoclonus.

Polygraphic recordings enable identification of myoclonus, either during the myoclonic attacks or at other times.

Coinciding with the onset of myoclonus, we also observed a *slowing down of psychomotor development,* particularly in the child's language, and the gradual appearance

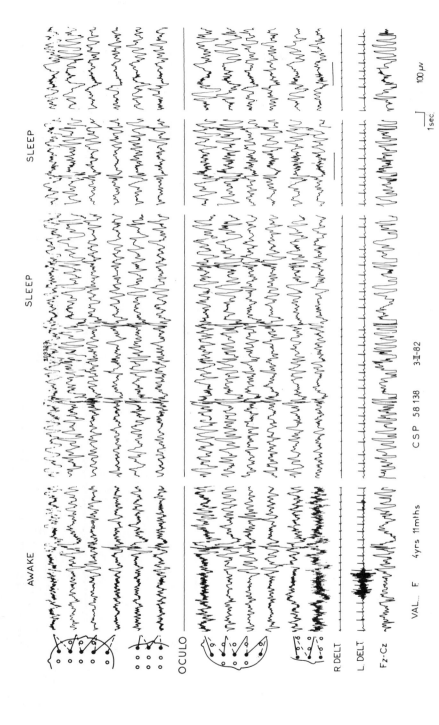

Fig. 2. Girl, 4 years 11 months old. *Left:* awake EEG showing a generalized spike-wave discharge, more evident on the left hemisphere. *Middle:* during sleep, either generalized or only left spikes and spike-waves. *Right:* the two last parts show rapid, low-voltage rhythms, higher on the left.

61

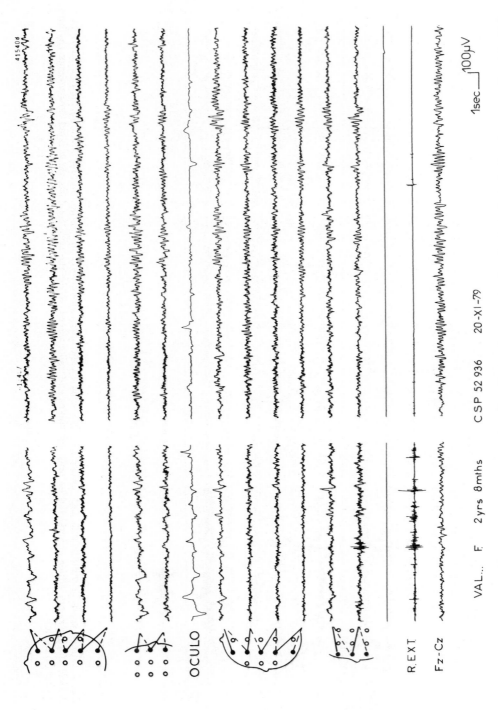

Fig. 3. Girl, 2 years 8 months old. *Left:* opened-eyes recording. *Right:* when eyes are closed a theta 5 c/s rhythm appears on the central areas and the vertex,

62

SEVERE MYOCLONIC EPILEPSY IN INFANTS

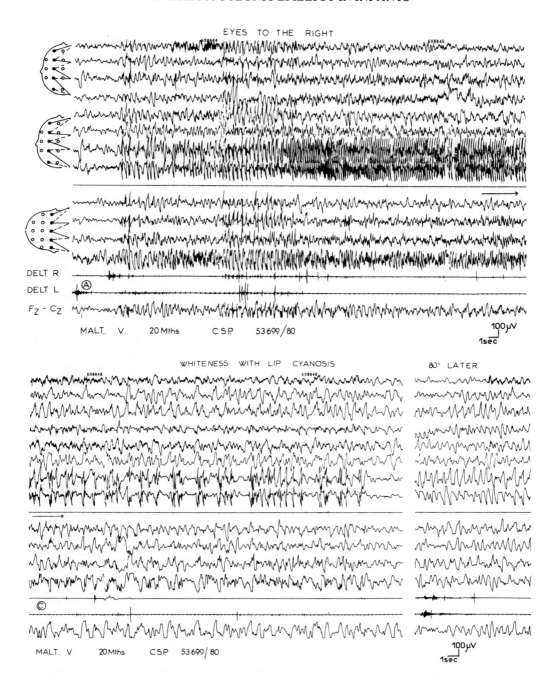

Fig. 4. Girl, 1 year 8 months old. A — Onset of a partial seizure, occurring on awakening, in the left mid and posterior areas. Clinically: right deviation of the eyes, loss of contact, arrhythmic myoclonias (of the two deltoids). The duration of this seizure was 1 min and 45 s. C — On the left, end of the seizure: after a hiccup, the child became pale, with cyanosis of lips and still presents rare myoclonias. On the right, 1 min and 20 s after the end, EEGs are still slow, particularly on the left hemisphere, in the region where the seizure started.

63

of neurological signs: ataxia (35 out of 42 cases), hyper-reflexia, fragmental and segmental myoclonus (21 out of 42 cases).

Biological and radiological investigations, on the other hand, remained negative in most cases. However, Dalla Bernardina *et al.* (1982) report four cases of dilatation of the cisterna magna in the 17 CT scans conducted.

Evolution

The seizures, whatever their type, are extremely resistant to any kind of treatment during the first year of the disease and often require hospitalization. In some children, seizures can be brought on not only by photic stimulation but even by closing the eyes; thus these children can carry out self-stimulation.

The period during which the epilepsy is particularly active varies greatly from one child to another (it sometimes continues up to the age of 11 or 12 years). Diurnal convulsive seizures and myoclonic jerks then tend to occur at less frequent intervals. Convulsive seizures occur mainly at night and are less dramatic in appearance. They take the form of clonic or tonic-clonic seizures of brief duration, often with a focal starting point. Nocturnal tonic seizures are rare (two children in our group and two in that of Dulac and Arthuis), and occur in the form of vibratory tonic seizures.

The myoclonic jerks may be transformed into very atypical absence seizures with slight disturbances in consciousness, more or less random myoclonus of limited proportions and modifications in muscular tonus tending towards hypertonia (Fig. 5). These absences may provoke states of obtundation of varying duration, sometimes maintained by photic stimuli from the environment or closing of the eyes.

We know less about evolution of EEG recordings. The generalized spikes and spike-wave become much less frequent during waking, photosensitivity diminishes and may even disappear altogether. But the generalized discharges are replaced by spikes, spike-waves and polyspike-waves involving the two central regions and the vertex, sometimes more diffuse in one hemisphere. Focal abnormalities vary greatly in their topography.

Background activity fluctuates greatly and appears to depend on the frequency of seizures. A posterior alpha rhythm can be identified, usually during the periods when

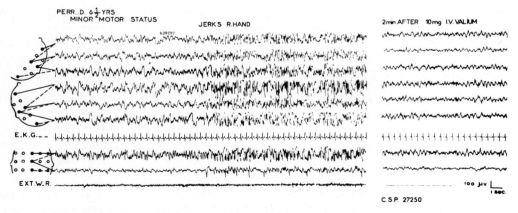

Fig. 5. Obtundation status with myoclonias recorded in a 6-year 6-month-old girl (minor motor status). *Left:* EEG shows mixed theta waves and spikes; EMG of the right wrist extensor shows sporadic myoclonias and an irregular tonic activity. *Right:* an intravenous injection of diazepam 10 mg has stopped this status and theta waves associated with rapid rhythms reappear.

seizures diminish, even in children whose epilepsy has existed for 14 years. We also observe changes related to drug-therapy.

The neurological signs which appeared with onset of the epilepsy seem to persist without getting worse. However, we have not yet studied the phenomenon over a sufficiently long period to be certain of this, since we have also seen adults with severe cerebellar and pyramidal syndromes and myoclonus, whose history was very similar to that of SME.

Psychological development varies greatly from one case to another. Some children manage to acquire language but remain intellectually deficient. Others acquire only a very rudimentary knowledge of language. Some develop psychoses.

The children in our group were followed up for 6 years 3 months on average and are aged between 2 and 14 years. The oldest are all in specialized institutions. Intellectual level was assessed in 20 cases: 7 children had an IQ of between 50 and 75 and 13 children had an IQ of less than 50. Six children died (14.2 per cent) either during a seizure, or due to infection, or by sudden death.

All the others still have seizures.

Differential diagnosis

Differential diagnosis begins with *febrile convulsions*. If an infant of less than 12 months with a family history of epilepsy suffers a prolonged and/or unilateral febrile seizure, evolution towards SME can be suspected. If the febrile convulsions are repeated at close intervals under the influence of a more or less high temperature, then the risk is even greater. But the diagnosis cannot be confirmed until myoclonic jerks occur, or spike-waves resulting from photic stimulation appear on the EEG because other febrile convulsions of the same kind never evolve towards SME, but rather towards a partial epilepsy which is also severe.

Diagnosis of benign myoclonic epilepsy does not appear to us to pose any particular problem apart from cases which begin with febrile convulsions. However, these occur later (between the ages of 1 and 2 years), are of brief duration, infrequent, and disappear after the onset of myoclonic jerks.

Lennox-Gastaut syndrome is completely different from SME: it begins later, in a much more varied manner, often in children with pre-existing cerebral lesions. It takes the form mainly of atypical absences and tonic seizures, during sleep, although these are associated with myoclonic or myoclono-atonic seizures (myoclonic variant). EEG recordings always show slow diffuse spike-waves occurring in bursts, and specific patterns during sleep (Gastaut *et al.*, 1966; Beaumanoir, chapter 11). Even in the few cases of SME where tonic seizures appeared later in the evolution of the epilepsy, these seizures had a specific form, with a long vibratory phase, and could be initiated, in one case, by photic stimulation. The EEG never showed slow spike-waves between seizures.

Nosological place

Because of the drug-resistant nature of the seizures, the appearance of neurological signs, the slowing down of psychomotor development, and the combination of generalized and focal abnormalities on the EEG, we placed SME in the category of secondary generalized epilepsies. However, it also presents certain characteristics of a primary generalized epilepsy: absence of etiological factors, high percentage of family history, initial ictal symptomatology and photosensitivity.

One could therefore consider that we are dealing with a serious form of primary generalized epilepsy and that the repeated occurrence of prolonged febrile convulsive seizures is responsible for the cerebral lesions, explaining later changes in characteristics. In some cases, however, localized abnormalities on the EEG were evident from the beginning. A more precise study of the evolution of EEG signs is needed to clarify this point.

Another hypothesis would be that the existence of unfavourable genetic factors may cause secondary aggravation of a primary epilepsy.

Anyway, the different authors who have studied myoclonic epilepsy in children have not characterized this group as such (Harper, 1968; Janz, 1969; Aicardi and Chevrie, 1971; Jeavons, 1977; Lagenstein, 1978; Giovanardi-Rossi et al., (1979); Aicardi, 1980). All admit, however, that myoclonic epilepsy may have either a favourable or an unfavourable outcome. Doose et al. (1970) distinguished, amongst cases of myoclonic-astatic petit mal, those which began with grand mal convulsive seizures and were generally of unfavourable outcome. This group appears to us to be similar to SME, although the absence of partial seizures and focal abnormalities on the EEG in the cases observed by Doose makes it impossible to identify them completely with our cases of SME. One element that all these cases do have in common is the existence of theta rhythms at 4 to 7 c/s which are specific to the centrencephalic form of myoclonic-astatic petit mal reported by Doose (Doose and Gundel, 1982) and which are also identified in our SME patients at the initial stages of the disease.

Thus SME would appear to represent a specific group of myoclonic epilepsy, beginning with convulsive seizures during the first year of life and always having unfavourable outcome.

References

Aicardi, J. (1980): Course and prognosis of certain childhood epilepsies with predominantly myoclonic seizures. In *Advances in epileptology:* The Xth Epilepsy International Symposium, ed J.A. Wada, J.K. Penry, pp 159-163, Raven Press: New York.

Aicardi, J., Chevrie, J.J. (1971): Myoclonic epilepsies of childhood. *Neuropädiatrie* 3, 177 - 190.

Dalla Bernardina, B., Capovilla, G., Gattoni, M.B., Colamaria, V., Bondavalli, S. Bureau, M. (1982): Epilepsie myoclonique grave de la première année. *Rev. EEG Neurophysiol.* 12, 21 - 25.

Dalla Bernardina, B., Colamaria, V., Capovilla, G., Bondavalli, S. (1983): Nosological Classification of epilepsies in the first three years of life. In *Epilepsy: an update on research and therapy,* ed G. Nisticó, R. Di Perri, H. Meinardi, pp 165 - 183, Alan R. Liss, Inc.: New York.

Doose, H., Gerken H., Leonardt R., Völzke E., Völz C. (1970): Centrencephalic myoclonic - astatic petit mal — clinical and genetic investigations. *Neuropädiatrie* 2, 59 - 78.

Doose, H., Gundel, A. (1982): 4 - 7 c/s rhythms in the childhood EEG. In *Genetic basis of the epilepsies,* pp 83 - 93, ed V.E. Anderson, W.A. Hauser, J.K. Penry, C.F. Sing. Raven Press: New York.

Dravet, C. (1978): Les épilepsies graves de l'enfant. *Vie Méd.* 8, 543-548.

Dravet, C., Roger, J., Bureau, M., Dalla Bernardina, B. (1982): Myoclonic epilepsies in childhood. In *Advances in epileptology:* the XIIIth Epilepsy International Symposium, pp 135 - 140, ed H. Akimoto, H.Kazamatsuri, M.Seino, A. Ward, Raven Press: New York.

Dulac, O., Arthuis, M. (1982): L'épilepsie myoclonique sévère de l'enfant. In *Journées Parisiennes de pédiatrie,* pp 259 - 268. Flammarion: Paris.

Gastaut, H., Roger, J., Soulayrol, R., Tassinari, C.A. Régis, H., Dravet, C., Bernard, R., Pinsard, N., Saint-Jean, M. (1966): Childhood epileptic encephalopathy with diffuse slow spike-waves. *Epilepsia* 7, 139 - 179.

Giovanardi Rossi, P., Pazzaglia, P., Cirignotta, F., Moschen, R., Lugaresi, E. (1979): Le epilessie miocloniche nell'infanzia. *Riv. Ital. Elettroencef. Neurofisiol. Clin,* 2, 321 - 328.

Harper, J.R. (1968): True myoclonic epilepsy in childhood. *Archs Dis. Child* 43, 28 - 35.

Janz, D. (1969): *Die Epilepsien. Spezielle Pathologie und Therapie.* Georg Thieme Verlag: Stuttgart.

Jeavons, P.M. (1977): Nosological problems of myoclonic epilepsies in childhood and adolescence. *Develop. Med. Child Neurol.* **19**, 3 - 8

Lagenstein, I. (1978): Das zentrencephale myoklonisch-astatische Petit Mal. Eine klinische und elektroenzephalographische Verlaufsuntersuchung an 52 Patienten. *Z. EEG. EMG,* **9**, 86 - 96.

*   *   *

Discussion pages 100-104

Epileptic syndromes in infancy, childhood and adolescence. J. Roger, C. Dravet, M. Bureau, F.E. Dreifuss and P. Wolf. John Libbey Eurotext Ltd ©1985.

Chapter 8
Myoclonic Epilepsy ('Myoclonic Status') in Non-Progressive Encephalopathies

Bernardo DALLA BERNARDINA, Emanuela TREVISAN, Vito COLAMARIA, Adriana MAGAUDDA*

*Neuropsichiatria Infantile, Università di Verona, Borgo Roma, 37100-Verona, and *Clinica Neurologica, Università di Messina, Italy*

Summary

The authors report the electroclinical study of 14 patients (eight girls and six boys) with hypotonic cerebral palsy and suffering from a peculiar type of myoclonic epilepsy. This syndrome is characterized by the repetition of long-lasting myoclonic status. These status, often displayed only polygraphically, induce an important worsening of neuropsychological impairment. The authors discuss the electroclinical limits of this epilepsy and its relationships with the other kinds of myoclonic epilepsy reported in the literature.

Introduction

The epilepsies characterized predominantly by myoclonic manifestations raise many nosological and clinical problems because they can be observed in widely different clinical contexts. In fact, in some cases myoclonic phenomena can characterize some forms of cryptogenetic epilepsies (Harper, 1968; Aicardi, 1980, 1981; Dalla Bernardina *et al.*, 1981, 1982*a*, 1983*a,b;* Dalla Bernardina, 1983; Dravet and Bureau, 1981; Dravet *et al.*, 1982). In other cases they belong to progressive encephalopathies of metabolic origin (Tassinari *et al.*, 1976; Dalla Bernardina *et al.*, 1982*b, c*). Finally in other cases they are associated with non-progressive encephalopathies (Aicardi and Chevrie, 1971; Pazzaglia *et al.*, 1979; Cavazzuti *et al.*, 1979; Giovanardi Rossi *et al.*, 1979; Dalla Bernardina *et al.*, 1980, 1983*b;* Dalla Bernardina, 1983).

The purpose of this work is to describe a particular form of myoclonic epilepsy appearing in infants affected by a non-progressive encephalopathy and characterized by the repetition of myoclonic status and by a particularly poor prognosis. The following description arises from the electroclinical longitudinal study of some personal observations.

Electroclinical Features

Fourteen subjects (eight girls and six boys) followed until the mean age of 4 years 6 months have been studied. Three children (one girl, two boys) died at the age of 18, 24, 30 months respectively.

In all cases a severe encephalopathy was clearly evident from the first months of life, surely before the appearance or the recognition of the epileptic manifestations. This encephalopathy is essentially characterized by a severe axial hypotonia and by polymorphous abnormal movements, giving a picture of a hypotonic cerebral palsy with a dystonic-dyskinetic syndrome and severe mental retardation. Only in two cases (14.2 per cent) were familial antecedents of epilepsy reported. In six cases (42.8 per cent) an important fetal or neonatal anoxic injury had occurred. In the other cases the aetiology was unknown but no progressive disease had been discovered in any case. Three children (21.4 per cent) showed a slight microcephaly at the onset of the fits, never present at birth. The CT scans, normal in seven cases (50 per cent), showed generally slight signs of cerebral atrophy, in the absence of any more important pathology (hydrocephaly, porencephaly, malformations) in the other seven.

The initial ictal manifestations were characterized by brief but frequent (several a day) 'absences' accompanied by jerks of eye-lids and/or of eyes and of distal muscles.

Because of severe mental retardation and continuous involuntary movements, both the paroxysmal attention disturbances ('absences') and the myoclonias can remain undiscovered for a long time; so it is frequently difficult to precisely assess the age of onset of fits, but they seem to appear during the first year of life. Frequently the polygraphic records only allow the detection of paroxysmal epileptic manifestations.

In the awake state the EEG is characterized by a slowed background activity with more or less frequent focal or multifocal abnormalities. The ictal manifestations are characterized by brief bursts of diffuse slow spike and waves, accompanied by myoclonias, often rhythmic and bilateral, mixed with other continuous and polymorphous abnormal movements. The myoclonias are frequently rhythmic and bilateral, continuous and strictly related to EEG discharges (Fig. 1). In many cases, in the same subject, myoclonias are continuous but asynchronous on the different muscles. In these cases it is more difficult to appreciate their relationship to paroxysmal EEG discharges. During all stages of slow sleep, in most cases, there is a great increase in frequency of the paroxysmal discharges, in some cases realizing an epileptic status; for these reasons in some cases the sleep record only permits to show the presence of paroxysmal discharges. Like the 'absences' the myoclonias are more easily recognized during drowsiness because of the disappearance of other abnormal movements.

The evolution is always poor because of the unresponsiveness of fits to the treatments and the high frequency of appearance and repetition of long-lasting myoclonic status. Also these myoclonic status can sometimes remain clinically unrecognized, but they are easily displayed by polygraphic records. These records in fact show a rhythmic discharge of diffuse, but frequently asynchronous, slow spike-waves accompanied by rhythmic myoclonias both continuous when awake and during sleep, and not, or only temporarily, stopped by iv benzodiazepines (Figure 1). Moreover these status are refractory to different treatments even to ACTH; generally they last several days or weeks and they are selflimited. Apart from some rare partial or generalized clonic fits, other types of seizures have never been observed; particularly neither atonic nor tonic fits have been observed. In spite of the important preexisting motor and intellectual deficits, myoclonic status and their recurrence are always accompanied by a worsened neuropsychological evolution. This worsening of the psychomotor impairment and of psychic disturbances can sometimes suggest a progressive disease, especially when

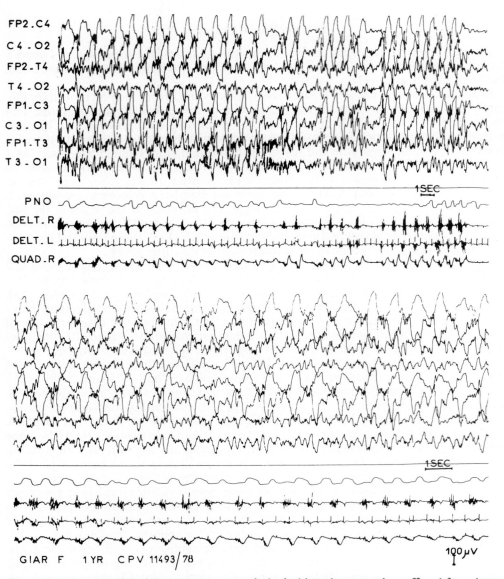

FP2.C4
C4.O2
FP2.T4
T4.O2
FP1.C3
C3.O1
FP1.T3
T3.O1

1SEC

PNO
DELT.R
DELT.L
QUAD.R

1SEC

GIAR F 1 YR C P V 11493/78

100 µV

Fig. 1. One year old girl with severe neuropsychological impairment, who suffered from important neonatal anoxia. From the age of 6 months, repeated epileptic status lasting several days. Top: note the continuous discharges of generalized SW accompanied by rhythmic bilateral myoclonias. Bottom: similar pattern recorded with higher speed (3 cms = 1 s).

epileptic status is not recognized. In reality such a hypothesis has been confirmed in no cases.

Discussion

In spite of the different reports concerning the myoclonic epilepsies of childhood (Harper, 1968; Doose *et al.*, 1970; Aicardi and Chevrie, 1971; Jeavons, 1977;

Giovanardi-Rossi *et al.*, 1979; Pazzaglia *et al.*, 1979; Cavazzuti *et al.*, 1979; Aicardi, 1980; Aicardi, 1981) in the literature, there are no similar observations. In fact, with the exception of Giovanardi-Rossi *et al.*, (1979) no authors have ever reported the existence of myoclonic epilepsies characterized by repeated status. Moreover the myoclonic epilepsy in non-progressive encephalopathy first described by Aicardi and Chevrie (1971) and later reported by Cavazzuti *et al.* (1979) does not correspond to a homogeneous entity. In fact neither this epilepsy nor the encephalopathy are described; moreover these authors include in their population some cases in which the myoclonus phenomena do not correspond to EEG paroxysmal abnormalities. Probably some similar observations are classified by different authors under the heading of 'minor epileptic status' (Brett, 1966) or myoclonic variant of the Lennox-Gastaut syndrome (Erba and Lombroso, 1973; Aicardi, 1981; Gastaut, 1981). But it is very difficult to recognize what cases are really similar because of the absence of detailed clinical descriptions of the neurological pictures of these cases and of the electroclinical descriptions of paroxysmal events.

Conclusion

As previously outlined (Dalla Bernardina *et al.*, 1980, 1983 *b*; Dalla Bernardina 1983) we conclude that this particular type of myoclonic epilepsy is characterized by the appearance of repeated atypical status combined with an impairment of the attention and continuous jerks, in an infant suffering from a hypotonic form of cerebral palsy. Although this condition is difficult to recognize only clinically (because of previous intellectual deficit and above all of continuous abnormal movements), it can be easily demonstrated by polygraphic records which show rhythmic discharges of diffuse slow spike-waves accompanied by rhythmic myoclonias, continuous in the awake state and during sleep. These conditions are accompanied by a worsened neuropsychological evolution sometimes mimicking a progressive disease.

We think that it is justified to consider this form separately for the following reasons:
- homogeneous electroclinical picture,
- neuropsychological systematic poor prognosis,
- occurrence in subjects affected by a non-progressive encephalopathy, never in infants suffering from a progressive disease.

References

Aicardi, J., Chevrie, J.J. (1971): Myoclonic epilepsies of childhood. *Neuropädiatrie* **3**, 177-190.
Aicardi, J. (1980): Course and prognosis of certain childhood epilepsies with predominantly myoclonic seizures. In *Advances in epileptology:* the Xth Epilepsy International Symposium, pp 159-163, ed J.A. Wada, J.K. Penry. Raven Press: New York.
Aicardi, J. (1981): Epilessie miocloniche benigne. In *Le epilessie infantili benigne,* pp 11-22, ed B. Dalla Bernardina, C.A. Tassinari, G. Beghini, Documenti Sigma-Tau.
Brett, E.M. (1966): Minor epileptic status. *J. Neurol. Sci.* **3**, 52-75.
Cavazzuti, G.B., Nalin, A., Ferrari, F., Mordini, B. (1979): Encefalopatie miocloniche nel primo anno di vita. *Riv. Ital. EEG. Neurofisiol. Clin.* **2**, 253-261.
Dalla Bernardina, B., Trevisan, C., Bondavalli, S., Colamaria, V., Bureau, M., Roger, J., Dravet, C. (1980): Une forme particulière d'épilepsie myoclonique chez des enfants porteurs d'encéphalopathie fixée. *Boll. Lega It. Epil.* **29-30**, 183-187.
Dalla Bernardina, B., Capovilla, G., Colamaria, V., Gattoni, M.B., Del Zotti, F., Dravet, C., Bureau, M., Roger, J. (1981): Nosological classification of myoclonic epilepsies of the first three years of life. *Riv. Ital. EEG Neurofisiol. Clin.* **1**, 19-20.
Dalla Bernardina, B., Capovilla, G., Gattoni, M.B., Colamaria, V., Bondavalli, S., Bureau, M.

(1982*a*): Epilepsie myoclonique grave de la première année. *Rev. EEG Neurophysiol.* **12,** 21-25.

Dalla Bernardina, B., Dulac, O., Bureau, M., Dravet, C., Del Zotti, F., Roger, J. (1982*b*): Encéphalopathie myoclonique précoce avec épilepsie. *Rev. EEG Neurophysiol.* **12,** 8-14.

Dalla Bernardina, B., Tassinari, C.A., Lombardi, A. (1982*c*): Aspetti EEG e neurofisiologici delle malattie dismetaboliche con epilessia dell'età pediatrica. *Boll. Lega It. Epil.* **39,** 143-149.

Dalla Bernardina, B. (1983): L'EEG nelle convulsioni e nelle epilessie della prima infanzia. In *Le convulsioni febbrili e le epilessie.* Attualità cliniche e terapeutiche, 43-63. ed R. Canger, e Pruneri C. Masson Ital.

Dalla Bernardina, B., Colamaria, V., Capovilla, G., Vanoli, D. (1983*a*): L'epilessia mioclonica grave del primo anno di vita. *Gior. Neuropsich. Età Evol.* **2,** 187-194.

Dalla Bernardina, B., Colamaria, V., Capovilla, G., Bondavalli, S. (1983*b*): Nosological classification of epilepsies in the first 3 years of life. In *Epilepsy an update on research and therapy. Progress in clinical and biological research,* pp 165-183, ed G. Nisticó, R. Di Perri et H. Meinardi. Alan R. Liss, Inc.: New York.

Doose, H., Gerken, H., Leonhardt, R., Völzke, E., Völz, C. (1970): Centrencephalic myoclonic-astatic petit mal. Clinical and genetic investigations. *Neuropädiatrie,* **2,** 59-78.

Dravet, C., Bureau, M. (1981): L'épilepsie myoclonique bénigne du nourrisson. *Rev. EEG Neurophysiol.* **11,** 438-444.

Dravet, C., Roger, J., Bureau, M., Dalla Bernardina, B. (1982): Myoclonic epilepsies in childhood. In *Advances in Epileptology,* pp 135-140, ed H. Akimoto, H. Katzamatzuri, M, Seino, A.A. Ward Jr. Raven Press: New York.

Erba, G., Lombroso, C.T. (1973): La sindrome di Lennox-Gastaut. *Prospettive in Pediatria* **3,** 145-165.

Gastaut, H. (1981): Individualisation des épilepsies dites "bénignes" ou "fonctionnelles" aux différents âges de la vie. Appréciation des variations correspondantes de la prédisposition épileptique à ces âges. *Rev. EEG. Neurophysiol.* **11,** 346-366.

Giovanardi Rossi, P., Pazzaglia, P., Cirignotta, F., Moschen, R., Lugaresi, E. (1979): Le epilessie miocloniche dell'infanzia. *Riv. Ital. EEG Neurofisiol. Clin.* **2,** 321-328.

Harper, R.Y. (1968): True myoclonic epilepsy in childhood. *Archs Dis. Child.* **43,** 28-35.

Jeavons, P.M. (1977): Nosological problems of myoclonic epilepsies in childhood and adolescence. *Develop. Med. Child. Neurol.* **19,** 3-8.

Pazzaglia, P., Giovanardi Rossi, P., Cirignotta, F., Moschen, R., Lugaresi, E. (1979): Nosografia delle epilessie miocloniche. *Riv. Ital. EEG Neurofisiol. Clin.* **2,** 245-252.

Tassinari, C.A., Coccagna, G., Dalla Bernardina, B. (1976): Dissinergia cerebellare mioclonica di Ramsay-Hunt — Epilessia mioclonica progressiva di Unverricht-Lundborg con corpi di Lafora, Neurolipidosi — Elementi di semiologia e diagnostica elettroclinica. In *Le epilessie,* pp. 131-135, ed E. Lugaresi, P. Pazzaglia. Aulo Gaggi: Bologna.

*　　　*　　　*

Discussion pages 100-104

Epileptic syndromes in infancy, child-
hood and adolescence. J. Roger,
C. Dravet, M. Bureau, F.E.
Dreifuss and P. Wolf. John Libbey
Eurotext Ltd ©1985.

Chapter 9
Epileptic Seizures in Inborn Errors of Metabolism

Jean AICARDI

INSERM — U12, Hôpital des Enfants Malades, 149 rue de Sèvres, 75743 Paris Cedex 15, France

Summary

Epileptic seizures revealing inborn errors of metabolism are of two different types. Some have
no specific features as in pyridoxine-dependency or adrenoleucodystrophy. Others, such as
ceroid lipofuscinosis, have more suggestive features, especially the prominence of myoclonus
and a clearly progressive course. Because of the frequent absence of specific features, the diagnosis can be made only by systematic inquiry.

Repeated epileptic seizures are a common manifestation of many CNS disorders resulting from proven or suspected inborn errors of metabolism.

*(I) In many of these conditions where epileptic seizures are only an occasional manifestation
of the disease or, even if they constitute an important, or even essential, symptom, no characteristic seizure pattern has been described.*

In such cases, the diagnosis of any particular metabolic disorder rests on the associated signs and symptoms and on the clinical course, not on peculiar characters of the
seizures. An incomplete list of some of the diseases in which 'unspecific' epileptic seizures may occur appears on Table 1. Among these disorders, however, mention
should be made of:

(1) *Pyridoxine-dependency,* which is marked by early (in the first days of life or even
in the days preceding birth) and intractable seizures that respond dramatically to the
IV injection of pyridoxine. In rare cases, however, the seizures may be delayed and
appear only after a few months in the form of status epilepticus or even, perhaps, as infantile spasms, hence the interest in trying IV pyridoxine in all cases of severe seizures
of obscure origin which occur during the first year of life.

(2) *Adrenoleukodystrophy* — often revealed by severe unilateral or generalized seizures.

Table 1. Epilepsy in inborn errors of metabolism

I — *Metabolic disorders in which epileptic manifestations have no characteristic features* (associated signs and time course may suggest the diagnosis)
  Pyridoxine-dependency; amino-acids and organic acids disorders; ammonia cycle disorders; poliodystrophies; Menkes disease; GM1 gangliosidosis; Leigh's disease; Krabbe's disease; Canavan-Van Bogaert; adrenoleukodystrophy; atypical leukodystrophies, etc...

II — *Metabolic disorders in which the clinical and/ or EEG pattern of epileptic manifestations may suggest the diagnosis*
  Nonketotic hyperglycinemia and D-glyceric acidemia
  Early infantile ceroid lipofuscinosis (Santavuori-Hagberg-Haltia)
  Tay-Sachs and Sandhoff diseases
  PKU variant (deficit in biopterins)
  Late infantile and juvenile ceroidlipofuscinoses
  Sialosidoses (mucolipidosis I, cherry red spot myoclonus syndrome)
  Juvenile Gaucher's disease
  Lafora's disease
  Myoclonus epilepsy with ragged-red fibers

The presence of a prominent myoclonic component in a seizure disorder should always raise the suspicion of a metabolic disease since this type of seizure is often present in such conditions.

(II) In a second group of CNS metabolic disorders, the pattern of epileptic seizures is relatively characteristic and may, in itself, suggest the correct diagnosis.

In such cases, however, several patterns (or syndromes) can be seen. The main ones will be described successively (Table 2).

(1) *Non-ketotic hyperglycinaemia* (glycine encephalopathy) presents as an early myoclonic encephalopathy with erratic myoclonus, partial seizures of limited expression and a suppression-burst EEG pattern. The rare d-glyceric acidemia presents with an identical pattern (Dalla Bernardina *et al.*, 1979; Brandt *et al.*, 1974; Grandgeorge *et al.*, 1980).

(2) *Early infantile type of ceroid-lipofuscinosis (Santavuori-Haltia-Hagberg disease)* is characterized by myoclonus mainly of the massive, bilateral type, starting during the 2nd semester of the first year of life or the 1st semester of the second year. Rapid mental deterioration with autistic features is associated. Although the clinical epileptic syndrome is not characteristic, the evolution of the EEG pattern is highly suggestive (the so-called vanishing EEG) (Santavuori, 1973; Pampiglione and Harden, 1974).

(3) *Tay-Sachs and Sandhoff diseases.* These two conditions are clinically indistinguishable. From the very first months of life, acoustic startle (or myoclonus) is prominent. Sudden flexion of the limbs (symmetrical) occurs in response to sudden noises of even low intensity. The latency of this startle response is long (>250 msec) and its recovery or refractory period may last many seconds. No EEG manifestation is associated. Polygraphic recordings show a relatively sustained 'tonic' contraction. In the second year of life, 'true' epileptic manifestations do appear. They include:
- myoclonic jerks which are spontaneous or induced by a variety of stimuli (touch, proprioceptive). They may occasionally trigger a seizure. Their relationship with EEG discharges is unclear;
- erratic, partial seizures.

Table 2. Characteristics of the epileptic manifestations in some metabolic disorders

---

Ceroid-lipofuscinoses
> Early infantile (Santavuori-Haltia-Hagberg)
>> Early massive and erratic myoclonus
>> Vanishing EEG
> Late infantile (Jansky-Bielschowski)
>> Myoclonic and atonic-astatic seizures
>> Characteristic response to IPS
> Juvenile (Spielmeyer-Vogt-Sjögren)
>> Late myoclonus especially involving face

Sialosidoses
> Mucolipidosis type I
>> Late myoclonus (intention and action)
>> Low-voltage fast EEG, sharp spikes
> Cherry red spot-myoclonus syndrome
>> Massive myoclonus exaggerated by active and passive movement, thought of movement, touch, etc. . .
>> Facial, stimulus, insensitive myoclonus
>> Vertex positive waves

Tay-Sachs disease
> Startle to sound from birth, slow recovery
> Myoclonus from 1 year, spontaneous and stimulus-induced, may trigger seizure

Juvenile Gaucher
> Myoclonus (spontaneous, intention), photosensitivity, SER $\geq$ VER

The EEG then shows marked slowing of background rhythms and multifocal paroxysmal abnormalities. The visual evoked response (VER) tends to disappear as the disorder progresses (Pampiglione *et al.*, 1974).

(4) *Variant of phenylketonuria with biopterins deficiency.* Although the paroxysmal manifestations of this condition have not been studied neurophysiologically, the clinical pattern of the seizures is fairly suggestive. They start in the 2nd semester of life in infants which have been hypotonic since birth or a few weeks of age. Generalized motor seizures occur but the most remarkable manifestations are erratic myoclonic jerks occurring spontaneously which have also been designated as choreic movements. Characteristically, they are associated with oculogyric fits with sudden upward deviation of gaze lasting from one to several seconds. The disorder is a progressive one but can be improved by the combined administration of neurotransmitter precursors (Smith *et al.*, 1975; Kaufman *et al.*, 1975; Rey *et al.*, 1977).

(5) *Late infantile ceroid-lipofuscinosis (Jansky-Bielschowski disease)* is probably the commonest metabolic disorder associated with epileptic seizures in Western Europe. The clinical and EEG picture is distinctive. The seizures usually start between 2 and 4 years of age and are as a rule the first manifestation of the disease. They include occasional generalized motor seizures, massive myoclonic jerks, atonic or astatic fits which often provoke repeated falls. On this account, the diagnosis of Lennox-Gastaut syndrome is often suspected. However, tonic fits with recruiting, low voltage, fast rhythms have not been reported. 'Atypical absences' associated with slow spike-wave complexes have been reported in atypical form (Andermann, 1967; Pinsard *et al.*, 1978). The

EEG is always abnormal from the onset, showing slow background rhythms with poor reactivity and multifocal spikes without true slow 'spike-wave' complexes. The response to IPS at a slow rhythm is characteristic: each flash evokes over the occipital areas (bilaterally) a giant abnormal VER with a spike-wave configuration. During sleep, the multifocal abnormalitites are activated, whereas bilateral synchronous paroxysms are not. The disease is rapidly progressive with the eventual appearance of visual disturbances and of neurological signs (pyramidal, extrapyramidal, cerebellar). The ERG is extinguished early, although we have seen its persistence for the first 10 months in one of our patients (Harden and Pampiglione, 1980; Pinsard *et al.*, 1978).

(6) *The juvenile type of the neuronal ceroid lipofuscinosis, Lafora's disease and the sialosidoses* are dealt with elsewhere. They certainly represent some of the most characteristic epileptic patterns associated with inborn errors of metabolism. Mucolipidosis type I is biochemically distinct from both the cherry-red spot-myoclonus syndrome and the Japanese-Italian type of sialosidosis with partial deficiency of B-galactosidase. An intention and action myoclonus (sometimes also spontaneous) occurs from 8 years onward. The EEG picture is characterized by very sharp mono, di or polyphasic spikes (unrelated to the myoclonus) supervening upon an irregular, low voltage, fast background activity. They may be symmetrical or asymmetrical and are not activated by IPS (Doose *et al.*, 1975).

(7) *Myoclonus epilepsy with ragged-red fibers* has been described by Tsairis *et al.*, (1972) and Fukuhara *et al.*, (1980). The clinical picture is quite similar to that in the Ramsay Hunt syndrome but mental deterioration, muscle atrophy and deformities of the feet are also observed. An increase of blood lactate and pyruvate levels may be observed. Muscle biopsy reveals subsarcolemmal aggregates of abnormal mitochondria, the so-called ragged-red fibers.

In this second group, myoclonus represents the most common type of seizures. All cases of myoclonic epilepsy should therefore be suspected of being of possible metabolic origin. The vast majority of the myoclonic epilepsies, however, are not due to recognizable metabolic diseases, even when ataxia is associated (Aicardi, 1982). It should be remembered that the most treatable of all epileptic conditions due to a metabolic derangement, pyridoxine-dependency, is manifested by seizures which have no suggestive characteristics (Goutieres and Aicardi, 1985) so that a high index of suspicion is the only effective means of recognizing metabolic abnormalities. Globally, however, convulsive seizures are only rarely the initial or main manifestation of neurometabolic diseases.

References

Aicardi, J. (1982); Les myoclonies dans les maladies dégénératives du système nerveux central chez l'enfant. *Rev. EEG Neurophysiol.* **12**, 15-20.

Andermann, F. (1967); Absence attacks and diffuse neuronal disease. *Neurology* **17**, 205-212.

Brandt, N.J., Rassmussen, K., Brandt, S., Schonheyder, F. (1974); D-glyceric acidemia with hyperglycinemia. A new inborn error of metabolism. *Br. Med. J.* **4**, 334.

Dalla Bernardina, B., Aicardi, J., Goutières, F., Plouin, P. (1979); Glycine encephalopathy. *Neuropädiatrie* **10**, 209-225.

Doose, H., Spranger, J., Warner, M. (1975); EEG in mucolipidosis I. *Neuropädiatrie* **6**, 98-101.

Fukuhara, N., Tokiguchi, S., Shirakawa, K., Tsubaki, T. (1980); Myoclonus epilepsy associated with ragged-red fibers (mitochondrial abnormalities). Disease entity or a syndrome? Light and electron-microscopic study of two cases and review of the literature. *J. Neurol. Sci.* **47**, 117-133.

Goutières, F., Aicardi, J. (1985): Atypical presentations of pyridoxine-dependent seizures: a treatable cause of intractable epilepsy in infants. *Ann. Neurol.* **17**, 117-120.

Goutières, F., Aicardi, J. (1985); Pyridoxine-dependency. A treatable cause of intractable epilepsy in infants. *Ann. Neurol.* **17**, 117-120.

Grandgeorge, D., Favier, A., Bost, M., Frappat, P., Bonjet, C., Garrel, S., Stoebnor, P. (1980): L'acidémie D-glycérique. A propos d'une nouvelle observation anatomo-clinique. *Arch. Franc. Pédiatr.* **37**, 577-584.

Harden, A., Pampiglione, G. (1982); Neurophysiological studies (EEG, ERG, VEP, SEP) in 88 patients with so-called neuronal ceroidlipofuscinosis. In *Ceroid lipofuscinosis (Batten's disease)*, pp 61-70, ed D. Armstrong, N. Koppany, J.A. Rider. Elsevier: Amsterdam.

Kaufman, S., Holtzman, N.A., Milstien S., Butler, I.J., Krumholz, A. (1975); Phenylketonuria due to a deficiency of dihydropteridine reductase. *New Engl. J. Med.* **293**, 785.

Pampiglione, G., Harden, A. (1974); An infantile form of neuronal 'storage' disease with characteristic evolution of neurophysiological features. *Brain* **97**, 355-360.

Pampiglione, G., Privett, G., Harden, A. (1974); Tay-Sachs disease: neurophysiological studies in 20 children. *Develop. Med. Child. Neurol.* **16**, 201-208.

Pampiglione, G., Harden, A. (1977): So called neuronal ceroid-lipofuscinosis. Neurophysiological studies in 60 children. *J. Neurol. Neurosurg. Psychiatr.* **40**, 323-330.

Pinsard, N., Livet, M.O., Saint Jean, M. (1978); Ceroïde-lipofuscinose à début atypique. *Rev. EEG Neurophysiol.* **8**, 175.

Rey, F., Harpey, J.P., Leeming, R.J., Blair, J.A., Aicardi, J., Rey, L. (1977); Les hyperphenylalaninémies avec activité normale de la phenylalanine-hydroxylase. *Archs. Franc. Pédiatr.* **34**, 109-120.

Santavuori, P. (1973): EEG in the infantile type of so-called neuronal ceroid lipofuscinosis. *Neuropädiatrie* **4**, 375-397.

Smith, I., Clayton, B.E., Wolff, O.H. (1975); New variant of phenylketonuria with progressive neurological illness unresponsive to phenylalanine restriction. *Lancet* **1**, 1108-1110.

Tsairis, P., Engel, W.K., Karr, P. (1973); Familial myoclonic epilepsy syndrome associated with skeletal muscle mitochondrial abnormalities. *Neurology* **23**, 408.

*   *   *

Discussion pages 100-104

Epileptic syndromes in infancy, childhood and adolescence. J. Roger, C. Dravet, M. Bureau, F.E. Dreifuss and P. Wolf. John Libbey Eurotext Ltd ©1985.

Chapter 10
Myoclonic Astatic Epilepsy of Early Childhood

Hermann DOOSE

Universitäts-Kinderklinik, Schwanenweg 20, 2300 Kiel 1, FRG

Summary

Myoclonic astatic epilepsy is characterized by primarily generalized seizures: myoclonic, astatic and myoclonic-astatic seizures, often in combination with absences, generalized tonic clonic and tonic seizures. A status of minor seizures is especially characteristic. Boys are affected more often than girls. The onset takes place between the first and fifth years of age. The EEGs show bilateral synchronous irregular and regular 2-3 c/s spikes and waves and/or polyspikes and waves. The background activity exhibits marked 4-7 c/s rhythms. The course of this epileptic syndrome is variable. Spontaneous remission as well as malignant course with dementia can be seen. Myoclonic astatic epilepsy is based on a genetic predisposition of a polygenic type. Primary organic brain lesions are rare. This type of epilepsy is considered as a nosologic entity in its own right, distinguishable from epilepsies with generalized minor seizures of multifocal type (most cases of the Lennox-syndrome).

Introduction

There is hardly another area of pediatric epileptology presenting such terminological uncertainty and confusion as is to be found in the domain of epileptic syndromes with generalized minor seizures of early childhood. Though a distinction between primarily and secondarily generalized seizures in adolescents and adults is regarded as a matter of course, the differentiation is not as clearly defined in generalized minor seizures of early childhood. The reason for that probably lies in the fact that the clinical and bio-electric reaction patterns of the immature brain are relatively uniform: the myoclonic flexor spasm, the astatic fit, the generalized tonic clonic seizure as well as the tonic seizure can occur as a symptom of pathophysiologically different mechanisms: they can be primarily or secondarily generalized in origin.

Those deliberations precipitated our own researches in 1964 (Doose, 1964*a*). At that time, we separated infantile spasms from primarily generalized myoclonic seizures which are not accompanied by hypsarrhythmia but by generalized irregular spikes and waves. In contrast to infantile spasms, it was impossible to prove a secondary generalization for this kind of epilepsy. Epilepsies with this seizure type have been designated as myoclonic *petit mal* of early childhood ('myoklonisches Kleinkind-Petit mal', Doose, 1964*a*) and attributed to the epilepsies presenting primarily generalized minor seizures (absences, impulsive *petit mal*). In the same way we later established (Doose, 1964*b*, Doose *et al.*, 1970) the difference between primarily generalized myoclonic-astatic petit mal of early childhood and the Lennox syndrome (Gastaut *et al.*, 1966). As it follows from the study of Gastaut *et al.* (1966), the Lennox syndrome comprises only a small subgroup which presents all the characteristics of an epilepsy with primarily generalized seizures, whereas the majority of the cases with this syndrome have to be classified as multifocal in origin.

Since 1951 we collected 117 cases with primarily generalized myoclonic and myoclonic-astatic seizures. This large number might be explained by the wide referral source of the Epilepsy Centre at Kiel. Based on these 117 observations, the clinical picture can be described as follows:

General

Prevalence. According to an epidemiologic study of Doose and Sitepu (1983), primarily generalized myoclonic and myoclonic-astatic seizures occur in 1-2 per cent of all childhood epilepsies up to age 9.

Sex ratio. The number of affected boys is twice as high as that of girls (in our group 86 boys and 31 girls).

Etiological factors. Brain defects are only of minor importance in the pathogenesis of this disease. Only 16 per cent of 117 children showed signs of a developmental retardation before the onset of epilepsy or indications of definite high-risk factors in their history.

Genetics. In 1983, we extended our genetic studies dating from 1970 (Doose *et al.*, 1970; Doose *et al.*, 1984). In 37 of 100 families seizure affected relatives could be detected (siblings, parents, parents' siblings, grandparents, Table 1). Onset of seizures before the age of 5 years (above all febrile convulsions) was twice as frequent as after this age. In detail, the prevalence turned out to be higher in siblings (16 per cent) than in parents (6 per cent). The prevalence was higher in relatives of female than of male probands. In siblings, definitely pathological EEGs were found in 46 per cent (4-7 c/s-rhythms, spikes and waves during rest, photosensitivity). There is a correlation between the course of the disease and the familial prevalence: in patients suffering from *grand mal* in addition to minor seizures, the prevalence of seizures in the ancestry (parents, parents' siblings) is higher than in patients who are only affected by minor seizures (36 per cent and 12 per cent of the families, Doose *et al.*, 1984).

Table 1. Familial prevalence of seizures in families of 100 cases with myoclonic-astatic epilepsy

	n	%	
Brothers	76	18 }	16
Sisters	78	13 }	
Fathers	98	7 }	6
Fathers' siblings	244	3 }	
Mothers	100	4	
Mothers' siblings	224	4	
Grandparents, paternal	180	1	
Grandparents, maternal	194	3	

In total, the demonstrated family prevalence of seizures is the highest ever found in different kinds of epilepsy. There can be no doubt that myoclonic astatic epilepsy of early childhood is based on a genetic predisposition of a polygenic type. Moreover, the myoclonic astatic epilepsy is genetically heterogeneous. The greater the genetic impact is, the more unfavourable is the course of the disease. Organic lesions, on the other hand, only act as factors of realization.

Age of onset. Epilepsy started in 94 per cent of our patients during the first 5 years, in 24 per cent during the first year of life (Fig. 1A). The first events are febrile convulsions, major afebrile seizures and minor seizures, each in about one third of the probands. The peak age for the manifestation of minor seizures turned out to be the 4th year of life (Fig. 1B).

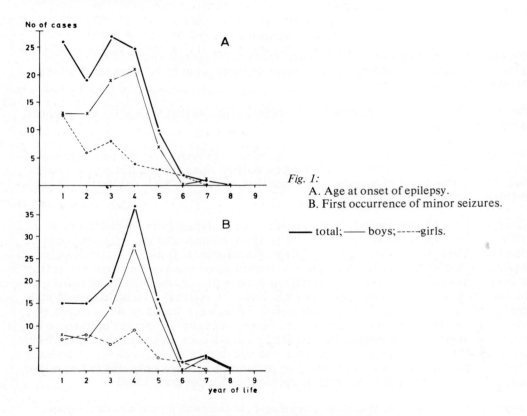

Fig. 1:
A. Age at onset of epilepsy.
B. First occurrence of minor seizures.

——— total; ——— boys; -----girls.

Seizure symptomatology (Table 2)

Myoclonic seizures consist of usually symmetrical jerking of the arms and shoulders, often with simultaneous nodding of the head. Some myoclonic jerks are violent, with arms being flung upwards, some are so mild that they are palpable rather than visible. Accompanying vocalization is rare. Violent generalized myoclonic jerks can lead to abrupt falling to the ground (drop attacks by myoclonias). Besides these symmetrical myoclonic jerks, irregular myoclonic twitching of the facial muscles, especially of the oral and ocular region may occur in severe cases. Rarely, myoclonic attacks are precipitated by fright or light stimuli.

Table 2. Seizure symptomatology in 109 cases

Myoclonic and/or astatic	100%
Absences	62%
Febrile convulsions	28%
Grand mal:	75%
at onset	34%
during course	41%
Status of minor seizures	36%
Tonic seizures	30%?

Astatic seizures. Real astatic seizures with abrupt loss of muscle tonus only rarely occur as the sole symptom of the disorder. Without any precursory signs, the patient suddenly falls to the ground. The direction of the fall depends on the position of the centre of gravity of the body when the seizure occurs. Mild astatic attacks may appear as brief head nodding and as a slight knee-bending of the erect child.

Myoclonic astatic seizures. More often than myoclonic and astatic seizures, a combination can be observed. The more or less pronounced loss of muscle tonus is preceded by symmetrical myoclonias of the arms or irregular twitching of the face (postmyoclonic amyotonia, Gastaut and Regis, 1961) (Fig. 2).

Absences. In more than half of the cases myoclonic and astatic symptoms are accompanied by a short lasting loss of consciousness: absences with myoclonic jerks and irregular myoclonias of the face and/or total or partial loss of postural tone.

Status of minor seizures. An accumulation of minor fits of different types to produce a status is especially characteristic for myoclonic astatic epilepsy (36 per cent of our cases). The condition is characterized by apathy or even stupor. Careful observation reveals irregular twitching of the facial muscles and the extremities. Astatic seizures and head nodding can appear serially. The facial expression is slack, saliva drools, and speach is slurred or disappears completely. The status may last for hours or even days. Mostly there is a marked dependence on the sleeping-waking cycle, as short status regularly occurs after awakening in the morning or in the afternoon. Status of pure myoclonic fits seem to be extremely rare.

(a)   (b)   (c)

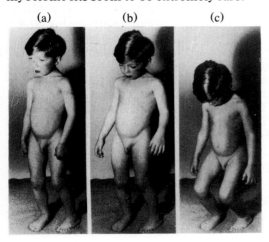

Fig. 2. Myoclonic astatic seizure in a 3-year-old boy: (a) before onset; (b) onset of the seizure with flexor myoclonias of the arms; (c) fall onto the ground.

Febrile and afebrile grand mal. In two-thirds of our cases epilepsy started with febrile or afebrile grand mal. Initially, the generalized tonic clonic or clonic seizures occur almost exclusively during daytime, and only in the later course also during night. In severe cases the tonic clonic seizures show an alternating lateralization.

Tonic seizures. Axial tonic seizures are to be seen only in the later stages of unfavourable cases. Characteristically they occur almost exclusively during night, especially between 4 and 6 o'clock in the morning. As can be demonstrated by long-term EEG, they are bounded on the non-REM-sleep and can then occur serially. A status of tonic seizures during daytime represents a rarity which can be observed only in the late course of the most unfavourable cases.

Focal seizures. Real focal seizures are not characteristic for myoclonic astatic epilepsy. They can occur as a facultative phenomenon in those rare cases with a primary brain lesion or, on the other hand, in the late course of unfavourable cases.

EEG findings

At onset of epilepsy, especially in cases wih febrile or afebrile *grand mal,* the EEG often shows only monomorphic theta rhythms with parietal accentuation (Fig. 3) as well as occipital 4 c/s-rhythms, constantly blocked by opening the eyes. During this early stage, irregular spikes and waves can often be found only during sleep. Later on, bilateral synchronous irregular spikes and waves appear, often with accentuation over the anterior regions. The type of hypersynchronous activity depends on the seizure type: in cases with predominantly or exclusively myoclonic seizures short paroxysms of irregular spikes and waves and polyspike waves are most typical (Figs. 4, 5). On the other hand, in children with astatic or myoclonic astatic seizures the record is characterized by 2-3 c/s spikes and waves and spike wave-variants (Fig. 6). Usually, they are of irregular shape, only rarely grouped in rhythmic sequences but interrupted by high amplitude slow waves. The background activity usually is dominated by a 4-7 c/s-rhythms with parietal accentuation (Fig. 3, for literature see Doose and Gundel, 1982). Often groups of theta rhythms immediately precede or follow the spike wave-paroxysms (Figs 6, 8). During stages with a high frequency of seizures, the theta rhythms are substituted by a polymorphous slowing. In unfavourable cases the 4-7 c/s-rhythms can persist until puberty and adulthood (Gundel *et al.,* 1981) (Fig. 7). During status, the EEG shows 2-3 c/s-spikes and waves (Fig. 8) and, especially in younger children, very irregular polymorphous hypersynchronous activity (Fig. 9) and polyspikes in the rare cases of myoclonic status (Fig. 10). Most cases show photosensitivity at least between the age of 5 and 15 years, i.e. at the age of maximal expressivity of this pattern. Whereas lateralization of spikes and waves can often be seen, focal abnormalities are not characteristic. They can occur especially in the rare cases with primary brain damage, but they never dominate the EEG for a longer time. During sleep, spikes and waves are regularly activated. The whole night record shows hypersynchronous activity predominantly during non-REM-sleep. Nocturnal tonic seizures are accompanied by typical 10-15 c/s-spike series.

Course and prognosis

A representative figure from the course of the disease cannot be derived from our material because the cases have been collected over 30 years and have been treated by different regimens. Furthermore, in our centre, we are confronted with a selection of unfavourable cases. Follow-up studies of 115 cases showed complete seizure control

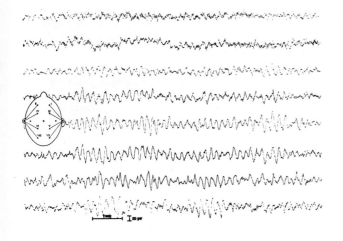

Fig. 3. 4-year-old boy with myoclonic astatic seizures. Parietally accentuated 5 c/s rhythms.

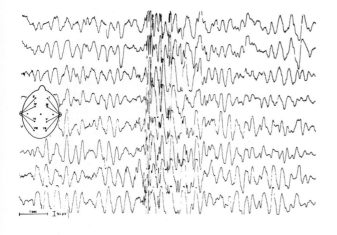

Fig. 4. 18-month-old girl with short myoclonic fits, mostly provoked by startle. Bilateral synchronous irregular spikes and waves.

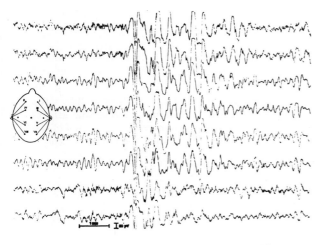

Fig. 5. 5-year-old girl. Myoclonic fits since the age of 11 months. Bilateral synchronous polyspike waves. Rhythmic slowing of the background activity.

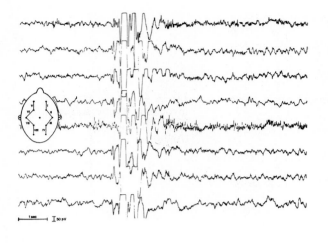

Fig. 6. 3-year-old boy with myoclonic astatic seizures. Paroxysmal bilateral synchronous slow spike waves and slow waves.

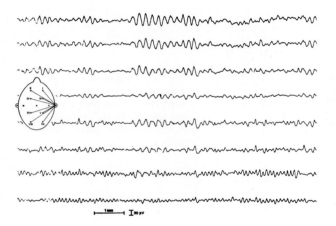

Fig. 7. 26-year-old male. Rare nocturnal grand mal. During early childhood myoclonic astatic epilepsy with frequent status. Mild dementia. Rhythmic slowing of the background activity.

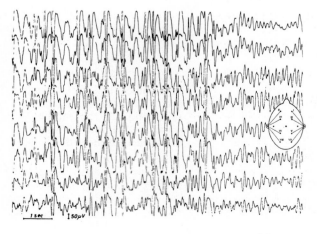

Fig. 8. 4-year-old boy. Status of myoclonic astatic seizures. Long series of irregular spikes and waves.

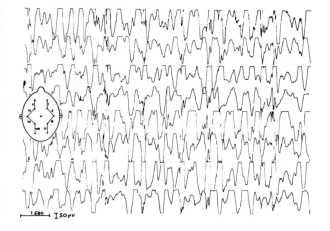

Fig. *9.* 2-year-old girl. Status of myoclonic astatic seizures. Polymorphic irregular hypersynchronous activity.

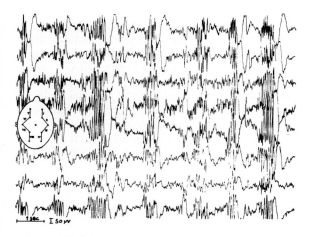

Fig. *10.* 7-year-old boy. Myoclonic status.

for at least two years in 54 per cent of the children beyond the age of 7 years.

Apparently, there is a wide range of possible developments.

In some cases the disease resolves spontaneously. After some months, myoclonic or myoclonic astatic seizures disappear without any therapy; the development of the children is quite normal. We observed such a benign course for instance in monozygotic twins who suffered from identical myoclonic fits at the age of 9 months; the seizures could be regularly provoked by startle. Without any therapy, both children were seizure-free at the age of 15 months and they developed normally. In other cases, minor seizures can disappear rapidly under valproate therapy.

The prognosis is more unfavourable if major seizures develop. By means of therapy with valproate, however, this development may be prevented to some extent. Generally the course of the disease is unfavourable if epilepsy starts during infancy with afebrile and febrile generalized tonic clonic or clonic seizures. Generalized tonic clonic seizures, often of long duration, can recur frequently. Their accentuation can change from one side of the body to the other, and after a short time they even appear during sleep, a prognostically unfavourable sign. Prognosis of children suffering from long-lasting states of minor seizures is particularly poor. A definite correlation between these states and dementia exists (Doose, 1970; Doose and Völzke, 1979). Unlike the *petit mal* status of older children and adolescents, recurring and long-lasting myoclonic astatic status during infancy and early childhood can cause permanent changes rapidly leading to dementia. The younger the children are when the status appear, the higher is the risk of dementia. In these cases and in children suffering from frequent major seizures even neurological defects can be observed in the later course: slight ataxia, poorly differentiated coarse motor dysfunction, clumsiness and speech disorder among others. Nocturnal tonic seizures are another characteristic of unfavourable courses. In those patients we detected this type of seizures almost regularly since we used long-term EEG monitoring. Often the tonic seizures had not even been noticed by the patient himself or by his parents.

As a rule, the following criteria can be identified as prognostically unfavourable: frequent febrile and afebrile tonic clonic seizures, *petit mal* status, onset of epilepsy during the first or second year of life with *grand mal,* continuance of 4-7 c/s-rhythms and spikes and waves during therapy, missing development of a stable occipital alpha-rhythm.

Differential diagnosis

The differentiation between myoclonic epilepsies of infancy and infantile spasms is essential. Normally this is possible without difficulty. Infantile spasms usually affect children with brain damage, the symptomatology of the seizures is more polymorphous, the seizures typically occur in series, and the EEG shows hypsarrhythmia.

The differentiation of epilepsies with generalized minor seizures of multifocal origin (Lennox syndrome) is more difficult. However, the discussion of differential diagnosis must take into account that the syndrome described by Gastaut *et al.* (1966) includes a subgroup with cases which show the above mentioned characteristics of primary generalized epilepsy. If those cases are excluded from the Lennox syndrome in the strict sense, the following criteria of differential diagnosis result:

- genetic predisposition,
- mostly normal development before onset,
- never neurometabolic or degenerative diseases,
- mostly no neurological deficits,
- primarily generalized myoclonic, astatic or myoclonic-astatic seizures and often *grand mal,*
- rarely focal seizures,
- no atypical absences,
- no tonic seizures during daytime,
- primarily generalized EEG pattern (spikes and waves, photosensitivity, 4-7 c/s-rhythms),
- no multifocal EEG abnormalities.

Of course, there may be an overlap with the multifocal type of the Lennox syndrome. If myoclonic astatic epilepsy is due to a genetic predisposition, such a disposition obviously is likely to also affect a number of children with brain defects too. In these rare cases a definite distinction may be impossible. Here, the same problems emerge as in, for instance, the rare absence epilepsy of brain-defected children. Primarily generalized and focal seizures are then co-existent or occur successively. Moreover, the EEG can no longer be classified exactly. There are analogous findings for the severe cases showing therapy resistant seizures and dementia. In the later course of these cases, clinical and EEG symptoms develop which defy classification.

Conclusion

Myoclonic astatic epilepsy of corticoreticular type of early childhood is a nosologically distinct group which has to be included in the category of primary epilepsies with minor seizures, together with absence epilepsy and epilepsy with massive bilateral myoclonus of later childhood and adolescence. Similar to these groups of corticoreticular epilepsies, myoclonic astatic epilepsy appears to be a rather comprehensive nosologic group. It can be subdivided into subgroups according to predominating symptoms or different course; for instance, epilepsies with prevailing myoclonic or myoclonic astatic seizures, epilepsies with or without grand mal as well as epilepsies with benign and severe evolution. However, the limits between these subgroups are indistinct. Their differencies seem to represent only variants of one basically, i.e. pathogenically uniform disease. The extent of the genetic impact seems to influence the clinical course and prognosis.

To a large extent, our report corresponds to the observations made by other authors or respectively includes as subgroups those types of epilepsy which have been described by these authors.

This concerns:

- cases of myoclonic and astatic *petit mal* of Lennox (1945), Lennox and Davis (1950),
- 'centrencephalic' subgroups of myoclonic astatic petit mal of Kruse (1968),
- some cases of the true myclonic epilepsy of Harper (1968),
- cryptogenic and true myoclonic epilepsy of Aicardi and Chevrie (1971), Aicardi (1980),
- myoclonic epilepsy (group B) of Loiseau *et al.* (1974),
- myoclonic epilepsy of childhood of Jeavons (1977),
- benign and severe myoclonic epilepsy of Dravet (1978), Dravet *et al.* (1982),
- 'Effondrements atoniques épileptiques' of Gastaut *et al.* (1966)

Without doubt, there is great variability of the clinical and electroencephalographic manifestations of the disease. The question may be posed whether in view of this variability it would be preferable to subdivide this syndrome into separate nosological entities. The research on the genetic origins of early childhood spike wave epilepsies with minor seizures shows more and more clearly that groups can be genetically non homogeneous, even if the EEG and the clinical picture are uniform (Doose *et al.* 1984). In an analogous way, this is also true for the apparently homogeneous group of absence epilepsy. Actually, the subgroups of early infantile epilepsies with primary generalized minor seizures, as they are described in this report, have in common a genetically determined corticoreticular hyperexcitability.

References

Aicardi, J. (1973): The problem of the Lennox syndrome. *Develop. Med. Child Neurol.* **15**, 77-81.

Aicardi, J. (1980): Course and prognosis of certain childhood epilepsies with predominantly myoclonic seizures. In *Advances in epileptology.* XII. Epilepsy International Symposium, ed J.A. Wada, J.K. Penry, pp 159-163. Raven Press: New York.

Aicardi, J., Chevrie J.J. (1971): Myoclonic epilepsies of childhood. *Neuropädiatrie* **3**, 177-190.

Doose, H. (1964a): Zur Nosologie der Blitz-Nick-Salaam-Krämpfe. *Arch. Psychiatr. Nervenkr.* **206**, 28-48.

Doose, H. (1964b): Das akinetische Petit Mal. *Arch. Psychiatr. Nervenkr.* **205**, 637-654.

Doose, H., Gerken, H., Leonhardt, R., Völzke, E., Völz Ch. (1970): Centrencephalic myoclonic-astatic petit mal. *Neuropädiatrie* **2**, 59-78.

Doose, H., Völzke, E. (1979): Petit mal-Status in early childhood and dementia. *Neuropädiatrie* **10**, 10-14.

Doose, H., Sitepu, B. (1983): Childhood epilepsy in a German city. *Neuropediatrics* **14**, 220-224.

Doose, H., Gundel, A. (1982): 4-7 cps rhythms in the childhood EEG. In *Genetic basis of the epilepsies,* ed V.E. Anderson, W.A. Hauser, J.K. Penry, C.F. Sing, pp 83-93. Raven Press: New York.

Doose, H., Reinsberg, E., Baier, W. (in press): Genetic heterogeneity of spike wave epilepsies. In *Advances in Epileptology.* XVth Epilepsy International Symposium|, ed. R. Porter *et al.* Raven Press: New York.

Dravet, C. (1978): Les épilepsies graves de l'enfant. *Vie Méd.* **8**, 543-548.

Dravet, C., Roger, J., Bureau, M., Dalla Bernardina, B. (1982): Myoclonic epilepsies in childhood. In *Advances in Epileptology.* XIIIth Epilepsy International Symposium, ed H. Akimoto *et al.* pp 135-140. Raven Press: New York.

Gastaut H., Régis, H. (1961): On the subject of Lennox's 'akinetic' Petit Mal. *Epilepsia* **2**, 298-305.

Gastaut, H., Roger, J., Soulayrol, R., Tassinari, C.A., Régis, H., Dravet, Ch., Bernard, R., Pinsard, N., Saint-Jean, M. (1966): Childhood epileptic encephalopathy with diffuse slow waves (otherwise known as 'petit mal variant' or Lennox syndrome). *Epilepsia* **7**, 139-179.

Gastaut, H., Tassinari, C.A., Bureau, M. (1966): Etude polygraphique et clinique des "effondrements atoniques épileptiques". *Riv. Neurol.* **36**, 5-21.

Gundel, A., Baier, W., Doose, H., Hoovey, Z. (1981): Spectral analysis of EEG in the late course of primary generalized myoclonic-astatic epilepsy. I: EEG and clinical data. *Neuropediatrics* **12**, 62-74.

Gundel, A., Baier, W., Doose, H. (1981): Spectral analysis of EEG in the late course of primary generalized myoclonic-astatic epilepsy. II: Cluster analysis of the power spectra. *Neuropediatrics* **12**, 110-118.

Harper, R.J., (1968): True myoclonic epilepsy in childhood. *Archs Dis. Child.* **43**, 28-35.

Jeavons, P.M. (1977): Nosological problems of myoclonic epilepsies in childhood and adolescence. *Develop. Med. Child. Neurol.* **19**, 3-8.

Kruse, R. (1968): *Das myoklonisch-astatische Petit mal.* Springer: Berlin.

Lennox, W.G. (1945): The petit mal epilepsies; their treatment with Tridione. *J. Am. Med. Ass.* **129**, 1069-1074.

Lennox, W.G., Davis, J.P. (1950): Clinical correlates of the fast and slow spike wave electroencephalogram. *Pediatrics* **5**, 626-644.

Loiseau, P., Legroux, H.M., Grimond, P., du Pasquier, P., Henry, P. (1974): Taxometric classification of myoclonic epilepsies. *Epilepsia* **15**, 1-11.

*   *   *

Discussion pages 100-104

Epileptic syndromes in infancy, childhood and adolescence. J. Roger, C. Dravet, M. Bureau, F.E. Dreifuss and P. Wolf. John Libbey Eurotext Ltd ©1985.

Chapter 11
The Lennox-Gastaut Syndrome

Anne BEAUMANOIR

Division de Neurophysiologie Clinique, Hôpital Cantonal Universitaire, Genève, Switzerland

Summary

The Lennox-Gastaut syndrome is characterized by epileptic seizures: atypical absences, axial tonic seizures and sudden falls (atonic or myoclonic), interictal diffuse slow spike-waves in the awake EEGs and bursts of rapid (10 c/s) rhythms during sleep, a slowing mental development associated with personality disturbances. In 60 per cent of cases it occurs in children suffering from a previous encephalopathy, but it is apparently primary in the other patients. Evolution is unfavourable in most cases, with regard to seizures (frequent epileptic status, essentially tonic status) as well as neuropsychiatric disorders. The author underlines the transitory occurrence of this symptomatology in some cases, particularly in the course of partial epilepsies.

General

In 1950, with their studies on the most common seizures in children whose EEG shows discharges of 'petit mal variant' (PMV) pattern, Lennox and Davis identified an epileptic syndrome that Sorel, in 1964 called 'myokinetic epilepsy' and that Doose, at the same time, included in the framework of 'petit mal akinétique'. However, the limits of the epileptic syndrome associated with PMV called: Lennox-Gastaut Syndrome (LGS) (Gastaut *et al.,* 1966) were defined only later by the works of Gastaut and his school first reported in Dravet's thesis: 'Encéphalopathie de l'Enfant avec pointes ondes lentes diffuses (Petit Mal Variant)' (1965). From the following extensive reviews (Gastaut *et al.,* 1966; Beaumanoir *et al.,* 1968; Kruse, 1968; Niedermeyer, 1969; Janz, 1969, 1972; Karbowski *et al.,* 1970; Chevrie and Aicardi, 1972; Aicardi, 1973; Ohtahara *et al.,* 1976; Markand, 1977) it seems that LGS was unanimously identified as a symptomatic triad:
- epileptic seizures: mainly axial tonic seizures, atonic seizures, atypical absences
- EEG abnormalities: diffuse slow spike and waves (SW) or PMV on waking, bursts of fast rhythms around 10 c/s in sleep.
- slow mental development with associated psychological disorders.

However some authors have extended the nosology of the LGS and published, under the heading of LGS, observations in which one or even two of the main symptoms were absent.

Prevalence: in fact, some authors consider that LGS includes all forms of severe child-hood epilepsy secondary to cerebral lesions or of unknown etiology in which the EEG, on waking, shows slow SW. This fact can explain the discrepancy regarding the LGS prevalence from 3 per cent to 10.7 per cent of children's seizures according to different authors (Gastaut, *et al.,* 1973; Alving, 1979; Beaumanoir, 1981).

Genetics: No family history of LGS has been reported in the literature and the frequency of family history of epilepsy ranges from 2.5 to 40 per cent (Chevrie and Aicardi, 1972; Doose *et al.,* 1970).

Sex: males are more frequently affected.

The mode of onset is variable. The syndrome can be observed in a normal child. More often it begins with epileptic seizures usually developing into the dominant forms of the syndrome. But in some cases, the first seizures are focal. Sometimes status epilepticus, with hemiconvulsions in some cases, more frequently stupor status with tonic seizures can be the first manifestations of the syndrome.

However, in most cases (60 per cent) LGS occurs in children presenting an encephalopathy showing epileptic seizures with or without psychomotor retardation and with or without neurological deficit. In some observations, the seizures are missing and the encephalopathy leads to a psychomotor retardation only. The etiology of pre-existing encephalopathies is very heterogeneous, and remains unknown in most cases. In about 20 per cent of the cases LGS is preceded, with or without a seizure-free interval, by a West syndrome.

The age of onset is before 8 years with a peak between 3 and 5 years. An early onset, before the age of 2, is not exceptional while a late onset, after 10 years, is uncommon.

Electro-clinical symptomatology

This can be summarized by a symptomatic triad.

Ictal symptomatology
The characteristic seizures are: (a) tonic seizures, (b) atypical absences and (c) myoclonias, myoclonoatonias and atonic seizures. These different seizures can be associated in the same child.

(a) From our point of view, *tonic seizures* and their EEG pattern are one of the main signs of the syndrome. Diurnal or nocturnal they can be axial, axorhizomelic or global. They can be symmetric but in some cases a marked unilateral predominance is possible. When the seizures are short and reduced to a *sursum vergens* of the eyeballs with modification of the breathing rhythm (which is a common feature during sleep) they can remain unnoticed. If they are lasting (up to 20s) they can develop a vibratory stage corresponding to extremely rapid clonias of small amplitude, of the whole body. The loss of consciousness is not a constant feature. The return to a normal consciousness corresponds always to the end of the EEG discharge. Enuresis is sometimes observed. A pupillary dilatation is commonly noted.

Tonico-automatic seizures have been described by Oller Daurella (1970). They are particularly frequent in the observations of late onset. They are characterized by a stage of gestural automatisms, ambulatory in some cases, following the tonic phase.

S... G. ♂ 1961

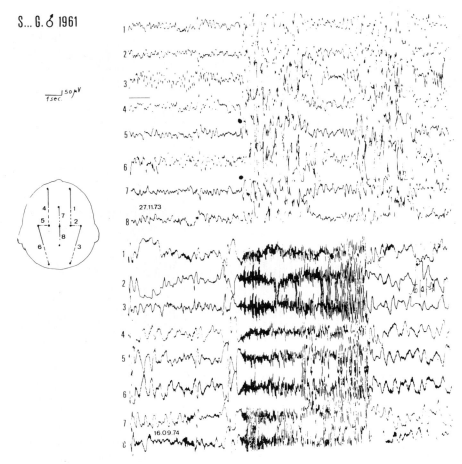

Fig. 1 Above: bursts of slow spike-waves in the EEG of a 12-year-old boy with a congenital right hemiplegia. *Below:* a tonic seizure in the same boy at 13 years.

Slow sleep facilitates the occurrence of tonic seizures which, during this stage, may be of short duration. They occur more frequently in the latter part of the night and, in the young child, often in series on waking.

As regards EEG, tonic seizures appear as a discharge of bilateral rapid rhythms, predominant in the anterior areas and on the vertex. These discharges are sometimes preceded by a short flattening period of the background rhythms or by a discharge of generaliz 1 slow SW. There is no postictal silence (Fig 1). Tonico-automatic seizures show rapid rhythms of the tonic stage followed by diffuse slow SW during the automatic stage. Rapid discharges are particularly frequent during sleep and mainly slow sleep during which they may be very short and look subclinical. This ictal pattern recorded during sleep was described by Gibbs under the unsuitable heading of 'grand mal pattern'.

(b) *Atypical absences* are also observed in the majority of cases. As they begin and end progressively, the clinical observation is often difficult. The loss of consciousness is incomplete and a slight activity remains possible. Eyelid and mainly mouth myoclonias

T... C. ♂ 1980

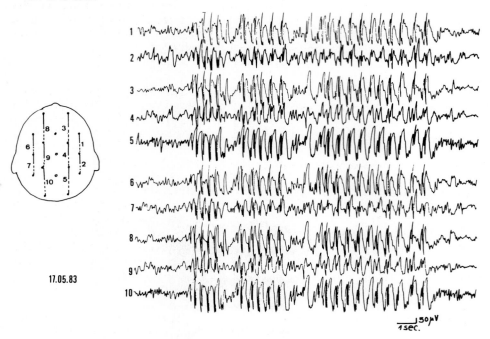

17.05.83

Fig. 2. An atypical absence consisting of a discharge of irregular, diffuse, slow spike-waves.

concomitant with the absences are frequent. However, most often atypical absences affect the musculature with a decrease of the muscular tonus up to a progressive collapse of the body, beginning or localized in the muscles of the face and neck; in such cases the head is leaning forward open-mouthed. This 'amyotonic absence' may be associated with a flow of saliva.

On the EEG, the pattern of atypical absences is a discharge of irregular, diffuse slow 2 - 2.5 c/s SW, more or less symmetrical on both hemispheres, sometimes difficult to differentiate from slow inter-ictal SW (Fig 2).

(c) A sudden fall of the head or of the body is a common sign of *massive myoclonias,* of *myoclono-atonias* and of *atonic seizures* which are very difficult to differentiate clinically. The diagnosis is based on the recording of muscular activity.

EEG shows slow polyspike and waves or diffuse SW or rapid rhythms with anterior predominance. In the last possibility, the seizure corresponds to a very short spasm which has a clinical manifestation very similar to myoclonia.

Most often the three forms of seizures are associated in the same subject. It seems that the predominance of one of them depends on several factors, specially the age of the patient (short spasms are more frequent in the young child), and the state of consciousness (atypical absences with fall and amyotonia are more frequent if the child is not stimulated, tonic short or lasting seizures are always observed during sleep). Tonic-clonic, clonic or partial seizures which are not specific of the syndrome may also be observed.

Status epilepticus (SE) are described in almost two-thirds of cases. Most often they correspond to a more or less marked clouding of mind with repeated tonic seizures, less frequently with myoclono-atonic seizures. The main characteristics of these SE are a long duration (several days, several weeks, even several months), their lack of response to therapy and their repetition in the same patient.

Interictal EEG symptomatology

The first EEG (except in some cases) is generally recorded when the child is already affected. On awaking, it is abnormal in almost all cases from the beginning of the evolution. The reactivity of the rhythms may be preserved but most often rhythms are slow and badly structured for the age. Even in the absence of seizures, the awake recording is dominated by 2-2.5 c/s discharges of slow SW, diffuse on both hemispheres (Fig 3). More often, spikes and multifocal SW predominant in the frontal and temporal areas are also observed.

The sleep stages and their cyclic organization are normal throughout the evolution but the tracings show discharges of rhythmic spikes of about 10 c/s, diffuse though predominant in the anterior areas ('grand mal pattern', Gibbs and Gibbs, 1952) (Fig 4). We think that these discharges of fast rhythms, accompanied or not by clinical tonic manifestations are the most significant element of a positive diagnosis of LGS. During slow sleep, spikes and diffuse slow SW have a tendency to increased bisynchronia compared with the awake state.

Neuropsychiatric symptomatology

LGS has no specific neurological symptomatology. Conversely, in any mode of onset, an intellectual deficit develops very soon. In the 3 to 5-year-old child, a slowing down of the psychomotor development with instability and psychic disorders is observed. In older children, attention disorders impair the school work and make further learning

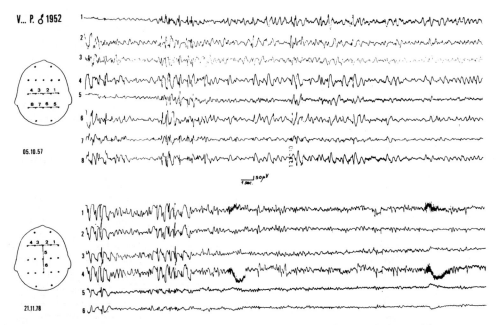

Fig. 3 Interictal slow spike-waves recorded in a boy, above, at 5 years, below at 16 years.

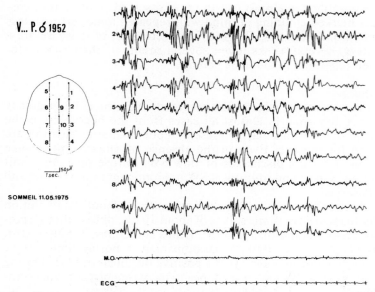

V... P. 6 1952

SOMMEIL 11.05.1975

Fig. 4 In the same boy as in Fig. 3, asleep recording at 23 years: more or less symmetrical spikes and multiple spikes, of higher voltage in the anterior areas.

difficult if not impossible. Psychic disorders and aggressive behaviour appear at the same time. In most cases, intellectual deterioration is associated with or expresses a disorder of the personality development with progressive dysharmonia. They are often severe from the onset and their expression varies according to the age of onset of the syndrome.

Clinical forms

Of course this symptomatic triad does not develop in all patients in the same way.

A subvariety, the myoclonic form of LGS corresponds to a predominance of massive myoclonias and myoclono-atonias (18 per cent of the cases of Chevrie and Aicardi, 1972). Tonic seizures are rare and mainly nocturnal, SE corresponds to an obtundation state with myoclonias. The inter-ictal EEG, when the patient is awake, does not have any special features but sleep does not always induce tonic seizures. The myoclonic form is often primary (64 per cent of cases) and the mental prognosis seems to be less severe than in the typical form.

The study of the forms in relationship to the age of onset suggests that primary forms occurring before the age of 1 year have a symptomatology and an evolution slightly different from the others, but this group has not been differentiated in the literature. Oller Daurella (1973) insisted on the severity of secondary forms occurring before the age of one year. However, late onset forms (after 10 years) have been studied more thoroughly. Oller Daurella differentiated the forms developing after an apparently primary generalized epilepsy, showing the co-existence of rapid and slow SW on EEG recordings, and the forms appearing directly as LGS. The seizures are often tonico-automatic seizures but also sudden falls. Intellectual slowing down appears progressively and above all behavioural and personality disorders develop to produce a psychotic condition in some cases. It must be noted that these late onset forms appear before 20 years of age, exceptionally between 20 and 30 years. (Lipinski, 1977; Stenzel and Pantelli, 1981; Bauer *et al.,* 1983).

Evolution

Recent studies on LGS have dealt mainly with the long-term evolution. The mortality rate is difficult to evaluate. In the observations with more than 10 years follow-up, it reaches about 5 per cent of cases (Gastaut et al., 1973; Loubier, 1974). However the death is rarely directly related to the evolution of the disease. Most often it is accidental. Generally, the disease tends to become chronic. While after a few years of evolution epilepsy is sometimes less active, intellectual and psychic disorders have a tendency to worsen. This aggravation is related to the additional effect of drugs and the lack of social stimulation as well as to still undetermined other factors. Development of a psychotic syndrome, whilst not universal, is not rare. Between 15 - 20 per cent of the observations showed some improvement after several years of evolution. There is a decrease of the frequency of seizures which allows a reduction of the antiepileptic therapy and therefore a better social adaptability of the subject. The cases published in the literature noted that, whatever the condition of the patient in adulthood, the evolution showed a succession of periods of improvement and regression. The regression corresponds to an aggravation of the epileptic symptomatology with SE (Kruse, 1976) often followed by a period during which the neurological symptomatology is characterized by cerebellar and sometimes extra-pyramidal disorders, possibly iatrogenic. A complete seizure-free recovery with a satisfactory psychological condition is exceptional (6.7 per cent of Gastaut's 1973 series, 4 per cent of Loubier's 1974 series).

Differential diagnosis

The electroclinical features of LGS are sufficiently well determined to allow a differential diagnosis. However, a retrospective study of 103 LGS observations, with an evolution of more than 10 years, (in four diagnostic centres) showed that the diagnosis was wrong in 38 cases (37 per cent) (Beaumanoir, 1982). In most observations the pseudo-LGS corresponded to a more or less severe epilepsy whose electroclinical symptomatology had been enlarged throughout the evolution by atonic, myoclonic or myoclono-atonic seizures and diffuse slow SW on EEG. This transient electroclinical syndrome was observed either in subjects with a partial epilepsy, more often frontal or of the mesial aspects of the hemispheres (the latter is sometimes associated with infantile hemiplegia), or in subjects with benign partial or generalized epilepsy who presented a deterioration of their clinical condition (Beaumanoir et al., 1979) during an intercurrent disease but more often on account of a therapeutic overdose. This transient picture may however have lasted for several months, even for several years and in the case of an iatrogenic etiology, yielded only after the reduction of the anti-epileptic therapy. Some observations of severe focal epilepsy in which EEG shows a focus associated with burst of spikes, polyspikes or generalized SW have sometimes been wrongly described as LGS.

The differential diagnosis between typical LGS and the syndrome described by Doose under the heading of 'Centrencephalic myoclonic Astatic Petit Mal' (Kruse, 1968; Doose et al., 1970; Doose, 1980) is still a subject for discussion. This syndrome appears between 2 and 5 years of age; like LGS it is more frequent in males. It always develops in a child who is healthy until the occurrence of the first epileptic signs, usually myoclonic or myoclonic-astatic seizures. A family history of epilepsy is frequently reported (37 per cent of cases). From the onset EEG shows posterior theta activities associated with generalized rapid SW. The condition improved quickly in some cases, while in others the neurological symptomatology is enlarged by tonic seizures and mental deterioration. The observations described by Doose look heterogeneous. The observations with a poor prognosis and tonic seizures throughout the evolution of the disease could correspond to particular forms of LGS onset, close to its myoclonic variety. But the other observations must be clearly differentiated from LGS and may rather be compared to benign and severe myoclonic epilepsies.

Prognosis

The main indicators of a poor prognosis are the following:
- symptomatic character of the syndrome, particularly following a West syndrome. (Ohtahara *et al.,* 1976)
- early onset before 3 years of age. The early onset is often related to the symptomatic character of the disease, but also to a worse prognosis in idiopathic cases (Chevrie and Aicardi, 1972)
- high frequency of seizures, long duration of aggravation periods, recurrence of SE
- existence of background activity constantly slow on the different EEG tracings, and association of localized abnormalities to diffuse slow SW.

Nosology

The symptomatology of LGS tending to become chronic corresponds to the data of Dravet's thesis (1965) specified by Gastaut *et al.,* (1966). As regards the epileptic symptomatology, the tonic seizures and their EEG pattern are almost always present (90 per cent of Dravet's 1965 observations — 87.2 per cent of Beaumanoir's 1982 observations).

SE clinically characterized by obtundation and tonic or myoclono-atonic seizures with EEG tracings close to hypsarrhythmia are also frequent (72 per cent of Dravet's observations in 1965 — 75.8 per cent of Beaumanoir's observations in 1982). Diffuse slow SW, although frequently wrongly selected as cardinal elements of diagnosis in all series (due to the belief that they are pathognomonic of the syndrome), are however required as a *sine qua non,* in spite of their non-specificity (Gastaut, 1982). Although CT scan showed evidence of supratentorial atrophy in about half of the cases (Lagenstein *et al.,* 1979) and although LGS often developed in subjects with a previous cerebral lesion (60 per cent of cases), the pathogenesis of the syndrome is still unknown. Although certain data concerning the mode of onset and the evolution of the syndrome directed research towards virology and immunology (Smeraldi *et al.,* 1975) so far no results allow the determination of the pathological process which generates LGS. Therefore it seems justified to classify LGS in the wide framework of 'generalized epilepsies secondary to non-specific or seemingly primary encephalopathies', as Roger *et al.,* have done (1984).

Case histories

No. 1 — Chronic LGS. (VP)
A male patient, born 17 October, 1952. No family nor personal history. Normal psycho-motor development until the age of 4 years. At this age, confusional state with very frequent falls, twisting of the hands, twitching of eyelids and hypersalivation. The patient was hospitalized at Brussels. The first EEG was performed after this confusional state and showed several discharges of 'petit mal variant' (Fig 3).

Therapy: diones and barbiturates. After a few months, there was an improvement of the seizures, then nocturnal tonic seizures appeared and in June 1957 onset of another SE with axial tonic seizures and complex absences frequently with micturition and hypersalivation.

Between 3 and 8 years of age, the child had no more social activity. The therapy was an association of: suxinutin, barbiturates and carbamazepine. The patient was treated three times with ACTH but seizure control was not complete. Since the age of 9, the evolution showed improvement and aggravation periods of the epilepsy as well as of the mental condition.

SE with mental confusion and successive tonic seizures, frequent at first, became less frequent later. From the age of 20 years, they occurred about every two years. Intellectual disorders were observed from the beginning. Psychotic disorders required a psychiatric assistance as from 16 years. At 26 years, the patient was still living in an institute for the epileptic mentally disabled.

No. 2 — (GS)

A male patient born on 30 October, 1961. No family history. Personal history: breech delivery, possible neo-natal anoxia. Right hemiplegia. The development was normal except in walking. First steps at the age of 18 months. The patient presented an infantile hemiplegia and was investigated at the Pediatric Clinic in Marseille in 1968. At that time, the intellectual coefficient was within normal values: mental age of 6 years and 9 months at the age of 7 years and 1 month.

In 1972 epilepsy started with diurnal tonic seizures. Several antiepileptic therapies were unsuccessful. In 1973, an evaluation in the Hospital of Nice mentioned the following treatment: 100 mg barbiturates, 300 mg phenytoin, 600 mg sulthiame a day. The latter drug had replaced the suxinimide given to the child for a few months.

EEG showed slow SW (Fig 1). The diagnosis was a LGS. Sulthiame was replaced by clonazepam. Tonic seizures were still noted. In 1974, EEG still showed evidence of spikes extending in the fronto-medio-central area of the left hemisphere (Fig 5). Tonic seizures (Fig 1), sometimes induced by unexpected contact, were sometimes recorded mainly during the day. Diazepam responsive SE were reported.

On 29 July, 1976, the child was transferred to the Pediatric Clinic of Geneva. The neurological examination showed a right hemiplegia, and marked dysarthria. Seizures were frequent: diurnal tonic seizures induced by noises or unexpected contacts, com-

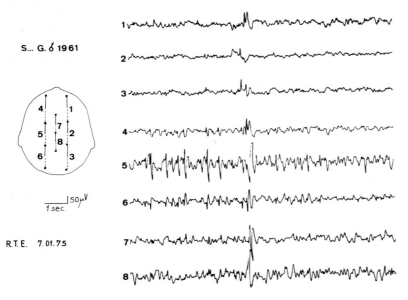

Fig. 5 In the same boy as in Fig. 1, bursts of spikes localized in the left rolandic area, associated with a discharge of diffuse spike-waves.

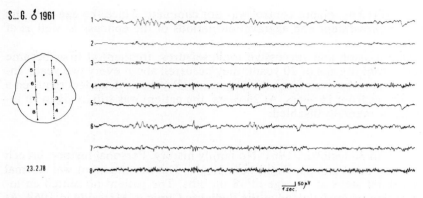

Fig. 6 In the same boy as in the Figs. 1 and 5, at 17 years the diffuse slow spike-waves have disappeared and some small spikes persist in the left rolandic area.

plex absences, focal seizures beginning by a tonic deviation of the eyes and head on the right. On his hospitalization in Geneva the child was given 100 mg barbiturates, 400 mg phenytoin and 800 mg sodium valproate per day. The plasma level of phenytoin was toxic.

CT scan revealed a cortical atrophy and a slight subcortical atrophy with a dilatation of the temporal horn more marked on the left.

Atypical SW associated with diffuse SW were always recorded on EEG. The deep sleep tracing showed tonic seizures mainly in stage II. In June 1977, a psychometric evaluation was performed giving the following results: about 13 years of age for Rey verbal memory test, 6 years of age for the spatial memory test, and about 6 years of age for Stambach motor test.

The therapy was changed. As from 9 November, 1976 the child received 1050 mg sodium valproate and 50 mg phenobarbital. Seizures obviously became better controlled. He was re-examined in February 1978 (Fig. 6). There were still tonic seizures induced by unexpected stimulations. EEG was still asymmetric. Discharges of diffuse SW had practically disappeared (Fig. 6). Except for a period of frequent seizures in the summer 1977, the condition of the patient was maintained at the improved level. The young man has been employed as a filing clerk in his uncle's company where he was still working in 1981.

References

Aicardi, J. (1973): The problem of the Lennox syndrome. *Develop. Med. Child Neurol.* **15**, 77-81.

Alving, J. (1979): Classification of the epilepsies. An investigation of 402 children. *Acta Neurol. Scand.* **60**, 157-163.

Bauer, G., Aichner, F., Saltuari, L. (1983): Epilepsies with diffuse slow spikes and waves of late onset. *Eur. Neurol.* **22**, 344-350.

Beaumanoir, A. (1981): Les limites nosologiques du syndrome de Lennox-Gastaut. *Rev. EEG Neurophysiol.* **11**, 468-473.

Beaumanoir, A. (1982): The Lennox-Gastaut syndrome: a personal study. *EEG Clin. Neurophysiol.* (Suppl. 35), 85-99.

Beaumanoir, A., Martin, F., Panagopoulos, M., Mundler, F. (1968): Le syndrome de Lennox. *Schweiz. Arch. Neurol. Neurochir. Psychiatr.* **102**: 31-62.

Beaumanoir, A., De Castro, R., Nahory, A., Zagury, S. (1979): A follow up study of four cases of subacute anti-epileptic drug encephalopathy. Abstracts 11th Epilepsy Int. Symp., Florence, p 234.

Chevrie, J.J., Aicardi, J. (1972): Childhood epileptic encephalopathy with slow spike-wave. A statistical study of 80 cases. *Epilepsia* **13**, 259-271.

Doose, H. (1964): Das akinetische Petit Mal. *Arch. Psychiatr. Nervenkr* **205**, 625-654.

Doose, H. (1980): Primary generalized myoclonic-astatic epilepsy. In *Advances in Epileptology*, ed R. Canger, F. Angeleri, J.K. Penry, pp 289-296. Raven Press: New York.

Doose, H. Gerken, H., Leonhart, R., Völzke, E., Völz, C. (1970): Centrencephalic myoclonic-astatic petit mal. *Neuropädiatrie.* **2**, 59-78.

Dravet, C. (1965): Encéphalopathie épileptique de l'enfant avec pointe-onde lente diffuse. Thèse, Marseille.

Gastaut, H. (1982): The Lennox-Gastaut syndrome. *EEG Clin. Neurophysiol.* (Suppl. 35), 71-84.

Gastaut, H., Roger, J., Soulayrol, R., Tassinari, C., Régis, H., Dravet, C., Bernard, R., Pinsard, N., Saint-Jean, M. (1966): Childhood epileptic encephalopathy with diffuse slow spike-waves (otherwise known as 'petit mal variant') or Lennox syndrome. *Epilepsia* **7**, 139-179.

Gastaut, H., Dravet, C., Loubier, D., Giove, C., Viani, F., Gastaut, J.A., Gastaut, J.L. (1973): Evolution clinique et pronostic du syndrome de Lennox-Gastaut. In *Evolution and Prognosis of Epilepsies,* ed E. Lugaresi, P. Pazzaglia, C. Tassinari, pp 133-154. Aulo Gaggi: Bologna

Gibbs, F., Gibbs, E. (1952): *Atlas of electroencephalography,* (Vol. 2), pp 31-54. Addison-Wesley: Reading, Mass.

Janz, D. (1969): *Die Epilepsien.* Georg Thieme: Stuttgart.

Janz, D. (1972): Lennox Syndrome plus akinetisches Petit Mal. Myoklonisches astatisches Petit Mal. Epilepsie mit langsamer Spike Wave Variante. In *Psych. des gegenwart. Forschung und Praxis,* pp 585-587. Springer: Berlin.

Karbowski, K., Vassella, F., Schneider, H. (1970): Electroencephalographic aspects of Lennox syndrome. *Eur. Neurol.* **4**, 301-309.

Kruse, R. (1968): *Das myoklonisch-astatische petit mal.* Springer: Berlin, Heidelberg.

Kruse, R. (1976): Absenzen-Status. *Acta Neurol. Scand.* **3**, 155-170.

Lagenstein, I., Kühne, D., Sternuwsky, H.J., Rothe, E. (1979): Computerized cranial transverse axial tomography (CTAT) in 145 patients with primary and secondary generalized West syndrome, myoclonic astatic petit mal, absence epilepsy. *Neuropädiatrie* **10**, 15-28.

Lennox, W.G., Davis, J.P. (1950): Clinical correlates of the fast and slow spike wave electroencephalogram. *Pediatrics* **5**, 626-644.

Lipinski. C.G. (1977): Epilepsies with astatic seizures of late onset. *Epilepsia* **18**, 13-20.

Loubier, D. (1974): Le Syndrome de Lennox-Gastaut: Modalités Evolutives. Thèse, Marseille.

Markand, O.N. (1977): Slow spike wave activity in EEG and associated clinical features often called 'Lennox' or 'Lennox-Gastaut' syndrome. *Neurology* **26**, 746-757.

Niedermeyer, E. (1969): The Lennox-Gastaut syndrome, a severe type of childhood epilepsy. *Dtsch. Z. Nervenheilk.* **195**, 263-282.

Oller-Daurella, L. (1970): Un type spécial de crises observées dans le syndrome de Lennox-Gastaut d'apparition tardive. *Rev. Neurol.* **122**, 459-462.

Oller-Daurella, L. (1973): Evolution et pronostic du syndrome de Lennox-Gastaut. In *Evolution and prognosis of epilepsies,* ed E. Lugaresi, P. Pazzaglia, C.A. Tassinari, pp 155-164. Aulo Gaggi: Bologna.

Ohtahara, S., Yamatogi, Y., Ohtsuka, Y. (1976). Prognosis of the Lennox syndrome. *Folia psychiat, Neurol. Jap.* **30**, 275-287.

Roger, J., Bureau, M., Dravet, C. (1984): Les Epilepsies Généralisées Secondaires, EMC, Paris (In press).

Smeraldi, E., Sorza Smeraldi, R., Cazzullo, C.L., Guareschi-Cazzullo, A., Fabio, G., Canger, R. (1975): Immunogenetics of Lennox-Gastaut syndrome: Frequency of H.L.A. antigenes and haplotypes in patients and first degree relatives. *Epilepsia,* **16**, 699-704.

Sorel, L. (1964): L'épilepsie myokinétique grave de la première enfance avec pointe-ondes lentes (petit mal variant) et son traitement. *Rev. Neurol,* **110**, 215-233.

Stenzel, E., Panteli, C. (1981): Lennox-Gastaut syndrom des 2. Lebensjahrzehntes. In *Epilepsie 1981,* ed Remschmidt, Rentz, Jungmann, pp 99-107, Thieme, Verlag: Stuttgart, New York.

*   *   *

Discussion pages 100-104

Epileptic syndromes in infancy, childhood and adolescence. J. Roger, C. Dravet, M. Bureau, F.E. Dreifuss and P. Wolf. John Libbey Eurotext Ltd ©1985.

Discussion of Myoclonic Epilepsies and Lennox-Gastaut Syndrome
(Chapters 6 to 11)

Summarized by Olaf HENRIKSEN

Aicardi: There is no specific epileptic syndrome characteristic of all the inborn errors of metabolism. The epileptic seizures are not specific enough to suggest any diagnosis.

Gastaut: I would like to discuss three of the presented papers:

(1) I agree entirely with C. Dravet when she describes the benign myoclonic epilepsy as an indisputable entity, known for a long time, but not at this age. In 1951 I proposed to name it 'myoclonic petit mal' in childhood and adolescence (impulsive petit mal of Janz). I have not seen it in infancy, so I suggest calling it 'myoclonic petit mal'? I do not agree with the definition of severe myoclonic epilepsy. In my opinion it is part of a group of myoclonic syndromes, and I am much less sure it is a true entity.

(2) Concerning the presentation of Dalla Bernardina, I would like to question the nosology. If a disease changes or becomes worse, it is evolutionary; if it does not change it is a stable disease; for example, evolutionary or stable tuberculosis. Rather than fixed encephalopathy, I would prefer to use the word 'stable'.

(3) My most important discussion is that concerning Lennox-Gastaut syndrome.

In my opinion there are three criteria: (a) mental retardation, not absolutely necessary at the onset; (b) diffuse slow spike and waves, present in 95% of cases, and the sleep recruiting rhythms. In some subjects there are diffuse spikes and no spike and waves; (c) seizures: myoclonias are very rare, and indeed there is no place for the Lennox-Gastaut syndrome in the taxonomic study of myoclonic epilepsies by Loiseau. At St Paul we found 14 per cent of myoclonias with polygraphic recordings. Without polygraphy I now find only 3 per cent by questioning patients and their families.

Why should we therefore call this syndrome a myoclonic epilepsy? In his classification of myoclonic epilepsies Pazzaglia did not include the Lennox-Gastaut syndrome. I also question the term 'minor motor seizures'. In my opinion seizures which make children fall and have injuries should not be named minor! Call them 'astatic seizures' like Lennox did. It is very difficult to know whether a subject falls because he becomes rigid or because he becomes floppy.

It seems to me that the Lennox-Gastaut is an extraordinarily precise syndrome, which could be called 'astatic epilepsy with slow spike waves'.

Concerning the epilepsy of Dr Doose, I find that it very much resembles the Lennox-Gastaut syndrome, especially the myoclonic variant of this syndrome, and the myoclonic epilepsy with slow spike and waves of Aicardi and Chevrie. But sometimes, it has to be put into the 'minestrone' of myoclonic syndromes.

Doose: In no other field of pediatric epileptology does there exist such a confusion regarding classification and terminology as in the epileptic syndromes of early childhood with generalized minor seizures. Probably this is due to the uniformity of the clinical phenomena in the different types of early childhood epilepsy. Until further clinical and genetic studies exist, these types of childhood epilepsy should probably be listed together in one logic group, rather than in syndromes.

The syndrome or the group of myoclonic astatic petit mal with all its variants should be strictly delineated from secondary epilepsies like the West and the Lennox syndrome. It is, however, impossible to avoid an overlap of borderline cases between the different syndromes. The cases of Dalla Bernardina I believe to be on the borderline between primary and secondary epilepsies. Most cases of myoclonic astatic epilepsies or the myoclonic epilepsies are primary in origin while most of the cases with the Lennox-Gastaut syndrome are secondary. I believe that the reaction of the immature brain is rather uniform so that we cannot judge from the clinical symptomatology alone. When there is evidence of brain damage or other focal signs we have a criterion for secondary generalized epilepsy, like the Lennox-Gastaut syndrome, while generalized paroxysm in EEG without such signs will be classified as 'centrencephalic' - myoclonic astatic petit mal.

The patients fitting into this syndrome represent a heterogeneous group and Dr Henriksen stated that although we today, because of our limited diagnostic tools, cannot pin point the etiology, we cannot automatically call all cases with generalized seizures without detectable etiology, for primary epilepsies.

Aicardi: Which criteria would you use to make the distinction between the 'centrencephalic' myoclonic astatic epilepsy and the Lennox-Gastaut syndrome?

Doose: The leading syndrome of the cortico-reticular type is a primary generalized seizure in an undamaged child with irregular spike and waves. The difference between the primary and secondary myoclonic astatic epilepsy may be compared with the difference between absences with 3 c/s. spike and waves and the absence-like psychomotor seizure with focal changes in the EEG.

Dravet: Atypical absences are a most important type of seizure in the Lennox-Gastaut syndrome. Have you observed such absences in your patients?

Doose: These patients never have the atypical absences that you have shown. It is also important to note that you can recognize the children with myoclonic-astatic epilepsy right away by their well shaped, sensitive faces. This is because of their normal development before onset of the seizures.

Tassinari discussed a type of epilepsy with only one type of seizure — atonic drop attacks without any other seizures like atypical absences, tonic seizures or partial seizures or myoclonic jerks. No further evidence of such an existing syndrome was given.

Doose described a minor group of patients with atonic or astatic seizures, but these patients had occasionally other seizures as well. These children were well developed, had

101

no signs of a brain lesion and did not belong to the Lennox-Gastaut syndrome. They respond well to valproate, sometimes in combination with ethosuccimide.

Gastaut: I disagree with this since I have seen 5 or 6 cases with such drop attacks and they were all cases with severe encephalopathy and a very poor prognosis.

Doose: If you observe these children closely you will find they have brain lesions with multifocal epilepsy. These children with violent drop attacks have a short initial tonic seizure phase as described by Stenzel in Bethel.

Aicardi: I would like to ask Dr Doose for his definition of Lennox-Gastaut syndrome of secondary type.

Doose: It is characterized by a brain lesion and the variation of focal seizures. As the children with Lennox-Gastaut syndrome develop, they will show a variety of focal seizures including psychomotor seizures in the later course. Very often these children will have generalized seizures with a focal start.

Aicardi: But what is the clinical picture which makes you think it is secondary?

Doose: It consists of children with a retarded development, with neurological deficits like hemiplegia, tetraplegia and so on.

Jeavons: Perhaps we could decide that there is nothing myoclonic in the Lennox-Gastaut syndrome, and there is something myoclonic in the myoclonic astatic epilepsy. I will also comment that the myoclonic epilepsy of childhood is not necessarily benign. Many of these children continue to have seizures as adults, and such a course cannot be called benign.

Doose: I would like to give an example of benign types of myoclonic as well as myoclonic astatic epilepsy. There are several of these benign types which do not belong within the Lennox-Gastaut syndrome. Last year we treated a pair of monozygotic twins with myoclonic epilepsy. They both experienced their first myoclonic seizure within the same week, provoked by startles. The EEG's showed bilaterally synchronous spike and waves and the myoclonic jerks were symmetrical. One of the twins was treated with valproate while the other twin received no treatment. After 14 days the latter was seizure free while the first twin receiving valproate became seizure free 14 days after withdrawal of the drug.

Henriksen: Whether an epilepsy proves to be benign or not is a poor criterion in the beginning of the disease. It is only later in the course that one can tell with some certainty what the prognosis is.

Lerman: In our everyday life we don't treat diseases or syndromes, we treat patients. And each patient behaves in their own individual way which sometimes is unpredictable. Patients may start out with a mild epilepsy and a good prognosis and later end up as an intractable malignant epilepsy. On the other hand it sometimes happens that a typical 'Lennox-Gastaut' recovers completely.

Beaumanoir's criteria for the Lennox-Gastaut syndrome were accepted by everyone — and *Jeavons* expressed relief since myoclonic attacks were included in the Lennox-Gastaut syndrome.

Henriksen: For many physicians myoclonic astatic epilepsy has been synonymous with the Lennox-Gastaut syndrome. We will therefore once again ask Dr Doose to specify his subgroup.

Doose: Normal development, at least in most cases. No neurological deficits. The clinical symptomatology often begins with primary generalized grand mal seizures. The first seizure may, or may not present itself as a febrile convulsion. There should be no focal seizures and never atypical absences. In the EEG there is usually 4-7 c/s background activity and seldom hypersynchronous activity in the beginning. The course of the epilepsy may differ in the myoclonic astatic petit mal, as there are benign cases with spontaneous remission or seizure control on valproate and normal psychomotor development. But there may be cases with seizure control and dementia, the dementia usually following a status epilepticus. Finally there may be unfavourable cases with predominantly absences and tonic seizures during night or nocturnal grand mal seizures, but never focal motor and never psychomotor seizures. The EEG never shows focal or multifocal changes. The genetic predisposition is higher in myoclonic astatic epilepsy and in myoclonic epilepsy than in all other types of childhood epilepsy. It is also noteworthy that the correlation of EEG patterns and the clinical symptoms is stronger in this group. Poly-spike and wave will be correlated with myoclonic seizures. And longer groups of 2-3 c/s spike and wave will give alteration of vigilance while patients with the Lennox-Gastaut syndrome may exhibit long sequences of 2-3 c/s spike and wave without any clinical symptoms.

Dalla Bernardina: I want to defend severe myoclonic epilepsy and benign myoclonic epilepsy.

Severe myoclonic epilepsy occurs in normal children; with a high rate of epilepsy in their family history; they always start having seizures in the first year of life; they resemble the cases of Dr Doose which begin in the first year and which also have a high incidence of epilepsy in their family history. They begin with clonic and often unilateral and long seizures, provoked by fever, and the EEG is normal.

The first diagnosis is febrile convulsions. These same clonic convulsions, febrile or not febrile, unilateral but which can change sides, are repeated before the end of the first year.

Psychomotor development is still normal. EEG is more or less normal, but can show the four to seven rhythms as described by Dr Doose, and there may be photosensitivity. This is important since it is exceptional to observe photosensitivity at this age (between one year and 18 months).

Then, 'absences' appear with myoclonias, and also non epileptic myoclonias may appear. Never are there tonic seizures and never slow spike and waves, as in the Lennox-Gastaut syndrome.

The evolution is always bad with persistence of seizures and mental retardation, without deterioration. If one considers the evolution the picture is very homogeneous. And it is completely different from the Lennox-Gastaut syndrome. But there is a relationship with some of the cases of Dr Doose.

Beaumanoir: In the Lennox-Gastaut syndrome the background activity in the EEG is abnormal for the age when the patient is awake, except at the very beginning. There are diffuse slow spike and wave discharges, predominantly in the anterior regions.

During sleep the EEG may be well organized in the beginning, but it quickly becomes abnormal. There are discharges of 10 c/s rapid rhythms (grand mal rhythms of Gibbs).

Bureau: In my opinion the percentage of the different stages of sleep is maintained and spindles persist.

Beaumanoir: I accept that the organization of sleep remains good enough — Stage II remains long enough, particularly the spindles — and I will not include in the definition the poor organization of sleep.

Dravet: It seems that in severe myoclonic epilepsies the criteria are more precise: early onset, clonic seizures, focal anomalies on the EEG, and that allows one to predict that there will be a bad prognosis.

Cavazzuti: I think that the group (severe myoclonic epilepsies) described by C. Dravet is different from the type described by Doose. It is truly an individual syndrome, with a characteristic succession of seizures: febrile seizures, early, numerous and prolonged, focal fits, myoclonias. I totally agree that this is a syndrome.

III
Epileptic syndromes in childhood

Epileptic syndromes in infancy, childhood and adolescence. J. Roger, C. Dravet, M. Bureau, F.E. Dreifuss and P. Wolf. John Libbey Eurotext Ltd ©1985.

Chapter 12
Childhood Absence Epilepsy

Pierre LOISEAU

Hôpital Pellegrin/ Tripode, Place Amélie-Raba-Léon, 33076 Bordeaux, France

Summary

Childhood absence epilepsy is a relatively rare form of primary generalized epilepsy, occurring in previously normal children with a strong genetic predisposition. Absence seizures of any kind apart from myoclonic absences are the initial type of attacks, with an onset between 3 and 12 years of age and a peak at 6-7 years of age. They are very frequent throughout the day, occurring spontaneously or precipitated by environmental factors. They are concomitant to a bilateral, synchronous and symmetrical spike-wave discharge in the EEG. Spike-waves are, in most patients, regular at a three per second rhythm but can sometimes be less regular. Electroencephalographic background activity is normal but may occasionally be slightly abnormal. Absence seizures tend to vanish spontaneously and are in 80 per cent of cases controlled by specific antiepileptic drugs. A durable remission is not infrequent but 40 per cent of patients develop during adolescence or later in life a mild generalized tonic-clonic epilepsy. Very few patients have only absence seizures when adults. A poor social adjustment is frequent. Childhood absence epilepsy must be carefully distinguished from other epilepsies with absence seizures.

Introduction

Absence childhood epilepsy should be a clear-cut epileptic syndrome. Its main character is the presence of absence seizures. Unfortunately absence seizures occur in other forms of epilepsy. A major difficulty arising in a survey of the literature is to distinguish absence childhood epilepsy from the multiplicity of conditions commonly referred to as petit mal.

Historical

The first description of childhood absence epilepsy is probably Tissot's (1770): 'La jeune malade avait eu fréquemment, dans l'intervalle des grands accès, de petits accès très courts, qui n'étaient marqués que par une perte instantanée de connaissance, qui lui coupait la parole avec un très léger mouvement dans les yeux; souvent, en revenant à elle, elle achevait la phrase au milieu de laquelle elle avait été interrompue; d'autres fois, elle l'avait oubliée'[1]. This girl was 14 years old. Her 'petits accès' had begun at 7 years of age. Some months later she also had had 'very intense and very frequent' tonic-clonic seizures.

Esquirol in 1815 proposed calling all non-convulsive epileptic seizures petit mal. The term absence is quoted for the first time by Calmeil (1824). In 1861 Reynolds considers two opposite forms of epilepsy: *epilepsia gravior* (convulsive seizures) and *epilepsia mitior*. Like Gowers (1881) he does not distinguish clearly typical absences and other seizures with a mild appearance. At the end of the nineteenth century absence seizures are well recognized and their epileptic nature is admitted. For a moment, at the beginning of the twentieth century, some authors try to separate petit mal from epilepsy: 'nicht epileptischen Absencen oder kurzen narkoleptischen Anfälle' (Friedmann, 1906). However, this heresy did not last. In 1916, Sauer introduced the term pyknolepsy and was of the opinion that it was an epileptic disease. In 1924, Adie summarized 'pyknolepsy, a form of epilepsy occurring in children with a good prognosis' as follows: 'A disease with an explosive onset between the age of 4 and 14 years, of frequent, short, very slight, monotonous minor epileptiform seizures of uniform severity which recur almost daily for weeks, months or years, are uninfluenced by antiepileptic remedies, do not impede normal mental and psychological development, and ultimately cease spontaneously never to return'.

However, even if childhood absence epilepsy is correctly described, the terms petit mal and pyknolepsy are often used improperly to name every form of absences. As the diagnosis is only based upon clinical observation, some partial seizures are involved in this group of epilepsies. In 1935, Gibbs, Davis and Lennox called petit mal absences brief interruptions of consciousness associated with a rhythmic 3 cycles per second discharge of regular spike and wave complexes on the EEG. Things were clear... for a moment. Unfortunately, eight years later, Gibbs, Gibbs and Lennox wrote: 'It is more accurate to apply to a particular electroencephalographic pattern the name of the clinical type of seizure with which it is associated than to use purely descriptive terms . . . There can be no question of the propriety of speaking of a petit mal type of dysrhythmia when it occurs during a clinical petit mal seizure . . . we believe that it is equally proper to speak of a petit mal type of dysrhythmia when the same pattern appears in a routine record in the absence of clinically obvious seizures, even if the particular patient has no history of petit mal or of epilepsy'. Furthermore 'The electroencephalographic classification of alternate spikes and waves brings together a triad of seizures having diverse clinical manifestations' (Lennox, 1945). It was the petit mal triad, with: (i) absences; (ii) myoclonic seizures; (iii) akinetic seizures. This triad is misunderstood and misused. All minor seizures accompanied by bilateral spikes and waves are considered as petit mal, despite Lennox's warning (1950): 'Minor seizures other than petits have to be called minor epilepsy or given their proper designation, such as myoclonic or atonic members of the petit mal triad'.

The International Classification of Epileptic Seizures (1970) opposes typical absences to atypical absences and the confusion becomes less severe. Nevertheless, clinical and EEG criteria for the diagnosis of petit mal remain till now somewhat imprecise. This lack of accuracy in definition explains the wide discrepancies observed in the published data on petit mal or on the prognosis of absences. Such an ambiguity is associat-

---

[1] 'In the intervals between major attacks, the young female patient had frequently had very short minor attacks which were recognized only by an instantaneous loss of consciousness which stopped the patient's speech, accompanied by a very slight movement in the eyes. Often, on recovery, she completed the sentence which was interrupted; on other occasions she had totally forgotten it.'

ed with the term petit mal that it is preferable to use this term no longer. In fact, childhood absence epilepsy is very close to the pyknolepsy of the German authors (Janz, 1955).

Definition

Childhood absence epilepsy should be a term restricted to an epilepsy characterized as follows:
(1) A form of epilepsy with an onset before puberty;
(2) Occurring in previously normal children;
(3) Absence seizures as the initial type of seizures;
(4) Very frequent absences of any kind apart from myoclonic absences.
(5) Absence seizures associated in the EEG with a bilateral, symmetrical and synchronous discharge of regular three-per-second spike and wave complexes on a normal background activity. Less regular spike-wave activity is possible, when compatible with a diagnosis of typical absences.

Description

Defined according to these criteria, childhood absence epilepsy is a rather homogeneous entity.

I. General
1. Frequency.
The annual incidence rate of absence seizures has been estimated 1/10 000 (Hauser and Kurland, 1975). Strong discrepancies exist in the literature concerning its prevalence among epileptic children: from 2.3 per cent (Livingston *et al.,* 1965) to 37.7 per cent (Lennox, 1945). The recruitment of patients was probably different. In fact, it probably represented 8 per cent of epilepsy in school-age children (Cavazzuti, 1980).

2. Sex ratio.
Childhood absence epilepsy is clearly more frequent in girls than in boys. Sixty to 76 per cent of affected children are girls (Lennox and Lennox, 1960; Hertoft, 1963; Weir, 1965; Gibberd, 1966; Dalby, 1969).

3. Genetics.
'Pour produire l'épilepsie, il faut nécessairement deux choses: (i) une disposition du cerveau à entrer en contraction plus aisément qu'en santé; (ii) une cause d'irritation qui mette en action cette disposition' (Tissot)[1]. These two factors (genetic factor and acquired factor) exist with a very unequal significance in childhood absence epilepsy.

(a) Positive family history of epilepsy. 'J'ai consulté une jeune dame, dont le père est épileptique, qui est prise de ses accès au milieu d'un cercle, à la promenade, à cheval: elle n'est point renversée, les yeux sont convulsifs, le regard est fixe; l'accès ne dure que peu de secondes et la malade reprend la conversation, la phrase où elle les a

---

[1] 'To produce epilepsy, two things are necessary: (i) a tendency for the brain to fall into spasm more readily than during health; (ii) a source of irritation that can precipitate this tendency.'

laissées sans se douter nullement de ce qui vient de lui arriver' (Esquirol, 1815)[2].

A positive family history of epilepsies is found in 15 per cent (Bergamini *et al.*, 1965; Lugaresi *et al.*, 1973), in 18 per cent (Lugaresi and Volterra, 1963), in 20 per cent (Holowach *et al.*, 1962), in 22 per cent (Lennox and Lennox, 1960; Gibberd, 1966), in 40 per cent (Sato *et al.*, 1976) and in 44 per cent (Currier *et al.*, 1963) of children with absence seizures. These seizures in parents and relatives are absence and tonic-clonic seizures. In the studies on twins, monozygotic twins develop absence attacks in 75 per cent of pairs (Lennox, 1951; Gedda and Tataralli, 1971) and dizygotic twins 16 times less often. Febrile convulsions are frequent in siblings of these children (Doose *et al.*, 1973).

(b) Acquired factors. Perinatal complications, postnatal head trauma and cerebral inflammatory disease are found in the case histories of 7 to 30 per cent of patients (Lugaresi and Volterra, 1963; Weir, 1965). The onset of absence seizures can be just after an infectious disease with and sometimes without cerebral complication (Dalby, 1969). A history of febrile convulsions is common: 15 per cent of cases (Penry *et al.*, 1975). However the role of these acquired factors is often of dubious significance. These cerebral aggressions are very common in infancy and childhood and are found in the same proportion in children without absences.

(c) Mode of inheritance. An autosomal dominant monogenic mode of inheritance with age-dependent penetrance has been suggested by the Metrakoses (1972). However polygenic factors have been suggested by others (Doose *et al.*, 1973). In fact, a multi-factorial origin with both genetic and environmental factors is likely (Andermann, 1980).

4. Age of onset. Absence seizures begin usually between 3 and 13 years of age. They peak at age 6-7 (Lennox and Lennox, 1960; Holowach *el at.*, 1962; Currier *et al.*, 1963; Livingston *et al.*, 1965; Dalby, 1969). An earlier onset is possible but is very rare (Beaumanoir, 1976). A second peak is noted at 11-12 years of age (Oller-Daurella and Sanchez, 1981). Absence seizures with a later onset do not belong to childhood absence epilepsy.

II. Seizures

Absence seizures are characterized as follows:

> a short duration;
> an abrupt onset and termination;
> an impairment of consciousness, with or without other signs;
> a high frequency.

(a) Absence duration. It ranges from 2 or 3 seconds to 1 or 2 minutes but is in most cases from 5 to 10 seconds (Penry *et al.*, 1975) or from 5 to 30 seconds (Lennox and Lennox, 1960). In a personal series it was: less than 5 seconds in 23 per cent of cases; 5 to 15 seconds in 39 per cent of cases; 15 to 30 seconds in 21 per cent of cases; more than 30 seconds, in 3 per cent of cases; and variable in 14 per cent of cases.

---

[2] 'I have visited a young lady, whose father is epileptic. She has attacks during meetings, and when walking or riding. She does not fall down, her eyes are convulsive, with a fixed stare. The attack lasts no longer than a few seconds and the patient takes up the conversation at the point she left it, without suspecting anything has happened to her.'

(b) Onset and termination. As a rule, the onset of absence seizure is sudden. 'If warning occurs, the diagnosis of petit mal may be questioned'. (Lennox and Lennox, 1960). However some authors admit in rare cases some warning sensation before the absence (Dalby, 1969). The frequency of a brief retrograde amnesia is controversial (Jus and Jus, 1962; Ounsted *et al.*, 1963). This amnesia lasts from 4 to 15 seconds, occurs when the patient is still fully conscious and has a normal EEG. It is partly reversible.

The attack ends as abruptly as it has commenced. The patient usually carries on with his on-going activity as if nothing had happened. However it can take a few seconds before returning to a normal behaviour. 'The occasional patient will 'come to' rather slowly over a period of seconds' (Lennox and Lennox, 1960). The child is very often unaware of his attack. An external stimulus (call, pain) can shorten the absence seizure (Schwab, 1947).

(c) Symptomatology of absence. The essential feature of the absence seizure is a loss of awareness and responsiveness with cessation of on-going activities. The patient stops talking, eating, walking. He remains motionless, with vacant eyes, staring straight ahead or drifting upwards. Breathing continues normally or slows, especially in long-lasting attacks.

However 'Observation of children suffering these brief attacks has disclosed that the seizures have a more complex character than the name petit mal or absences implies' (Dalby, 1969).

Different degrees of involvement of consciousness were described. A complete abolition of awareness, responsiveness and memory is usual in seizures of childhood absence epilepsy. However 'The occasional patient is dimly aware of what is taking place or he can hear but he cannot respond' (Lennox and Lennox, 1960). The level of consciousness is sometimes difficult to ascertain without special devices (for details, see Penry, 1973 and Browne and Feldman, 1983).

The International Classification of Epileptic Seizures (1981) distinguishes six types of absence seizures, according to their associated clinical features. These features have very often been described, with some discrepancies on their frequency or importance. They can be missed by casual observation. Their most accurate description based on simultaneous recording with videotape and electroencephalography was given by Penry, Porter and Dreifuss (1975). The varieties of absence seizures are:

— *simple absences,* with only an impairment of consciousness. They are rare: less than 10 per cent of the observed seizures;

— *absences with mild clonic component.* The term mild must be emphasized. Marked clonic components - clonic jerks of the head, of the shoulders and arms - characterize myoclonic absences. Myoclonic absences do not belong to childhood absence epilepsy. In childhood absence epilepsy, clonic movements are restricted to eyelids (blinking at a rhythm of 3 per second), they more rarely involve the chin and the lips, resulting in twitching of the face. Mild clonic components exist in approximately half the absences.

— *absences with atonic components.* A diminution in tone of muscles subserving posture rather than a complete atonia is observed. It results in a gradual lowering of head and/or arms, often rhythmic, because of mixed clonic jerks. In these cases, the patient may drop what he is holding in his hands. Very rarely tone is sufficiently diminished to cause the patient to fall. Absences with a sudden fall are usually atypical absences. An atonic component is present in about 20 per cent of absences seizures. It is most frequently combined with other components.

— *absences with tonic components.* An increase in postural tone affects mainly the extensor muscles. It is most often limited to the eyes, which rotate upwards and to the head, which draws backwards. It can be more diffuse leading to retropulsion of the trunk. If this increase in postural tone occurs asymmetrically, the patient's head or trunk will be pulled to one side. Sometimes a mild clonic component is mixed with the tonic contraction. This variety of absence is frequent according to Janz (1955) but not according to Penry *et al.* (1975).

— *absences with automatisms.* Two categories of ictal automatisms exist: perseverative and *de novo* automatisms. In perseverative automatisms, the patient persists in what he is doing, i.e. eating, walking, handling objects. These activities can be correctly done. 'I have known these seizures to occur in a gentleman while hunting, and yet he has maintained his seat' (Reynolds, 1861, p.83). However they are often distorted: walking more slowly, pouring water in a full glass. *De novo* automatisms are in the great majority of cases very simple: lip licking, swallowing, face rubbing, scratching, fumbling with clothes. They can be more complex: catching objects, grunting, mumbling, humming or singing. Some automatisms are clearly determined by reaction to environmental stimuli (Penry *et al.,* 1975). Automatisms, as a sole component or often associated with other components are very frequent, occurring in more than 60 per cent of attacks (Penry *et al.,* 1975). They are related to the duration of seizures. Their frequency increases with increasing seizure duration, ranging from 22 per cent in a seizure lasting less than 3 seconds to 95 per cent in a seizure lasting more than 16 seconds.

— *absences with autonomic components.* Autonomic components are either easily recognized, when leading to urinary incontinence or need a careful observation, when consisting of pupil dilatation, pallor, flushing, tachycardia, change in blood pressure and so on.

These six types of absence seizures do exist but two important comments have to be made: (i) in many cases several components are noted during a given absence seizure (Dreifuss, 1972; Penry *et al.,* 1975); (ii) even if the tendency for individual patients to have attacks of the same type is statistically significant, many patients have several types of absence seizures (Penry *et al.,* 1975).

(d) Repetition and precipitating factors. Attacks are usually very frequent throughout the day. 'If attacks do not recur daily, the diagnosis may be questioned' (Lennox and Lennox, 1960). 'They begin in driblets, the parents noting short episodes of immobility or eye-rolling but passing it off as day-dream or an emotional display.... In time, however, the blackout periods increase in frequency or in duration and cannot be disregarded any longer' *(Ibid.).* At this moment, they range from 10 to 200 per day.

They occur spontaneously but are particularly influenced by environmental factors. Precipitating factors are very numerous. It is worth noting that in a given patient the absences are often triggered by the same factor. The main factors are: emotional (anger, sorrow, fear, surprise, embarrassment), intellectual (lack of interest, release of attention, meal-time for some children, school-time for others), nycthemeral (evening or awakening), metabolic (hypoglycaemia, hyperventilation). Hyperventilation deserves a special comment. It is the easiest way to provoke an absence seizure and 'with a few exceptions, a diagnosis of petit mal should be seriously questioned in the untreated patient who does not have an attack on hyperventilation' (Holowach *et al.,* 1962). On the other hand, absences generally do not occur when a child is busy and stimulated by a physical or psychic activity, or has a sustained attention (Bureau *et al.,* 1968). However in certain cases an emotional or conflicting situation provokes absences: epilepsia arithmetices (Ingvar and Nyman, 1962), learning difficulties (Bureau *et al.,* 1968).

Absence status are relatively rare in childhood absence epilepsy: 10 per cent of cases (Livingston *et al.,* 1965).

III. Electroencephalography

Absence seizures are associated with a bilaterally synchronous and symmetrical discharge of rhythmic spike and wave complexes (Fig. 1). This paroxysmal activity occurs bilaterally, begins abruptly and synchronously in both hemispheres. The spike-waves have the same shape and amplitude at homologous points in the two hemispheres. They have their highest amplitude under the fronto-central leads. This point appears to be important: 'The distribution of potential is so constant in all true petit mal that deviations as, for example, a maximum potential at the frontal pole instead of in mid-frontal regions should suggest another form of epilepsy' (Jasper, 1951). 'Termination of the spike-and-wave sequence is less abrupt than its onset. The slow waves may take several seconds to decelerate and decrease in amplitude before merging with the pre-seizure form of record' (Lennox and Lennox, 1960). The frequency of the spike-wave complexes is three-per-second at the beginning of the discharges and may slow to 2.5-2 per second towards the end. An individuality of 'fast spike-wave' discharges for particular patients was noted as well as many individual variations from patient to patient. The relative amplitude of the spike-waves, the leads which are first involved (usually the anterior ones), the shape of the patterns vary. Toposcopic examinations on spatial and temporal changes of spike and wave fields demonstrated these variations better than routine records (Petsche, 1962). More irregular spike-wave discharges (polyspike-waves, changing rhythm inside a discharge) are compatible with a diagnosis of childhood absence epilepsy (Livingston et al., 1965). In an unpublished study we compared two groups of patients with either regular three-per-second or irregular spike-waves. No difference in evolution and prognosis was found.

The interictal EEG background activity is usually normal. Mild background abnormalities may be accepted (Sato et al., 1976). Interictal paroxysmal activity, consisting of single or brief discharges of bilateral spike-waves are frequent. These paroxysmal abnormalities are more numerous during non-REM sleep, with important morphologic changes (Sato et al., 1973). Some children exhibit a rather particular posterior delta rhythm, usually as long bursts of sinusoïdal activity at three-per-second high activity, either symmetrical or more often asymmetrical on occipital and occipito-parietal areas

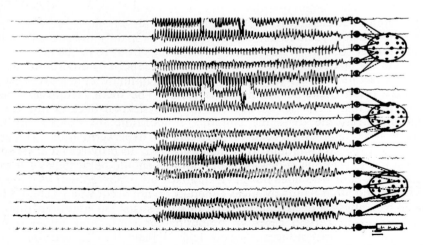

Fig. 1: Absence seizure with automatisms. Duration: 14 seconds. At the fourth and eighth seconds, mouth movements displace some leads or give rise to a muscular artefact. At the eleventh second, note the artefact on the ECG record, due to hand movement.

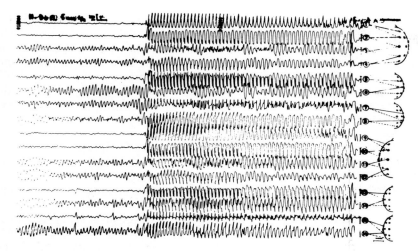

Fig. 2: Absence seizure with interictal delta posterior rhythms.

(Fig. 2). This slow posterior rhythm is blocked by eye-opening and is enhanced by hyperventilation (Subirana and Oller-Daurella, 1953; Cobb *et al.,* 1961).

Evolution

As said in the introductory remarks different forms of epilepsy have been studied under the heading petit mal. As a consequence the evidence present in the literature is inconclusive concerning evolution and prognosis of the absence epilepsy of childhood. However some of the published data are detailed enough to allow an identification of cases with childhood absence epilepsy and to select these cases. Another difficulty arises from too short a follow-up period, casting doubts on the long-term outcome of the syndrome. As pointed out by Lugaresi et al. (1973) two prognosis parameters must be considered: (a) evolution of the seizures, (b) interictal state.

I. Seizure prognosis
The follow-up of patients with childhood absence epilepsy indicates three outcomes:
1. *Patients become seizure-free.* A wide range of remission rates has been given: 79.3 per cent (Dalby, 1969); 78.6 per cent (Livingston, *et al.,* 1967, with a follow-up between 5 and 28 years, 55 per cent only of patients beyond 15 years of age); 78.3 per cent (Sato *et al.,* 1976, follow-up 5.8 to 8 years); 57.5 per cent (Loiseau *et al.,* 1983, follow-up 5 to 25 years, mean - 16 years); 44 per cent (Currier *et al.,* 1966, mean follow-up 15 years, patients' ages 15 to 36 years, mean - 26 years) and 33 per cent (Oller-Daurella and Sanchez, 1981, follow-up 1 to 51 years, mean 16 years). The longer the follow-up, the smaller is the percentage of controlled patients. This is due to a late occurrence of tonic-clonic seizures which may occur many years after the cessation of absence seizures (see below). Thus a control of absence seizures is not an absolute proof of good prognosis. A prolonged follow-up is mandatory to ascertain the prognosis of childhood absence epilepsy. A rapid onset of therapy and the quality of anti-epileptic drugs are important (Oller-Daurella and Sanchez, 1981). With an early and adequate therapy, 70 per cent of patients were controlled and only 18 per cent with an incorrect therapy (Bergamini *et al.,* 1965). Absence seizures may disappear soon after onset of therapy

or persist for a time. A shorter duration of illness tends to favor cessation of seizures (Loiseau *et al.*, 1966; Sato *et al.*, 1976). Its average duration was 6.6 years (Currier *et al.*, 1963). 'The tendency for petit mal to cease is present at all ages and not just at puberty. In about a quarter of patients the attacks cease before the age of 15 and by the age of 30 years petit mal had ceased in about three quarters of the patients' (Gibberd, 1966). In this survey, with a follow-up of nearly 5 years, only 3 per cent of patients experienced absence seizures beyond 50 years of age. In another survey (Livingston *et al.*, 1965), of the 92 controlled patients, 89 were aged 20 or younger at the time of cessation of absence seizures.

2. *Absence seizure persist*. This is a rare occurrence which is reported to occur in about 6 per cent of patients (Oller-Daurella and Sanchez, 1981). Attacks become less frequent and are most apt to occur when patients are tired, excited, sleep-deprived or during a menstrual period (Currier *et al.*, 1963). Absence seizures tend to be very short, and not very troublesome to the patient.

3. *Tonic-clonic seizures develop*. Subsequent to the onset of absence seizures, tonic-clonic seizures occur in about 40 per cent of patients (35.6 per cent, Livingston *et al.*, 1965; 37 per cent, Currier *et al.*, 1963; 40 per cent, Loiseau *et al.*, 1983; 56 per cent, Charlton and Yahr, 1967; 60 per cent, Oller-Daurella and Sanchez, 1981). The development of tonic-clonic seizures is not in itself of grave significance for the patient: it is usually easily controlled (Currier *et al.*, 1963; Charlton and Yahr, 1967; Oller-Daurella and Sanchez, 1981; Loiseau *et al.*, 1983). Seizures are infrequent. They begin in most cases between 10 and 15 years of age (Livingston *et al.*, 1965; Charlton and Yahr, 1967) but may appear in some patients beyond 20 and 30 years of age (Oller-Daurella and Sanchez, 1981). Onset of tonic-clonic seizures was mainly 5 to 10 years after the onset of absences (Loiseau *et al.*, 1983), but the lag time can be shorter or longer. Absence seizures either persist or have disappeared for several years. Predisposing factors for tonic-clonic seizures are: (a) absence seizures occurring after 8 years of age. The later the onset of attacks, the more likely it is that the patient will develop convulsive seizures (Lennox and Lennox, 1960; Lees and Liversedge, 1962; Livingston *et al.*, 1965; Bergamini *et al.*, 1965; Charlton and Yahr, 1967; Oller-Daurella and Sanchez; 1981; Loiseau *et al.*, 1983); (b) sex: boys are more often affected than girls (Oller-Daurella and Sanchez, 1981); (c) response to initial treatment: when absence seizures disappear promptly, tonic-clonic seizures occur rarely (Currier *et al.*, 1963; Bergamini *et al.*, 1965; Gibberd, 1966; Oller-Daurella and Sanchez, 1981); (d) prescribed drugs. In absence seizures treated with an anti-absence and a major anti-epileptic drug, such as phenobarbital, 35.6 per cent of patients developed tonic-clonic seizures, whereas 86 per cent did so when treated with an anti-absence drug only (Livingston *et al.*, 1965). In patients treated early and correctly, tonic-clonic attacks appeared in 30 per cent of patients, and in 68 per cent if incorrectly treated (Bergamini *et al.*, 1965). Pure anti-absence drugs, such as oxazolidine-diones or ethosuximide do not prevent tonic-clonic seizures. Sodium valproate is an active drug both in absence and in tonic-clonic seizures. It is the first choice drug for childhood absence epilepsy; (e) in the EEG, abnormal background activity (Gibberd, 1966; Sato *et al.*, 1976) and a photosensitive response; conversely, when delta posterior rhythms are present, tonic-clonic seizures will seldom occur (Cobb *et al.*, 1961; Oller-Daurella and Sanchez, 1981; Loiseau *et al.*, 1983). No general agreement exists for many other clinical or EEG signs.

An evolution of absence seizures to psychomotor seizures has been described. It corresponds to erroneous diagnosis: prolonged absence attacks with automatisms may mimick complex partial seizures (Currier *et al.*, 1963; Sato *et al.*, 1976).

114

II. Social prognosis

Childhood absence epilepsy occurs mostly in neurologically and intellectually normal children (Lennox and Lennox, 1960; Currier *et al.,* 1963; Livingston *et al.,* 1965; Beaumanoir, 1976). This fact means that it is not due to brain damage. However it may occur in children with an idiopathic mental subnormality (they belong to the normal population). Patients' IQ, whatever are their initial abilities, often falls during evolution. Social adaptation of patients having had this illness is often poor, even if they are in remission (Hertoft, 1963; Pazzaglia *et al.,* 1969; Lugaresi *et al.,* 1973; Loiseau *et al.,* 1983). An impairment of intelligence may be produced by large dose of antiepileptic drugs (Beaumanoir, 1976). Behavioural problems may be a consequence of frequent attacks, of the parent's attitude and of therapy. One-third of patients appear to have such troubles (Loiseau *et al.,* 1983).

Diagnosis

Childhood absence epilepsy is an epileptic syndrome which has to be distinguished from a variety of conditions, most of them having been referred to as petit mal epilepsy. According to the above definition one must exclude:

1. *Absence seizure with a late onset.* Absence seizures may appear during adolescence and, very seldom, in adults. Attacks are less frequent and in most cases do not have the same EEG pattern. According to Janz' terminology (1969) they belong to a group of non-pyknoleptic absences, i.e., to adolescence absence epilepsy, which is another syndrome (chapter 27).

2. *Absence seizures occurring in brain-damaged children.* Acquired factors may precipitate absence seizures in patients with an age-related predisposition. Petit mal epilepsy (i.e. absence seizures) has been observed in fixed encephalopathies: congenital microcephaly, tuberous sclerosis, Sturge-Weber syndrome, craniosynostosis, neonatal hemorrhage, postencephalomyelitis (Holowach *et al.,* 1962), and operated *tumor cerebri* (Niedermeyer, 1965). Neurological (pyramidal or cerebellar) impairment and/or mental insufficiency are the consequences of these encephalopathies. This group accounts for 16 per cent (Lennox and Lennox, 1960) to 58 per cent (Dalby, 1969) of petit mal epilepsy. It can be concluded that about one-third of children presenting absence seizures do not have an idiopathic petit mal, i.e. a childhood absence epilepsy, but a symptomatic, i.e. a mixed, genetic and acquired, epilepsy, with a poorer prognosis.

The occurrence of absence seizures in patients with frontal lesions deserves special attention. Absence seizures concomitant with more or less regular bilateral spike-waves discharges may arise from frontal foci, located in the mesial cortex (Tükel and Jasper, 1952; Marossero and Bergamini, 1953; O'Brien *et al.,* 1959; Fegersten and Roger, 1961). These frontal foci may have a traumatic origin with medico-legal problems. At least for a time frontal epilepsies may give rise to absence seizures, either without special features or with some peculiarities: a focal motor component, asymmetrical ictal discharges or an interictal focus in the EEG (Fig. 3). When these peculiarities are lacking, it is very difficult to differentiate these frontal epilepsies from childhood absence epilepsy, except by stereo-electroencephalographic records (Bancaud and Talairach, 1965). Later partial motor and generalized tonic-clonic seizures will appear (Loiseau and Cohadon, 1971).

On very rare occasions absences are due to an evolutive encephalopathy: lipidosis (Andermann, 1967), brain tumors (Madsen and Bray, 1966; Loiseau and Cohadon, 1971).

3. *Other types of seizures prior to the onset of absence seizures.* Partial motor seizures,

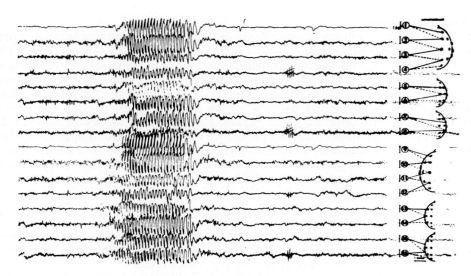

Fig. 3: Absence seizure with a focal onset. The regular at 3 c/s spike-wave discharge is preceded by a short burst of irregular spikes and slow waves recorded on the left fronto-temporal area.

but mostly generalized tonic-clonic seizures precede absence seizures in a certain number of children: 5 per cent of patients (Weir, 1965), 8.6 per cent (Gibberd, 1966), 14 per cent (Livingston *et al.,* 1965), 33 per cent (Lugaresi and Volterra, 1963). These patients do not have a childhood absence epilepsy but a more severe form of epilepsy, with a poorer prognosis: only 32 per cent of controlled cases (Dalby, 1969; Sato *et al.,* 1976).

4. *Myoclonic absences.* Absence seizures characterized clinically by rhythmic jerks of the proximal muscles of the upper limbs are a rather rare condition. They are usually associated with impaired mental development and are resistant to treatment (Tassinari *et al.,* 1969; Lugaresi *et al.,* 1973). They constitute a homogeneous group, different from childhood absence epilepsy (chapter 13).

5. *Absence seizures with unusual EEG patterns.* In patients with atypical absences and a secondary generalized epilepsy both ictal and interictal EEG abnormalities are very different from the ones recorded in childhood absence epilepsy.

More difficult to discard is the group of absence epilepsies called intermediate petit mal (Lugaresi *et al.,* 1973). Absence seizures are clinically similar to these of childhood absence epilepsy but they are associated with consistantly atypical spike-waves: irregularity of the rhythm, frequency lower than 3 or 2.5 c/s, asymmetry in the discharge. These EEG criteria are insufficient because of atypical ictal patterns in true childhood absence epilepsy. Other parameters are of diagnostic value: early age at onset, prevalence in male patients, brain-damage and mental deficiency, tonic-clonic seizures preceding absence seizures, and drug resistance. Errors remain possible.

Interictal focal abnormalities always cast a doubt on diagnosis. In the great majority of cases a diagnosis of childhood absence epilepsy must be discarded (Gordon, 1959). Some exceptions exist: an asymmetry of slow frequencies on background activity, very common in children, a transient asymmetry of ictal or interictal spike-waves, mainly noted in treated patients. Because of the known link existing between childhood absence epilepsy and benign epilepsy of childhood with centro-temporal (rolandic) focus, the existence of unilateral central spike-waves may be accepted (Fig. 4).

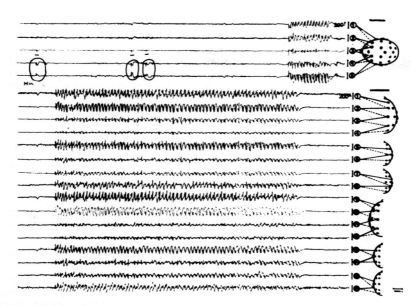

Fig. 4: Childhood absence epilepsy with absence seizures of various duration. Interictal spike-waves are recorded on the fronto-central left area.

Conclusion

Absence attacks are age-dependent epileptic seizures. Therefore they disappear spontaneously in most cases. This outcome explains why some authorities stated that pyknolepsy or petit mal were epilepsies with a good prognosis. A great deal of misunderstanding came in the past from the fact that all epilepsies with absence seizures were called petit mal. Absence seizures are only a type of epileptic seizures and do not constitute an epileptic syndrome. Conversely childhood absence epilepsy, a form of primary generalized epilepsy, is a real syndrome. An early prescription of anti-absence drugs - ethosuximide or sodium valproate - suppresses attacks in about 80 per cent of patients. The prognosis of the syndrome does not actually depend on the control of absence seizures. It depends on the further occurrence of tonic-clonic seizures, which occur in half the cases. Their prognosis is usually good, but the patients remain epileptic patients during an important part of their life, beyond childhood and adolescence. This chronicity is mainly responsible for interictal neuropsychological troubles. It has been proven that the quality of therapy is able to modify the evolution. With an early prescription of potent anti-epileptic drugs (such as sodium valproate controlling both absence and tonic-clonic seizures) childhood absence epilepsy could be a relatively benign form of epilepsy.

References

Adie, W.J. (1924): Pyknolepsy: a form of epilepsy occurring in children, with a good prognosis. *Brain* **47**, 96-102.

Andermann, F. (1967): Absence attacks and diffuse neuronal disease. *Neurology* **17**, 205-212.

Andermann, E., (1980): Genetic aspects of epilepsy. In *Epilepsy updated: causes and treatment* (ed. P. Robb). pp. 11-24. Year Book Medical Publishers: New York.

Bancaud J., Talairach J. (1965): *La stéréo-électro-encéphalographie dans l'épilepsie.* Masson, Paris.

Beaumanoir A. (1976): *Les épilepsies infantiles. Problèmes de diagnostic et de traitement.* Editions Roche: Bâle.

Bergamini L., Bram S., Broglia S., Alessandro R. (1965): L'insorgenza tardive di crisi Grande Male nel Piccolo Male puro. Studio catammestico di 78 casi. *Arch. Suisses Neurol. Neurochir. Psychiat.*, **96**, 306-317.

Browne T.R., Feldman R.L. (1983): Absence (petit mal) seizures. In *Epilepsy, diagnosis and management.* pp51-74. eds T.R. Browne, R.G. Feldman. Little, Brown and Company. Boston.

Bureau M., Guey J., Dravet C., Roger J. (1968): Etude de la répartition des absences Petit Mal chez l'enfant en fonction de ses activités. *Rev. Neurol.* **118**, 493-494.

Cavazzuti G.B. (1980): Epidemiology of different types of epilepsy in school-age children of Modena, Italy. *Epilepsia* **21**, 57-62.

Calmeil L.F. (1824): De l'épilepsie étudiée sous le rapport de son siège et de son influence sur la production de l'aliénation mentale. Thèse: Paris.

Charlton M.H., Yahr M.D. (1967): Long term follow-up of patients with petit mal. *Archs Neurol.* **16**, 595-598.

Cobb W.A., Gordon N., Matthews C., Nieman E.A. (1961): The occipital delta rhythm in petit mal. *Electroenceph. Clin. Neurophysiol.* **13**, 142-143.

Commission on classification and terminology of the International League against Epilepsy. Proposal for revised clinical and electroencephalographic classification of epileptic seizures. (1981): *Epilepsia* **22**, 489-501.

Currier R.D., Kooi K.A., Saidman L.J. (1963): Prognosis of pure petit mal. A follow-up study. *Neurology* **13**, 959-967.

Dalby M.A. (1969): Epilepsy and 3 per second spike and wave rhythms. A clinical, electro-encephalographic and prognostic analysis of 346 patients. *Acta Neurol. Scand.* **45**, suppl. 40.

Doose H., Gerken H., Horstmann T., Völzke, E. (1973): Genetic factors in spike-wave absences. *Epilepsia* **14**, 57-75.

Dreifuss F.E. (1972): The prognosis of petit mal epilepsy. In *The epidemiology of epilepsies: a workshop* (ed. M. Alter, W.A. Hauser). NINDS Monograph no. 14, pp. 129-132. Washington.

Esquirol J. (1838): De l'épilepsie. In *Traité des maladies mentales,* Tome 1, pp, 274-335. Baillière Publ.: Paris.

Fegersten L., Roger A. (1961): Frontal epileptogenic foci and their clinical correlations. *Electroencephal. Clin. Neurophysiol.* **13**, 905-913.

Friedmann M. (1906): Über die nichtepileptischen Absencen oder kurzen narkoleptischen Anfälle. *Dtsch. Z. Nervenheilk.* **30**, 462-492.

Gedda L., Tatarelli R. (1971): Essential isochronic epilepsy in MZ twin pairs. *Acta Genet. Med.* **20**, 380-383.

Gibberd F.B. (1966): The prognosis of petit mal. *Brain* **89**, 531-538.

Gibbs F.A., Davis H., Lennox W.G. (1935): The EEG in epilepsy and in conditions of impaired consciousness. *Archs Neurol. Psychiat.* **34**, 1134-1148.

Gibbs F.A., Gibbs E.L., Lennox W.G. (1943): Electroencephalographic classification of epileptic patients and control subjects *Archs Neurol. Psychiat.* **50**, 111-128.

Gordon N. (1959): Petit mal Epilepsy and cortical epileptogenic foci. *Electroenceph. Clin. Neurophysiol.* **11**, 151-153.

Gowers W.R. (1881): *Epilepsy and other chronic convulsive diseases: their causes, symptoms and treatment.* J.A. Churchill: London.

Hauser W.A., Kurland L.T. (1975): The epidemiology of epilepsy in Rochester, Minnesota, 1935 through 1967. *Epilepsia* **16**, 1-66.

Hertoft P. (1963): The clinical electroencephalographic and social prognosis in petit mal epilepsy. *Epilepsia* **4**, 298-314.

Holowach J., Thurston D.L., O'Leary J.L. (1962): Petit mal epilepsy. *Pediatrics* **30**, 893-901.

Ingvar D.H., Nyman E.G. (1962): Epilepsia arithmetices. *Neurology* **12**, 282.

Janz D. (1955): Die klinische Stellung der Pyknolepsie. *Dtsch. Med. Wschr.* **80** 1392-1400.

Janz D. (1969): *Die Epilepsien.* G. Thieme Verlag: Stuttgart.

Jasper, H. (1949): Anatomo-physiological study of epilepsies. *Electroenceph. Clin. Neurophysiol.* Suppl. **2**, 123-131.

Jus A., Jus K. (1962): Retrograde amnesia in petit mal. *Archs Gen. Psychiat.* **6**, 163-167.

Lees F., Liversedge L.A. (1962): The prognosis of petit mal and minor epilepsy. *Lancet* **2**, 797-799.

Lennox W.G. (1945): The petit mal epilepsies. *J. Am. Med. Ass.* **129**, 1069-1073.

Lennox W.G. (1951): Heredity of epilepsy as told by relatives and twins. *J. Am. Med. Ass.* **146**, 529-536.

Lennox W.G., Davis J.P. (1950): Clinical correlates of the fast and slow spike-wave electroencephalogram. *Pediatrics* **5**, 626-644.

Lennox W.G., Lennox M.A. (1960): *Epilepsy and related disorders.* Vol. I. Little, Brown and Co: Boston.

Livingston S., Torres I., Pauli L.L., Rider R.V. (1965): Petit mal epilepsy. Results of a prolonged follow-up study of 117 patients. *J. Am. Med. Ass.* **194**, 113-118.

Loiseau P., Cohadon F., Cohadon S. (1966): Le petit mal, qui guérit, guérit rapidement. *J. Méd. Lyon* **1108**, 1557-1565.

Loiseau P., Cohadon F. (1971): *Le petit mal et ses frontières.* Masson: Paris.

Loiseau P., Pestre M., Dartigues J.F., Commenges D., Barbeger-Gateau C., Cohadon S. (1983): Long-term prognosis in two forms of childhood epilepsy: typical absence seizures and epilepsy with rolandic (centrotemporal) EEG foci. *Ann. Neurol.* **13**, 642-648.

Lugaresi E., Pazzaglia P., Franck L., Roger J., Bureau-Paillas M., Ambrosetto G., Tassinari C.A. (1973): Evolution and prognosis of primary generalized epilepsy of the petit mal absence type (eds. Lugaresi E., Pazzaglia P., Tassinari C.A.). In *Evolution and prognosis of epilepsy,* pp 2-22 Aulo Gaggi: Bologna.

Lugaresi E., Volterra V. (1963): Considerazioni cliniche ed EEG sull'assenza Piccolo Male. *Clin. Paediat. (Bologne)* **45**, 3-18.

Madsen J.A., Bray P.F. (1966): The coincidence of diffuse electroencephalographic spike-wave paroxysms and brain tumours. *Neurology* **16**, 546-555.

Marossero F., Bergamini V. (1953): EEG records with bursts of spike and wave typical and atypical with evidence of lateralisation. Clinical and EEG correlations. *Electroenceph. Clin. Neurophysiol.* **5**, 618.

Metrakos J.D., Metrakos K. (1972): Genetic factors in the epilepsies. In *The epidemiology of epilepsy: a workshop* (eds. Alter R., Hauser W.A.). NINDS Monograph, no. 14, pp.97-102. US Government Printing Office: Washington D.C.

Niedermeyer E. (1965): Sleep EEG in petit mal. *Archs Neurol.* **12**, 625-630.

O'Brien J.L., Goldensohn E.S., Hoefer P.F. (1959): Electroencephalographic abnormalities in addition to bilaterally synchronous 3 per second spike and wave activity in petit mal. *Electroenceph. Clin. Neurophysiol.* **11**, 747-761.

Oller-Daurella L., Sanchez M.E. (1981): Evolucion de las ausencias tipicas. *Rev. Neurol. (Barcelone)* **9**, 81-102.

Ounsted C., Hutt J.J, Lee D. (1963): The retrograde amnesia of petit mal. *Lancet* **1**, 671.

Pazzaglia P., Franck L., Orioli G., Lugaresi E. (1969): L'evoluzione elettro-clinica del piccolo male tipico. *Riv. Neurol.* **39**, 557-566.

Penry J.K. (1973): Behavioural correlates of generalized spike-wave discharge in the electroencephalogram. In *Epilepsy, its phenomena in man,* UCLA Forum in Medical Sciences, number 17, pp.171-188. Academic Press, Inc.: New York.

Penry J.K., Porter R.J, Dreifuss F.E. (1975): Simultaneous recording of absence seizures with video tape and electroencephalography. A study of 374 seizures in 48 patients. *Brain* **98**, 427-440.

Petsche H. (1962): Pathophysiologie und Klinik des Petit Mal. Toposkopische Untersuchungen zur Phänomenologie des Spike-Wave-Musters. *Wien. Z. Nervenheilk* **19**, 345-352.

Reynolds J.R. (1861): *Epilepsy, its symptoms, treatment.* Churchill, London.

Sato S., Dreifuss F.E., Penry J.K. (1973): The effect of sleep on spike-wave discharges in absences seizures. *Neurology* **23**, 1335-1345.

Sato S., Dreifuss F.E., Penry J.K. (1976): Prognostic factors in absence seizures. *Neurology* **26**, 788-796.

Sauer H. (1916): Über gehäufte kleine Anfälle bei Kindern (Pyknolepsie). *Mschr. Psychiat. Neurol.* **40**, 276-300.

Schwab R.S. (1947): Reaction time in petit mal epilepsy. *Ass. Res. Nerv. Ment. Dis. Proc.* **26**, 339-341.

Subirana A., Oller-Daurella L. (1953): Contribution to certain clinical and electroencephalographic aspects of petit mal. Third Intern. Congress of EEG and clinical neurophysiology, *Electroenceph. Clin. Neurophysiol.,* suppl. **3, 83.**

Tassinari C.A., Lyagoubi S., Santos V., Gambarelli G., Roger J., Dravet C., Gastaut H. (1969): Etude des décharges de pointe-ondes chez l'homme. II: Les aspects cliniques et électroencéphalographiques des absences myocloniques. *Rev. Neurol.* **121,** 379-383.

Tissot S.A. (1770): *Traité de l'épilepsie, faisant le Tome Troisième du traité des nerfs et de leurs maladies.* Paris.

Tükel K., Jasper H. (1952): The EEG in parasagittal lesions. *Electroenceph. Clin. Neurophysiol.* **4,** 481-494.

Weir B. (1965): The morphology of the spike-wave complex. *Electroenceph. Clin. Neurophysiol.* **19,** 284-290.

*   *   *

Discussion pages 237-241

Epileptic syndromes in infancy, childhood and adolescence. J. Roger, C. Dravet, M. Bureau, F.E. Dreifuss and P. Wolf. John Libbey Eurotext Ltd ©1985.

Chapter 13
Epilepsy with Myoclonic Absences

Carlo Alberto TASSINARI* and Michelle BUREAU‡

*Clinique Neurologique, Via Ugo Foscolo 7, Bologne, Italy and ‡Centre Saint-Paul, 300 Boulevard Sainte-Marguerite, 13009 - Marseille, France

Summary

Epilepsy with myoclonic absences is characterized clinically by absences accompanied by severe bilateral rhythmical myoclonias, often associated with a tonic contraction. On the EEG they are always accompanied by bilateral, synchronous and symmetrical discharge of rhythmical SW at 3 c/s similar to that observed in the childhood absence epilepsy. These seizures occur many times a day. Associated seizures are rare. The age of onset is about 7 years. There is a male preponderance. The evolution has a poor prognosis because of the unresponsiveness of the seizures to therapy, mental deterioration and the possible evolution into a secondary generalized epilepsy similar to Lennox-Gastaut syndrome. The myoclonic absences seem to be a type of intermediary epilepsy between primary generalized epilepsy and secondary generalized epilepsy.

Definition of the seizures: Myoclonic absences (MA) are absence seizures clinically characterized by rhythmical bilateral diffuse myoclonias of severe intensity, accompanied on the EEG by bilateral, synchronous and symmetrical spike and wave discharges repeated at 3 c/s (as usually observed in absences of childhood absence epilepsy).

Definition of epilepsy with myoclonic absences: It is a childhood epilepsy characterized by the recurrence of myoclonic absences which constitute the only or the preponderant seizure type through the evolution of the epilepsy.

Historical review: Absence seizures have been known for a long time (the historical review is found in the chapters on childhood and juvenile absence epilepsy). The 1970 and 1981 seizures classification proposed by the International League Against Epilepsy does not refer to MA; these classifications refer only to generalized absences with mild clonic components indicated by an occasional slight twitching of the eyelids or face. The myoclonias of MA are on the contrary severe and diffuse.

Material

Although several studies in the literature mention MA (Gibberd, 1966; Tassinari *et al.*, 1969; Aicardi and Chevrie, 1971; Loiseau and Cohadon, 1971; Lugaresi *et al.*, 1973;

Loiseau *et al.,* 1974; Jeavons, 1977; Giovanardi-Rossi *et al.,* 1979) none of them contains detailed observations of these absences. Consequently our description is based on observations of 28 patients from the Centre Saint-Paul, (some of whom have been previously described: Tassinari *et al.,* 1969; Lugaresi *et al.,* 1973).

General

(1) Incidence: MA seem to constitute a very rare seizure type, 0.5 to 1 per cent of epilepsies observed in the selected population of epileptics of the Centre Saint-Paul.

(2) Sex ratio: There is a male preponderance (65 per cent) — at variance with the female preponderance in childhood absence epilepsy.

(3) Etiological factors are of the same nature and frequency as in childhood absence epilepsy.

(4) Genetic factors: a family history of epilepsy is found in 25 per cent of the cases; no evidence of febrile convulsions in the family.

(5) Age of onset: mean 7 yrs (range from 2 to 12.5 years).

(6) Mental retardation was present before the onset of epilepsy in 13 of the 28 cases.

Characteristics of myoclonic absences

(1) Duration of the MA ranges from 10 to 60 seconds (longer than usually observed in childhood absence epilepsy).

(2) Frequency is usually very high (several daily seizures), as in childhood absence epilepsy.

(3) Onset and end of MA are abrupt without any warning.

(4) Clinical symptomatology

(a) Consciousness impairment is of variable degree (although it was not systematically studied in our patients). From direct clinical observation and from anamnestic recall of the patients we found that there can be either a complete loss of consciousness or a simple disruption of consciousness: for example, the myoclonias, at times, are felt as a very disturbing experience; and the subject frequently holds himself, giving the impression of attempting to control the intensity of the jerking.

(b) The motor manifestations: The myoclonias constitute the constant characteristic feature, while a tonic contraction is often associated.

The clinical motor manifestations at times give a complex, albeit constant and recognizable pattern. The myoclonic movements mainly involve the muscles of shoulders, arms and legs. The muscles of the face are less frequently involved; when facial myoclonias occur they are more evident around the chin and the mouth.

The patient shows a rhythmic and striking jerking of the shoulders, head and arms, staggering (rarely falling) if he is standing. Head and body deviation (without concomitant ocular or oculoclonic deviation) can be a present feature in some patients.

In some cases slight automatic movements were observed.

(c) Autonomic manifestations: an arrest or change of respiratory movement (in relation either with the myoclonias and the tonic contraction or with the impairment of consciousness) was observed during MA. In six patients the MA could be accompanied by urine loss.

(5) EEG and polygraphic symptomatology:
The ictal EEG is a rhythmic spike and wave (SW) discharge at 3 c/s, bilateral, synchro-

nous and symmetrical, the same as those observed in the absences of childhood absence epilepsy, (vide infra for detailed analysis of the discharge). Polygraphic recording allows a better definition of the relationships between the ictal discharge on the EEG and the EMG recording of various muscles. Analysis of the ictal events with high speed records (oscilloscope and ink jet recording) shows the following concerning (a) the myoclonias and the SW and (b) the tonic component.

(a) There is a strict and constant relation between the spike onset of the SW discharge and the myoclonia. The detailed morphology of the spike is somewhat peculiar since it is a positive transient (Weir, 1965) of high amplitude, in strict relationship with the appearance, latency and amplitude of the myoclonias (Tassinari et al., 1969). At times, the SWs in the first second of the beginning of the discharge are of smaller amplitude (because the early positive component of the spike is of small amplitude) and are not accompanied by myoclonias (Fig. 1).

(b) A tonic contraction which appears after the first myoclonias and which increases progressively is frequently (but not constantly) observed (Figs. 1 and 2).

This tonic contraction is maximal on shoulder and deltoid muscles and it is responsible for the arm-elevation. The tonic contraction can mask and render clinically less evident the myoclonias and then, the motor manifestations are more complex. The EMG recording shows a sequence of the following events: each spike on the EEG is followed on the EMG by a myoclonia with a latency of 15 to 40 ms for the more proximal muscles and up to 50 to 70 ms for the more distal muscles; this myoclonia is itself followed by a brief silent period (60 to 120 ms) which breaks the tonic contraction (Tassinari et al., 1971).

The tonic contraction, as the myoclonias, can be asymmetrical (Fig. 3) this being responsible for versive lateral or antero-posterior motions of the head and body.

(6) Myoclonic absences and sleep:
The MA can occur during stage I of sleep, awakening the subject (Fig. 3). During stage II the SWs are less regular in frequency, occurring in bursts either of the same duration as the awake state (Fig. 3) or briefer (2-3 s). Bursts of myoclonias can be in relation with these discharges. With slow sleep the SW discharges are exceptionally accompanied by myoclonias. During sleep the evolution of the interictal SW discharges is similar on the whole to that observed in childhood absence epilepsy (Tassinari et al., 1974).

During sleep no other ictal discharges were observed and particularly no discharges of 10 c/s fast rhythmic activity (as observed in the 'tonic' seizures in the Lennox-Gastaut syndrome).

(7) Precipitating factors:
MA were provoked by hyperventilation in 19 cases; ILS facilitated MA in 13 cases. Awakening was also a facilitating factor in 13 cases.

Other seizures than myoclonic absences

In 12 patients, MA were the only seizures through the evolution. In 16 patients other seizures occurred.

(1) Seizures before the onset or the diagnosis of MA:
These were found in six cases. In one case there was history of tonic-clonic seizures. In the other five cases, some convulsive seizures and absences were mentioned. It was difficult however to ascertain whether they were not in fact MA in which either the 'absence' was overlooked (allowing the diagnosis of convulsive, usually clonic,

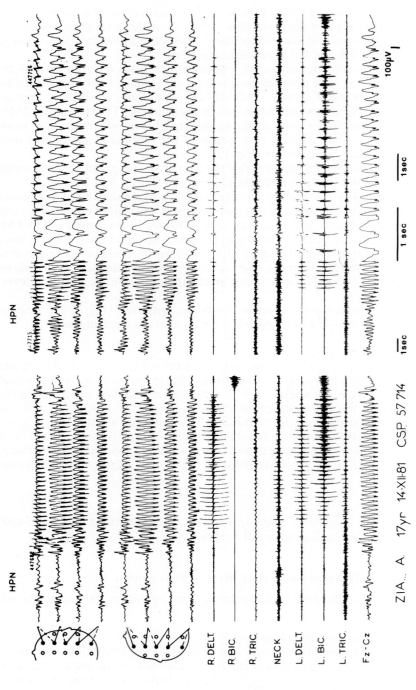

Fig. 1. Myoclonic absences elicited by hyperventilation. *On the left:* MA characterized by a 3 c/s spike and waves discharge. Note that the rhythmic jerks (recorded on the right and left deltoid, biceps and triceps muscles and on the neck) appear 1–2 s after the onset of the SW discharge and that the tonic contraction appears 3–4 s later. *On the right:* a variable speed record of an other MA. Note the left preponderance of motor manifestation.

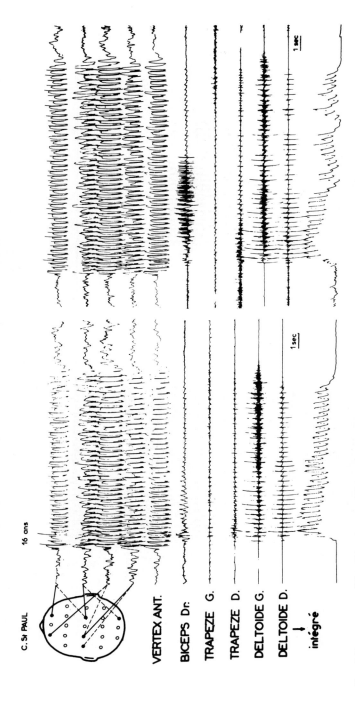

Fig. 2. Spontaneous MA. Rhythmical SW discharge at 3 c/s. Rhythmical myoclonias are progressively associated with a tonic contraction.

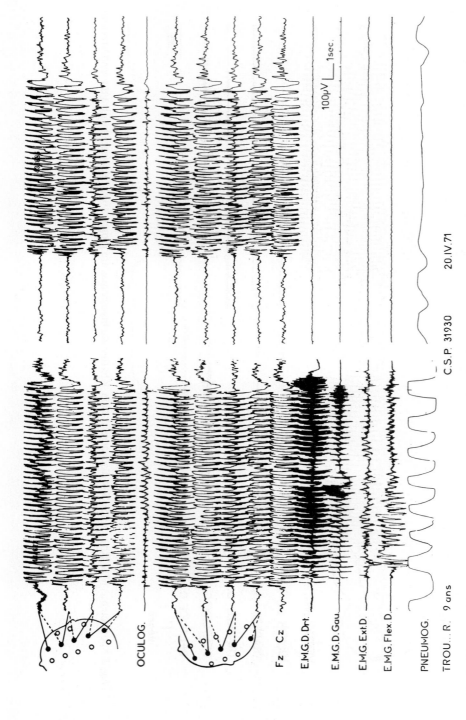

Fig. 3. On the left: MA occurring at drowsiness, awaking the patient. Note the asymmetry of the myoclonias and the tonic contraction on the left and right deltoïd muscles. *On the right:* Sleep stage II, more irregular SW bursts, not accompanied by myoclonias. Note the apnea.

126

seizures) or the motor manifestations were not considered (allowing the diagnosis of absence seizure). In no case was there a history of febrile convulsions.

(2) Seizures associated with MA

(a) Tonic-clonic seizures: six patients had a single (one case) or repeated (rare <1per year) tonic-clonic seizures. In two of these cases tonic-clonic seizures persisted after the end of MA.

(b) Absences without severe myoclonias were mentioned in the history of six cases; in our patients however, we never recorded absences without myoclonias.

(c) Status: one of our patients has presented a status with diffuse SWs and rhythmic myoclonias interrupted after 20 min by an IV injection of diazepam. Another case has had a prolonged status with SWs on the EEG but without myoclonias. Two other cases have had at times MA repeated at close intervals (1 min).

Evolution

Seizures

MA were still present after 10 years of evolution in 16 cases; in 12 cases the seizures have persisted for a mean duration of four years, then disappeared (mean follow-up after the disappearance of MA is 4.5 years).

The presence or absence of tonic-clonic seizures does not apparently affect the evolution of MA. Tonic seizures and atypical absences occurred in five cases after the end of MA.

Epilepsy

Generally, one can say that the evolution of epilepsy in 23 observations was mainly related to the evolution of MA *(vide supra)*. In five cases however there was a particular evolution of the epilepsy, characterized by the disappearance of MA while other seizures appeared, namely absences with atypical slow SWs, clinical and subclinical 'tonic' seizures. In these cases, the interictal EEG abnormalities consisted of slow SWs. These features suggested that the epilepsy was evolving toward a secondary generalized epilepsy similar to the Lennox-Gastaut syndrome.

Intellectual evolution

We have already pointed out that 13 patients had intellectual impairment before or at the time of the onset of MA. The 15 others patients were of normal intelligence prior to the onset of MA. Eight of them were still normal throughout the evolution (MA still present — five cases; or not — three cases).

The other seven who were normal at the onset showed significant mental deterioration through the evolution with MA still persisting (five cases) or not (two cases). Overall, either because of mental retardation before MA (13 cases) or because mental impairment appeared during the evolution (seven cases) we have a total of 20 out of 28 patients with mental deficiency. These data constitute a very significant difference as compared with mental status observed in childhood absence epilepsy.

Treatment

In our cases we can say that all antiepileptic drugs were used in the attempt to control the MA. Frequent MA persisted in 16 cases despite the treatment. Ten patients were treated with a combination of valproate and ethosuximide. In seven cases MA were controlled by this treatment; in three other cases MA persisted. This combined treatment seems the most effective one (Jeavons *et al.,* 1977).

127

Diones and benzodiazepines in association with valproate were effective in few cases. It was difficult to ascertain however, if the treatment was effective or if the MA ended independently.

Diagnosis

MA should not be confused with myoclonias of benign myoclonic epilepsy of childhood and adolescence, because in this type of epilepsy myoclonic jerks do not occur in rhythmic clusters, they are accompanied by polyspike discharges and not by rhythmic SWs at 3 c/s, and there is no strict relation between myoclonia and cerebral discharge.

Diagnosis of MA based only on the anamnestic description can be extremely difficult: (a) the motor manifestations, namely the rhythmic myoclonic movements, can be overlooked, particularly when there is a tonic contraction associated with myoclonias; (b) during the evolution and possibly under the effect of treatment the myoclonias can be of reduced intensity (c) when the motor manifestations (myoclonias and tonic contraction) are asymmetrical (with head and body turning) or predominant on one side, the MA seizures can be misdiagnosed as partial seizures and (d) at times, the motor pattern can be rendered more complex by the occurrence of automatisms during the absence. For these reasons, in some instances, the MA are extremely difficult to diagnose even when seizures are directly observed or reviewed on video tape.

On the other hand, the ictal EEG recording of the seizures alone does not allow the diagnosis of MA (indeed the diagnostic conclusion is: 'absence with 3 c/s typical SWs').

The polygraphic recording (EEG + EMG of various muscles, particularly the deltoïd muscles bilaterally) can be (as it was in some of our cases) the only way to obtain the correct positive diagnosis of MA. In this respect, we strongly suggest that in any case of 'absences' with concomitant 3 c/s SW which is resistant to correct treatment, the possibility of diagnosing MA should be considered. A specific and polygraphic recording should be made in search of the features of MA.

Conclusion

Is it justified from a particular type of seizures (MA) to propose the individualization of a particular type of childhood epilepsy? We think so for the following reasons:

— the very remarkable electroclinical aspect of the MA.
— the characteristics associated with MA are different from those of childhood absence epilepsy: male preponderance, frequency of associated mental retardation or consecutive deficit, resistance to treatment, non-exceptional evolution (18 per cent of the cases) toward an epilepsy similar to a secondary generalised epilepsy.
— the individuality of MA as for other epilepsies with myoclonias has been pointed out by the taxonomic study of Loiseau (Loiseau *et al.,* 1972, 1974).
— the MA seem to be an intermediary type of epilepsy between primary generalized epilepsy and secondary generalized epilepsy.

References

Aicardi, J., Chevrie J.J. (1971): Myoclonic epilepsies of childhood. *Neuropädiatrie* 3, 177-190.
Commission on Classification and Terminology of the International League against Epilepsy. (1981): Proposal for revised clinical and electroencephalographic classification. *Epilepsia* **22,** 489-501.

Gastaut, H. (1970): Clinical and electroencephalographic classification of epileptic seizures. *Epilepsia* 11, 102-113.

Gibberd, F.B. (1966): The clinical features of Petit Mal. *Acta Neurol. Scand.* 42, 176-190.

Giovanardi Rossi, P., Pazzaglia, P., Cirignotta, F., Moschen, R., Lugaresi, E. (1979): Le epilessie miocloniche nell'infanzia. *Riv. Ital. EEG Neurofisiol.* 2, 321-328.

Jeavons, P.M. (1977): Nosological problems of myoclonic epilepsies in childhood and adolescence. *Develop. Med. Child. Neurol.* 19, 3-8.

Jeavons, P.M., Clark, J.E., Maheshwari, M.C. (1977): Treatment of generalized epilepsies of childhood and adolescence with sodium valproate ('Epilim'). *Develop. Med. Child Neurol.* 19, 9-25.

Loiseau, P., Cohadon, F. (1971): *Le Petit Mal et ses frontières*. Masson: Paris

Loiseau, P., Legroux, M., Grimont, P., Henry, P., du Pasquier, P. (1972): Application de la taxonomie numérique au classement des myoclonies épileptiques, *Rev. Neurol.* 127, 587-596.

Loiseau, P., Legroux, M., Grimont, P., du Pasquier, P., Henry, P. (1974): Taxometric classification of myoclonic epilepsies. *Epilepsia* 15, 1-11.

Lugaresi, E., Pazzaglia, P., Franck, L., Roger, J., Bureau-Paillas, M., Ambrosetto, G., Tassinari, C.A. (1973): Evolution and prognosis of primary generalized epilepsies of the Petit Mal absence type. In *Evolution and prognosis of epilepsy,* ed E. Lugaresi, P. Pazzaglia, C.A. Tassinari, pp 2-22. Aulo Gaggi: Bologna.

Tassinari, C.A., Lyagoubi, S., Santos, V., Gambarelli, F., Roger, J., Dravet, C., Gastaut, H. (1969): Etude des décharges de pointes ondes chez l'homme, II-Les aspects cliniques et électroencéphalographiques des absences myocloniques. *Rev. Neurol.* 121, 379-383.

Tassinari, C.A., Lyagoubi, S., Gambarelli, F., Roger, J., Gastaut, H. (1971): Relationships between EEG discharge and neuromuscular phenomena. *Electroenceph. Clin. Neurophysiol.* 31, 176.

Tassinari, C., Bureau-Paillas, M., Dalla Bernardina, B., Mancia, D., Capizzi, G., Dravet, C., Valladier, C., Roger, J. (1974): Generalized epilepsies and seizures during sleep. A polygraphic study. In *Brain and sleep,* ed H.M. Van Praag, H. Meinardi pp 154-166. De Erven Bohn: B.V. Amsterdam.

Weir, B. (1965): The morphology of the spike-wave complex. *Electroenceph. Clin. Neurophysiol.* 19, 284-290.

*   *   *

Discussion pages 237-241

Epileptic syndromes in infancy, child-
hood and adolescence. J. Roger,
C. Dravet, M. Bureau, F.E.
Dreifuss and P. Wolf. John Libbey
Eurotext Ltd ©1985.

Chapter 14
Epilepsy with Generalized Convulsive Seizures in Childhood

Luis OLLER-DAURELLA

Escuelas Pias, 89, Barcelona, 17, Spain

Summary

Epilepsy with generalized convulsive seizures having all the characteristics of primary generalized epilepsy rarely appears in children (92 of 310 cases). Grand mal seizures rarely occur in
isolation; they are more often associated with absences (48 of 92). If a child suffers from grand
mal *alone,* prognosis is excellent (93 per cent were well controlled by treatment). Prognosis is
less favourable when they are associated with absences.

From our data bank containing information on 3000 epileptics, we conducted a study
on all cases of generalized tonic-clonic seizures without local onset (grand mal
seizures) in children aged between 3 and 11 years (Oller-Daurella and Oller Ferrer-
Vidal, 1978-1981).

Using the criteria given below, we found a total of 310 cases of primary generalized
epilepsy of the grand mal type including: 169 cases of pure grand mal epilepsy; 119
cases of grand mal seizures associated with absence seizures and 22 cases of grand mal
seizures associated with myoclonus.

In 92 of the 310 cases, grand mal seizures had begun between the ages of 3 and 11
years: of these 92 patients, 40 presented pure grand mal epilepsy, 48 presented grand
mal seizures associated with absence seizures and four presented grand mal seizures
associated with myoclonus.

There was an equal number of boys and girls.

We excluded from the study those cases where epilepsy had begun with absence
seizures, since we consider that they should be studied as part of childhood epilepsy of
the absence type.

We adopted the *criteria for inclusion* proposed in the International Classification for
primary generalized epilepsies of the grand mal type (Merlis, 1970; Niedermeyer,
1972; Gastaut, 1973). We included only tonic-clonic seizures, generalized from the
beginning, with initial loss of consciousness and without any initial focal clinical or
EEG manifestations. Contrary to other proposals for classification, we therefore eliminated secondarily generalized tonic-clonic seizures (secondary grand mal: Janz, 1969;
Wolf, 1979). The focal onset of the seizure can only be identified if the seizure has

Table 1. Grand mal syndrome (3 to 11 yr). Age at onset.

Grand mal ($n = 169$)		*(%)*
Before 3 yr	19 cases	11.2
From 3 to 11 yr	40 cases	23.7
After 11 yr	110 cases	65.1
Grand mal with absences ($n = 119$)		
Before 3 yr	11 cases	9.2
From 3 to 11 yr	48 cases	40.3
After 11 yr	60 cases	50.4

been recorded (Fig. 1). Abnormalities on the interictal EEG were restricted to generalized, bilateral and synchronous discharges of spike-waves or polyspike-waves, with a normal background rhythm.

In general, there were no apparent lesions, nor permanent neurological disorders. Slight intellectual deficiency existed in a few cases.

Results

We can see from Table 1 that only 23 per cent of primary generalized epilepsies of the pure grand mal type begin during childhood, and that 40 per cent of grand mal seizures associated with absence seizures begin at this age. It is our opinion that a certain number of cases are wrongly classed with the pure grand mal group, since the absence seizures may be of very short duration and detected only be EEG examination revealing short discharges or bilateral synchronous spike-waves accompanied by a very brief impairment of consciousness. To demonstrate this, we used hyperventilation: simultaneous recording of the EEG and respiration showed that many children stopped hyperventilation during the brief spike-wave discharges, and that we are therefore dealing with true absence seizures (Figs 2 and 3). Another possibility, referred to by Janz, is that the absences are grouped into the period immediately preceding a grand mal seizure (Fig. 4).

We made a comparison, based on a number of factors, between cases of pure grand mal and cases of grand mal seizures associated with absence seizures. There were no permanent neurological disorders in either group. Mental deficiency was rarely observed and was always slight. We found no obvious acquired etiological factor. Genetic factors were identified in 25 per cent of cases; the proportion was identical for the two groups.

We concentrated essentially on factors of prognosis in the 71 cases where the follow-up study was continued over a sufficiently long period (Table 2).

Table 2. Grand mal syndrome (3 to 11 yr). Prognosis (followed cases = 71), percentages in parentheses

	Good prognosis (Without seizures for > 1 yr)	Bad prognosis (Uncontrolled seizures)
1. Seizures		
Grand mal ($n = 31$)	29 (93.6)	2 (6.4)
Grand mal with absences ($n = 40$)	26 (65)	14 (35)
2. Mental evolution		*Deterioration*
Grand mal ($n = 31$)		1 (3.2)
Grand mal with absences ($n = 40$)		7 (17.5)

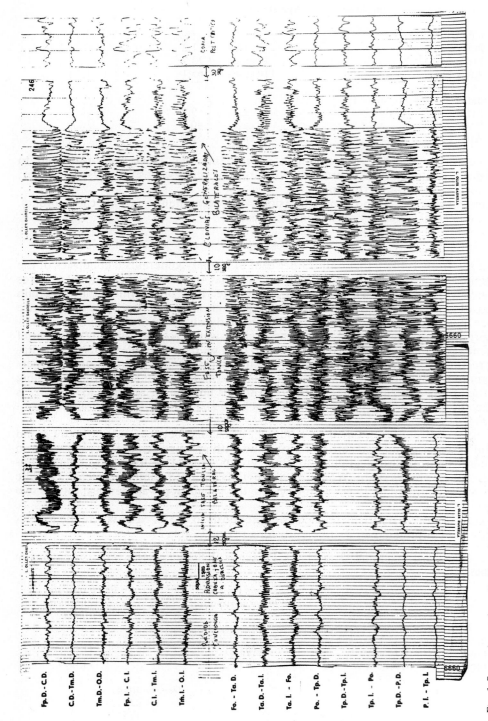

Fig. 1. Secondary generalized tonic-clonic seizure: before and at the end of the seizure, we observe a discharge of rhythmic spikes in the left temporal region. During the seizure, we can see the tonic and the clonic phases which coincide with a discharge or rapid rhythms and spike-waves, apparently bilateral and synchronous.

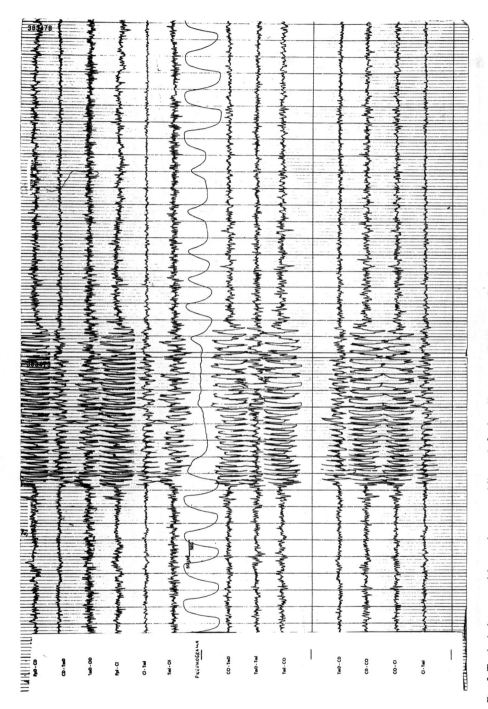

Fig. 2. Typical absence with synchronous, bilateral, 3 c/s spike-wave discharges. On the pneumogram, we can see that the patient stops hyperventilation because he forgets the instructions he has been given as a result of a disturbance in consciousness.

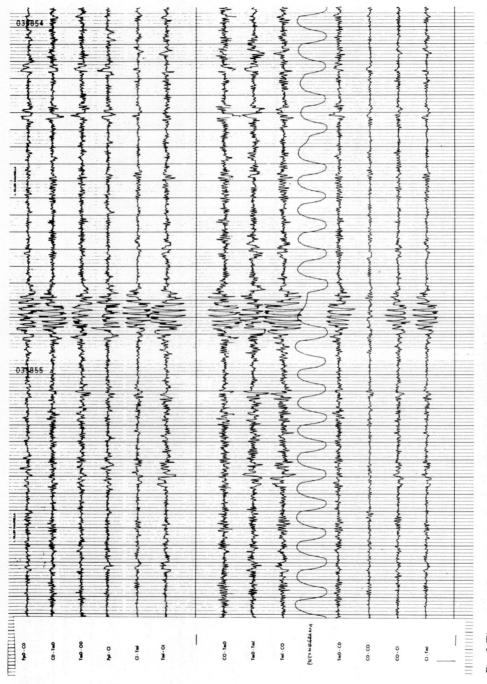

Fig. 3. The same phenomenon observed during a shorter discharge, lasting 2 s.

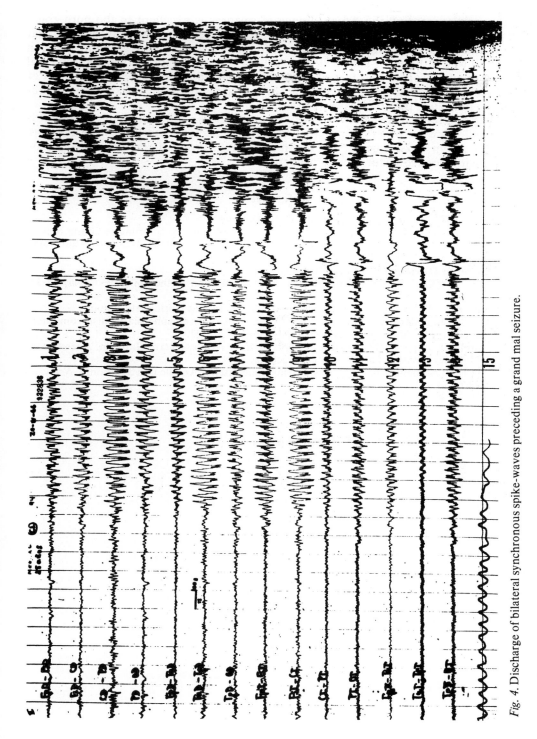

Fig. 4. Discharge of bilateral synchronous spike-waves preceding a grand mal seizure.

Prognosis concerning the disappearance of seizures is excellent in the pure grand mal group: 29 of the 31 cases (93.6 per cent) had been seizure-free for at least one year at the time of the final check-up. Prognosis for epilepsy of the pure grand mal type in childhood would therefore appear to be excellent, better than prognosis for grand mal epilepsy in adolescence. This fact was already mentioned by Gastaut *et al.* (1973). For grand mal seizures associated with absence seizures, disappearance of seizures was observed in only 26 of the 40 cases (65 per cent).

Similar differences exist between the two groups when intellectual development is concerned, since we observed only one case of intellectual deterioration in the pure grand mal group (3.2 per cent), and seven cases in the group of grand mal seizures associated with absence seizures (17.5 per cent).

References

Gastaut, H. (1973): *Dictionnaire de l'épilepsie.* OMS: Genève.
Gastaut, H., Gastaut, J.A., Gastaut, J.L. (1973): Epilepsie généralisée primaire Grand Mal. In *Evolution and prognosis of epilepsies,* pp 25-41, ed Lugaresi, Pazzagilia, Tassinari. Aulo Gaggi: Bologna.
Janz, D. (1969): *Die epilepsien.* Thieme: Stuttgart.
Merlis, J.K. (1970): Proposal for an international classification of the epilepsies. *Epilepsia* **11**: 114-119.
Niedermeyer, E. (1972): *The generalized epilepsies,* Ch. C. Thomas: Springfield, Illinois.
Oller-Daurella, L., Oller Ferrer-Vidal, L. (1978): Banco de datos de epilepsia: analisis computerizado de 3000 enfermos epilépticos. *Bol. Lega It. Epil.* **17**, 15-21.
Oller-Daurella, L., Oller Ferrer-Vidal, L. (1981): *Atlas de crisis epilépticas.* 2nd edn, Apéndice pp 319-343. Geigy Division Farmacéutica: Barcelona.
Wolf, P. (1979): Nomenklatur und Klassifikation epileptischer Anfälle und Syndrome. *Nervenarzt* **50**, 547-554.

* * *

Discussion pages 271-273

Epileptic syndromes in infancy, child-
hood and adolescence. J. Roger,
C. Dravet, M. Bureau, F.E.
Dreifuss and P. Wolf. John Libbey
Eurotext Ltd ©1985.

Chapter 15
Benign Partial Epilepsies
in Childhood

Bernardo DALLA BERNARDINA, Claudio CHIAMENTI, Giuseppe CAPOVILLA,
and Vito COLAMARIA

Neuropsichiatria Infantile, Università di Verona, Borgo Roma, 37100 Verona, Italy

Summary

From 260 personal observations, the authors describe the characteristics common to the various
forms of benign partial epilepsy of childhood. The study of anamnestic, clinical and EEG characteristics allows early diagnosis and differentiation from lesional partial epilepsies.

The rate of partial epilepsies ranges between 37 and 66 per cent of childhood
epilepsies, depending on the age-range considered and the modality of recruiting
(Gastaut *et al.,* 1975; Pazzaglia and Franck, 1976; Joshi *et al.,* 1977; Cavazzuti, 1977;
Dalla Bernardina *et al.,* 1983). In spite of this high incidence, studies concerning the
prognosis of partial epilepsies are rare and they have been carried out either by including partial epilepsies with other types of epilepsy — often independent of age —
(Gastaut *et al.,* 1975; Bergamini *et al.,* 1977; Laplane *et al.,* 1977; Salbreux, *et al.,*
1977; Cavazzuti, 1980; Okuma and Kumasuiro, 1981) or by analysing the prognosis of
partial epilepsies all together (Holowach *et al.,* 1972; Degen, 1976; Pazzaglia *et al.,*
1982; Scarpa and Carassini, 1982; Fusco *et al.,* 1983). Finally, other studies consider
only 'Psychomotor Epilepsy' or 'Temporal-Lobe Epilepsy' (Glaser and Dixon, 1956;
Holowach *et al.,* 1961; Chao *et al.,* 1962; Gamstorp, 1975; Blume, 1977; Lindsay *et al.,*
1979; Aicardi, 1983).

As recently outlined by Roger *et al.* (1981) and by Pazzaglia *et al.* (1982), the
parameters of prognosis resulting from these works are more or less the same as previously described by Rodin (1968), Annegers *et al.* (1979) and by Okuma and Kumasuiro (1981) concerning all the epilepsies. On the other hand, there are numerous
papers concerning the electroclinical and prognostic delineation of a peculiar form of
benign partial epilepsy: the benign childhood epilepsy with rolandic or centro-temporal
spikes (Nayrac and Beaussart, 1958; Bancaud *et al.,* 1958; Faure and Loiseau, 1960;
Gibbs and Gibbs, 1960; Smith and Kellaway, 1964; Lombroso, 1967; Aicardi and
Chevrie, 1969; Beaussart, 1972; Blom *et al.,* 1972; Beaussart and Loiseau, 1973; Heij-

bel *et al.*, 1975; Lerman, 1975; Dalla Bernardina *et al.*, 1981; Blom and Heijbel, 1982).

More recently some authors have suggested the possible existence of other forms of benign partial epilepsies of childhood, particularly one form, characterized by seizures with an affective symptomatology (Dalla Bernardina *et al.*, 1980*a,b;* Plouin *et al.*, 1980; Dulac and Arthuis, 1980; Dalla Bernardina *et al.*, 1984). But studies trying to discover the electroclinical patterns eventually common to all Benign Partial Epilepsies of Childhood (BPEC) are rare and incomplete (Roger *et al.*, 1981; Roger and Bureau, 1983; Dalla Bernardina *et al.*, 1982, 1984).

The aim of the present study is the description, on the basis of the literature and on personal data, of the electroclinical criteria which should permit an early recognition of the epilepsies of childhood with partial seizures and often focal EEG abnormalities — which are age-dependent, without anatomical lesion and recover spontaneously.

The follow-up study concerns 260 children (142 boys-54.6 per cent and 118 girls-45.4 per cent) ranging in age from 5 to 18 years and suffering from a benign form of partial epilepsy, with a mean age of onset of 4 years and 6 months (range 1-11 years). The average period of observation was 5 years and 9 months (range 3-15 years). None of the children had neurological disorders or abnormal psychomotor development. Neuroradiological investigations (CT scan) performed in 147 subjects (56.5 per cent) were completely normal. All the cases had repeated awake and one or more p.m. (early afternoon) EEG records; moreover in 150 children (76 boys, 74 girls) at least one nocturnal sleep record was performed.

The 260 subjects include:

(a) Benign partial epilepsy with rolandic spikes (BERS): 162 subjects

(b) Benign psychomotor epilepsy (BPE): 26 subjects

(c) Benign partial epilepsy with occipital spike-waves (BEOSW): 19 subjects

(d) Other benign partial epilepsies ('others'): 53 subjects. The subjects suffering from a partial epilepsy — having the fundamental patterns of a benign form of epilepsy and a favourable evolution without showing the peculiar feature of any of the above listed forms — are classified in this last group.

Clinical features

(a) *Absence of neurological deficit.* This condition represents not only a parameter of good prognosis, common to all forms of epilepsy, but it constitutes a specific part of the definition of all the BPEC described up to now. Among our 260 cases, the subjects with neurological and/or intellectual deficit have been excluded. Obviously in a subject with a fixed neurological or intellectual deficit, the diagnosis of BPEC must not be *a priori* excluded but it must be considered with reserve and only when the other diagnostic parameters are all present.

(b) *Absence of intellectual deficit.* The same remarks can be made.

(c) *Familial antecedents of epilepsy.* All the authors interested in the different forms of BPEC outline the particularly high incidence of familial antecedents of epilepsy in their population: BERS: Blom *et al.* (1972) 17 per cent, Beaumanoir *et al.* (1974) 26.9 per cent, Heijbel *et al.* (1975) 47 per cent, Blom and Heijbel (1975) 59 per cent; BPE: Dulac and Arthuis (1980) 36 per cent; BEOSW: Gastaut (1982*a*) 47 per cent, Beaumanoir (1983) 33 per cent. In our cases, familial antecedents of epilepsy are present in 32 per cent of BERS, 38 per cent of BPE, 19.3 per cent of BEOSW and 35.8 per cent of the 'others'. Moreover, in most cases there were familial antecedents of a benign type of epilepsy with seizures recovering during puberty.

(d) *Age of onset.* In all the described types of BPEC, the mean age of onset ranges between 4 and 8 years and there are very rare cases showing the first seizure before the age of two. The seizures appeared before the age of two in only 8 per cent of our observations and during the first year of life in 3 per cent of cases. This appears more important if we consider that an earlier onset corresponds to an organic aetiology. In fact, in a population of partial epilepsies beginning during the first three years of life (Dalla Bernardina *et al.,* 1983) the organic forms and the benign forms represent respectively, 91.4 and 8.6 per cent in the first year, 65 and 35 per cent in the second year, 45.5 and 54.5 per cent in the third year. So, the diagnosis of BPEC must be considered with reserve when the seizures appear, without fever, before the 18th month of life.

(e) *Frequency of seizures.* The seizures are usually rare during the later evolution of BPEC, but early in the course there can be a high frequency of seizures — several a day and this frequency can remain high for some days. This high frequency of attacks at onset is mentioned in some of the cases of BEOSW reported by Gastaut (1982*a*), Beaumanoir (1983), and in many cases of BPE reported by Dalla Bernardina *et al.* (1980*a, b*) and in some cases reported by Dulac and Arthuis (1980).

In our population this particular modality of onset was present in 50 of all 260 cases, that is 20.3 per cent (11.1 per cent of BERS; 50 per cent of BPE; 3.7 per cent of BEOSW; 30.1 per cent of 'others'). Even when the seizures occur many times a day on onset, they are quickly controlled by treatment, and the evolution is never characterized by a progressive increase of seizure frequency, even when the subjects are not treated.

(f) *Semiology of seizures.* In the majority of cases the seizures are partial with elementary motor (BERS) or sensory (BEOSW) symptomatology. But in many cases the seizures are of partial complex type. In our population, 60 subjects (23 per cent) had experience of partial complex seizures (4.3 per cent of BERS; 100 per cent of BPE; 47.3 per cent of BEOSW; 34 per cent of 'others'). In about a third of cases there can be associated unilateral motor seizures or, more rarely, generalized seizures. In a few cases typical absence seizures can appear during the evolution. In no case is the evolution characterized by a true polymorphism of attacks, — no tonic nor atonic fits have ever been observed or reported. In some cases, not included in our population, throughout the evolution frequent atypical absences, often with head drops or a massive myoclonia, sometimes accompanied by a variable level of intellectual impairment can appear. This condition raises different problems from the differential diagnostic point of view and will be considered later in the EEG analysis.

In conclusion, the existence of seizures with partial complex symptomatology and the eventual coexistence of rare generalized fits are not in contrast with the diagnosis of BPEC; on the contrary the diagnosis must be excluded when the fits are polymorphous or of tonic and atonic type. Moreover, as outlined by Roger *et al.* (1981), Roger and Bureau (1983), in BPEC we never observed seizures characterized by a complex symptomatology followed by an elementary symptomatology nor reflex seizures.

(g) *Postictal deficit.* In some cases, especially after unilateral clonic seizures, a mild homolateral deficit, generally not including the face, can be present for some minutes but in no cases is the deficit prolonged. No other postical deficits are observed even when the seizures occur in series: in these cases there is no impairment of consciousness between the seizures.

(h) *Neurological and pyschological development*. The evolution is invariably characterized by neurologically and intellectually normal development. No psychiatric disorders
have been observed. As previously outlined by Lerman (1975), psychological or behavioral problems can be observed when the diagnosis is not correct and the children and
their parents are not reassured about the absolute benignity of these forms of epilepsy.

EEG criteria

(a) *Background activity*. During waking it is symmetrical, well organized and reacts
normally in all cases of BPEC previously reported and in our 260 personal cases. As already reported (Dalla Bernardina and Beghini, 1975; Dalla Bernardina *et al.*, 1982,
1984) the cyclic organization of sleep and the percentages of different stages are also
quite normal; moreover the physiological patterns of sleep are normally represented
— even in the presence of seizures.

(b) *Focal abnormalities*. The peculiar EEG finding of BPEC is the presence of focal
paroxysmal abnormalities, often changing in frequency during the evolution, characterized by some typical features.

The typical paroxysmal abnormality is a focal slow spike followed by a slow wave,
like the rolandic spike (RS) characterizing the BERS (Fig. 1: awake). Most frequently
they are located on the centro-temporal or the parieto-temporal or parieto-occipital
areas. When they involve the frontal areas or the vertex they must be considered as

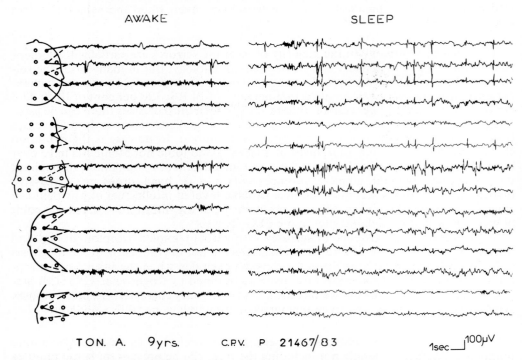

AWAKE   SLEEP

T ON. A.   9yrs.   C.P.V. P   21467/83   1sec 100μV

Fig. 1. Boy: 9 years old, neurologically normal, whose father had few seizures during childhood.
The boy suffered from one nocturnal brief unilateral clonic fit at the age of five, and, at the age
of ten, from some typical diurnal and nocturnal orofacial fits. Note the typical RS (slow spike -
slow wave complex) increasing in frequency during sleep without change in morphology.

less typical even if some cases of benign epilepsies with frontal spikes have been reported (Beaumanoir and Nahory, 1983).

As previously reported by many authors (Ambrosetto and Dalla Bernardina, 1976; Blom and Heijbel, 1975; Calvet, 1978; Dalla Bernardina and Beghini, 1975; Dulac and Arthuis, 1980; Dalla Bernardina et al., 1981, 1982, 1984; Beaumanoir, 1983) the most striking finding is their significant increase in frequency during drowsiness through all the stages of sleep (Fig. 1: sleep). This important increase in frequency has been observed in all subjects of our population, either when the interictal abnormalities were present on wakefulness or when they appeared only during drowsiness. When the frequency of paroxysmal abnormalities decreases abruptly during sleep an organic aetiology must be suspected (Fig. 2). As reported by Nishiura and Miyazaki (1976) the amplitude of these paroxysmal abnormalities increases during NREM sleep but decreases during REM sleep. During NREM sleep these abnormalities sometimes involve adjacent areas of the same hemisphere and sometimes the homologous area of the contralateral hemisphere but never attain a significant bilateral diffusion. If such a generalization develops, similar to electrical status epilepticus of sleep (ESES) or continuous generalized spike waves (Patry et al., 1971; Tassinari et al., 1977, 1982, 1984; Calvet, 1978) then it is a different form, recently reported as 'electrical status epilepticus during sleep in benign partial epilepsy' (Dalla Bernardina et al., 1978). In all forms of partial epilepsy we find some cases representing a continuous generalized spike waves syndrome (Dalla Bernardina et al., in preparation) but these cases are not included in this study. For this reason we do not agree with Aicardi and Chevrie (1982) who consider this type of electroclinical entity as a separate form of 'atypical benign partial epilepsy of childhood'. We think that the phenomenon of bilateral diffusion during waking and sleeping, can appear, for unknown reasons, in any type of partial epilepsy

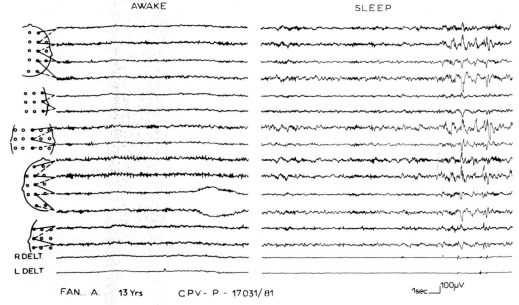

Fig. 2. Boy: 13 years old, without neurological deficit, who suffered between 9 and 11 years of life from two partial motor fits, later well controlled by carbamazepine treatment. Note the disappearance of the left frontocentral spikes, characteristic of the awake state, from the onset of drowsiness. The CT scan shows an irregular calcification on the left fronto-temporal area.

of childhood, leading to a clinical situation which requires special management to avoid, if possible, a poor mental prognosis. In our experience, a similar picture also characterized some cases of acquired epileptic aphasia, evoking the cases previously reported by Shoumaker *et al.* (1974), Kellerman (1978), Billard *et al.* (1981), Rodriguez and Niedermeyer (1982), Dulac *et al.* (1983).

As described above, in most cases RS are followed by a sharp wave. These sharp waves are particularly evident during REM sleep because of the low amplitude of rolandic spikes. According to Dalla Bernardina *et al.* (1982, 1984), in the waking state similar sharp waves were already present on the centro-parietal or centro-temporal areas in all subjects of our population who failed to show typical spikes either initially or for a period from 1-3 years after the spike disappearance. These sharp waves are the only interictal EEG abnormality in 24.5 per cent of subjects of group (d) ('others').

We think that they can be considered the 'phantom' or 'rudiment' of the typical slow-spike slow-wave. For this reason the diagnosis of benign partial epilepsy must be considered when both sharp waves and typical clinical features are present, even if typical spikes are absent.

(c) *Mutifocal abnormalities.* From the first EEG record or during the evolution, in the waking state or during sleep, independent foci with a similar morphology appear in about a third of our cases. During sleep they display the same behaviour. As we have previously pointed out (Dalla Bernardina *et al.,* 1984), in spite of their increase in frequency, the focal abnormalities show the same morphology described during wakefulness (Fig. 1); in particular, fast spikes or polyspikes never appear during sleep (Fig. 1). Likewise during sleep we never observed the appearance of an electrical depression or of a marked increase of the slow component, evoking a brief burst-suppression, following spikes. In our experience the appearance of fast polyspikes (Fig. 3) or brief burst-suppression corresponds to an organic aetiology even if the awake EEG and the initial clinical features could suggest a possible picture of BPEC.

(d) *Generalized spike waves (SW).* During the evolution brief and rare discharges of generalized spike waves appear in 1/3 or 1/2 of the cases of our groups. They can be present during the awake state or they can appear only during drowsiness. When present at the awake state, contrary to the opinion of Beaumanoir *et al.* (1974), these discharges last very rarely longer than 2-3 seconds and rarely have a clinical expression; they never increase in frequency during sleep, contrary to the SW observed in primary generalized epilepsy (Sato *et al.,* 1973; Tassinari *et al.,* 1974).

This absence of generalized spike wave activation during sleep is incongruent with the hypothesis that benign partial epilepsies constitute a particular form of primary generalized epilepsy as proposed by Beaumanoir and Nahory (1982). On the other hand, the coexistence of generalized spike waves does not influence the frequency of attacks (Dalla Bernardina *et al.,* 1982).

(e) *Seizures.* In the literature there are relatively many descriptions of recorded seizures concerning BEOSW (Gastaut, 1982*a, b;* Beaumanoir, 1983) and BPE (Dalla Bernardina *et al.,* 1980*a*), but rarely concerning BERS (Dalla Bernardina and Tassinari, 1975; Ambrosetto and Gobbi, 1975; Morikawa *et al.,* 1980; Dalla Bernardina *et al.,* 1982). Moreover the majority of recorded seizures seem quite similar from the EEG point of view.

The ictal pattern is characterized generally by a sequence of rhythmic sharp waves or spikes, remaining quite monomorphous through all the discharge, not followed by significant signs of postictal abnormality. Furthermore the ictal discharge remains quite

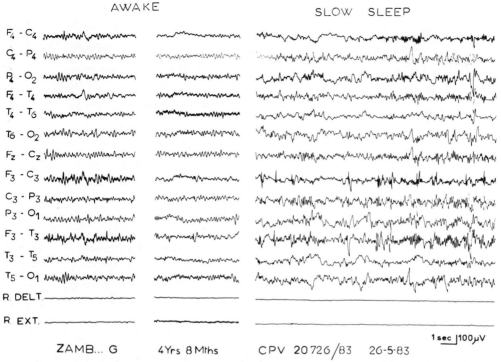

AWAKE   SLOW SLEEP

ZAMB... G   4Yrs 8Mths   CPV 20726/83   26-5-83

1 sec ⏐100μV

Fig. 3. Girl: 4 years 7 months old, without familial or personal antecedents, neurologically normal, who suffered from three brief partial fits from the age of 4 years. The focal abnormalities during the awake state can evoke typical RS. During sleep the paroxysmal abnormalities show a clear change in morphology into fast spikes. CT scan shows a small calcification surrounded by hypodensity evoking a previous inflammatory lesion.

similar when the fit occurs during the awake state and during sleep. In particular the onset of fits is never characterized by an important EEG depression followed by a fast rhythm and the ictal discharge never shows any change of the pattern during the same fit (Fig. 4). When the fits are polymorphous and when there are severe signs of postictal abnormality, an organic aetiology must be suspected (Figs 5, 6). In 63 per cent of our 'others' cases numerous fits have been recorded when awake and/or during sleep; in these cases the EEG pattern of fits is similar to those described above characteristic of the more typical forms of BPEC. The absence of polymorphism of ictal EEG pattern in the same subject, even when the seizures are frequent, seems to be in agreement with the absence of polymorphism on the clinical point of view.

Conclusions

Certainly BPEC represents one of the most important groups of childhood epilepsies. From the practical point of view, in spite of this great frequency, the cases which do not correspond to a well-defined electroclinical form are relatively numerous.

On the other hand, the good response to treatment alone is not a sufficient parameter of definition. Moreover the absence of neurological and neuroradiological signs of lesion is also not sufficient to assess the diagnosis of BPEC. It appears evident that only

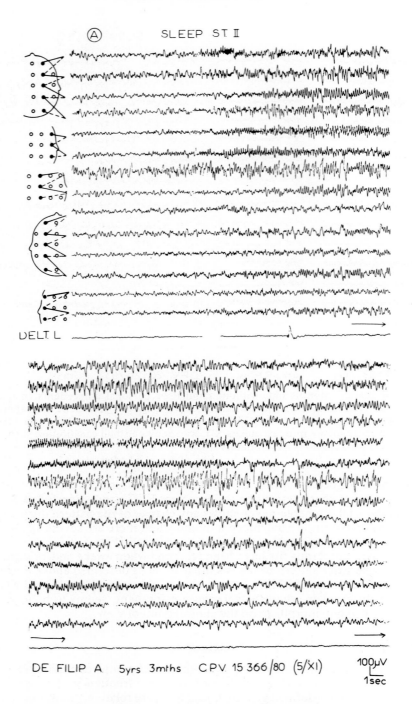

Fig. 4. Boy: 5 years 3 months old, neurologically normal. He presented several partial fits per day for 2 months. Note the monomorphic pattern of the ictal discharge. The fits have been completely controlled by carbamazepine therapy.

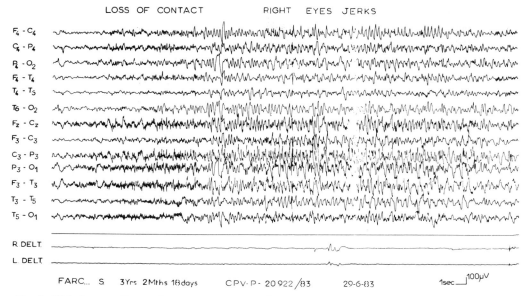

Fig. 5. Girl: 3 years 2 months old, has been suffering for one month from frequent partial fits with rare myoclonias of the face and significant autonomic symptoms. There are neither familial nor personal antecedents and the neurological picture is normal. The EEG pattern of seizure is polymorphous; in fact, the onset is characterized by a fast rhythm, increasing progressively in amplitude, followed by slow waves associated with fast spikes involving the whole of the left hemisphere. In spite of different treatments frequent fits persist 6 months later.

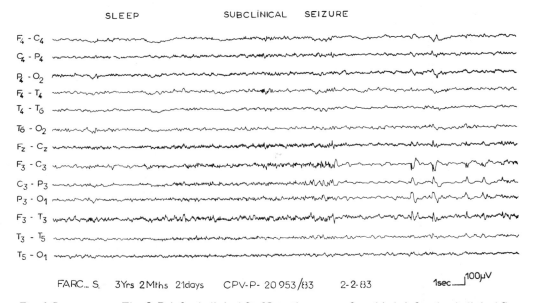

Fig. 6. Same case as Fig. 5. Brief subclinical fit. Note that even after this brief and subclinical fit a severe EEG depression involving the left centro-parietal area appears. The end of the fit is also characterized by the repetition of brief EEG depressions following repeated slow spikes.

the coexistence of different anamnestic, clinical and EEG features can allow an early diagnosis of BPEC, defined as the epilepsies of childhood with predominant partial seizures and focal EEG abnormalities which are age-dependent, without anatomical lesion, probably of functional rather than organic aetiology and which recover spontaneously.

We suggest that the most important criteria of diagnosis are the following:

Clinical criteria
- absence of neurological deficit
- absence of intellectual deficit
- family history of epilepsy, especially if of benign type
- onset of fits after 18 months of life
- seizures usually brief and rare, sometimes frequent at the onset, but only for a short period, with a good response to the treatment and no increase in frequency after
- seizures variable in symptomatology but not polymorphous in the same child (neither tonic nor atonic fits)
- absence of postictal prolonged deficit
- absence of impairment of neurological and psychological development through the evolution.

EEG criteria
- persistence of a normal background activity
- normal sleep organization
- focal abnormalities with 'like rolandic spikes' morphology, or focal sharp waves evoking the slow wave of the typical complex
- possible appearance of multifocal similar independent abnormalities
- possible appearance of brief bursts of generalized spike waves discharges, not increasing during slow sleep and generally without clinical expression
- increased frequency of focal abnormalities during sleep but without morphological changes, particularly without fast polyspikes, without bilateralization evoking the continuous generalized spike waves syndrome
- absence of polymorphism of ictal pattern at the awake state and during sleep.

Obviously a number of these criteria may lack in certain cases but the diagnosis of BPEC is all the more probable in a patient as the greatest number of these criteria are present.

References

Aicardi, J. Chevrie, J.J. (1969): Epilepsie partielle avec foyer rolandique de la seconde enfance. *Journées parisiennes de Péd.*, pp 125-142. Flammarion: Paris.

Aicardi, J., Chevrie, J.J. (1982): Atypical benign partial epilepsy of childhood. *Develop. Med. Child. Neurol.* 24, 281-292.

Aicardi J. (1983): Complex partial seizures in childhood. In *Advances in epileptology:* XIVth Epilepsy international Symposium, pp. 237-242, ed M. Parsonage, R.H.E. Grant, A.G. Craig, A.A. Ward Jr. Raven Press: New York.

Ambrosetto, G., Gobbi, G. (1975): Benign epilepsy of childhood with rolandic spikes or a lesion? EEG during a seizure. *Epilepsia* 16, 793-798.

Ambrosetto, G., Dalla Bernardina, B. (1976): Attività intercritica e critica durante il sonno notturno nella epilessia benigna dell'infanzia a parossismi EEG rolandici e/o medio-temporali. In *Le Epilessie,* pp 101-107, ed E. Lugaresi, P. Pazzaglia, R. Canger. A. Gaggi: Bologna.

Annegers, J.F., Hauser, W.A., Elveback, L.R. (1979): Remission of seizures and relapse in patients with epilepsy. *Epilepsia* **20**, 729-737.

Bancaud, J., Colomb, D., Dell, M.B. (1958): Les pointes rolandiques: un symptôme EEG propre à l'enfant. *Rev. Neurol.* **99**, 206-209.

Beaumanoir, A., Ballis, T., Varfis, J., Ansari, K. (1974): Benign epilepsy of childhood with rolandic spikes. *Epilepsia* **15**, 301-315.

Beaumanoir, A., Nahory, A. (1982): Etude évolutive clinique et EEG (plus de 10 ans d'observation) de 64 cas d'épilepsie avec foyer EEG "fonctionnel". *Boll. Lega Ital. Epil.* **39**, 9.

Beaumanoir, A. (1983): Infantile epilepsy with occipital focus and good prognosis. *Eur. Neurol.* **22**, 43-52.

Beaumanoir, A., Nahory, A. (1983): Les épilepsies bénignes partielles: 11 cas d'épilepsie partielle frontale à évolution favorable. *Rev. EEG Neurophysiol.* **13**, 207-211.

Beaussart, M. (1972): Benign epilepsy of children with rolandic (centro-temporal) paroxysmal foci. A clinical entity. Study of 221 cases. *Epilepsia* **13**, 795-811.

Beaussart, M., Loiseau, P. (1973): Evolution et pronostic de l'épilepsie à paroxysmes rolandiques. In *Evolution and prognosis of epilepsies,* pp 215-288. ed E. Lugaresi, P. Pazzaglia, C.A. Tassinari. A. Gaggi: Bologna.

Bergamini, L., Bergamasco, B., Benna, P., Gilli, M. (1977): Acquired etiological factors in 1785 epileptic subjects: clinical anamnestic research. *Epilepsia* **18**, 437-444.

Billiard, C., Autret, A., Laffont, F., Degiovanni, E., Lucas, B., Santini, J., Dulac, O., Plouin, P. (1981): Aphasie acquise de l'enfant avec épilepsie: à propos de 4 observations avec état de mal électrique infraclinique du sommeil. *Rev. EEG. Neurophysiol.* **11**, 457-467.

Blom, S., Heijbel, J., Bergfors, P.G. (1972): Benign epilepsy of children with centro-temporal EEG foci. Prevalence and follow-up study of 40 patients. *Epilepsia* **13**, 609-619.

Blom, S., Heijbel, J. (1975): Benign epilepsy of children with centro-temporal foci. Discharge rate during sleep. *Epilepsia* **16**, 133-140.

Blom, S., Heijbel, J. (1982): Benign epilepsy of children with centro-temporal EEG foci: a follow-up study in adulthood of patients initially studied as children. *Epilepsia* **23**, 629-632.

Blume, W.T. (1977): Temporal lobe seizures in childhood: Medical aspects. In *Topics in child neurology,* pp 105-125, ed M.E. Blaw, I. Rapin, M, Kinsbourne. Spectrum Publication Inc.: New York, London.

Calvet, U. (1978): Epilepsie nocturnes de l'enfant: épilepsies bénignes. Thèse, Toulouse.

Cavazzuti, G.B. (1977): Epidémiologie de l'épilepsie de la seconde enfance (âge scolaire). In *Congr. Soc. de Neurologie infantile,* pp 219-227. Marseille: Diffusion Générale de Librairie.

Cavazzuti, G.B. (1980): Epidemiology of different types of epilepsy in school age children of Modena, Italy. *Epilepsia* **21**, 57-62.

Chao, D., Sexton, J.A., Sautos Pardo, L. (1962): Temporal lobe epilepsy in childhood. *J. Pediatr.* **60**, 686-693.

Dalla Bernardina, B., Beghini, G. (1975): Rolandic spikes in children with or without epilepsy. (20 subjects polygraphically studied during sleep). *Epilepsia* **17**, 161-167.

Dalla Bernardina, B., Tassinari, C.A. (1975): EEG of a nocturnal seizure in a patient with benign epilepsy of childhood with rolandic spikes. *Epilepsia* **16**, 497-501.

Dalla Bernardina, B., Bureau, M., Dravet, C., Dulac, O., Tassinari, C.A., Roger, J. (1980*a*): Epilepsie bénigne de l'enfant avec crises à sémiologie affective. *Rev. EEG Neurophysiol.* **10**, 8-18.

Dalla Bernardina, B., Colamaria, V., Bondavalli, S., Tassinari, C.A., Dulac, O., Dravet, C., Roger, J., Bureau, M. (1980*b*): Epilepsie partielle bénigne de l'enfant à sémiologie affective. *Boll. Lega It. Epil.* **29-30**, 131-137.

Dalla Bernardina, B., Tassinari, C.A., Dravet, C., Bureau, M., Beghini, G., Roger, J. (1978): Epilepsie partielle bénigne et état de mal électroencéphalographique pendant le sommeil. *Rev. EEG Neurophysiol.* **8**, 350-353.

Dalla Bernardina, B., Beghini, G., Bondavalli, S., Colamaria, V. (1981): L'Epilessia parziale benigna dell'infanzia a parossismi rolandici e/o centrotemporali (EPR). In *Documenti Sigma-Tau,* pp 23-35.

Dalla Bernardina, B., Bondavalli, S., Colamaria, V. (1982): Benign epilepsy of childhood with rolandic spikes (bers) during sleep. In *Sleep and epilepsy,* pp 495-506. ed M.B. Sterman, M.N. Shouse, P. Passouant. Academic Press: New York and London.

Dalla Bernardina, B., Colamaria, V., Capovilla, G., Bondavalli, S. (1983): Nosological Classification of Epilepsies in the first three years of life. In *Epilepsy: an update on research and therapy. Progress in clinical and biological research,* pp 165-183. ed G. Nisticó, R. Di Perri, H. Meinardi. Alan R. Liss, Inc: New York.

Dalla Bernardina, B., Colamaria, V., Capovilla, G., Bondavalli, S. (1984): Sleep and benign partial epilepsies of childhood. In *Epilepsy sleep and sleep deprivation,* pp 119-133, ed R. Degen, E. Niedermeyer. Elsevier Science Publishers B.V.: Amsterdam.

Degen, R. (1976): *Die kindlichen Anfallsleiden Epileptische und nichtepileptische anfälle.* Hippokrates Verlag: Stuttgart.

Dulac, O., Arthuis, M. (1980): Epilepsie psychomotrice bénigne de l'enfant. *Journées parisiennes de Péd.* pp 211-220. Flammarion: Paris.

Dulac, O., Billard, C., Arthuis, M. (1983): Aspects électro-cliniques et évolutifs de l'épilepsie dans le syndrome aphasie-épilepsie. *Archs Fr. Pédiatr.* **40,** 299-308.

Faure, Y., Loiseau, P. (1960): Une corrélation clinique particulière des pointe-ondes rolandiques sans signification focale. *Rev. Neurol.* **102, 399-406.**

Fusco, L., Manfredi, M., Vigevano, F., Mallagnani, F., Bondavalli, S., Dalla Bernardina, B., Attolini, C., Calasso, E., Caldana, A., Giovanardi,Rossi, P., Gobbi, G., Mazzotta, G. (1983): Predittività della resistenza delle epilessie parziali. Revisione di una casistica multicentrica: dati preliminari. *Riv. Ital. EEG Neurofisiol. Clin.* (Suppl. 1), 163-169.

Gamstorp, I. (1975): Complex Partial seizures and their treatment. Treatment with carbamazepine: children. In *Advances in neurology,* 237-248, ed J.K. Penry, D.D. Daly. Raven Press: New York.

Gastaut, H., Gastaut, J.L., Gonçalves e Silva, G.E., Fernandez Sanchez, G.R. (1975): Relative frequency of different types of epilepsy: a study employing the Classification of International League against Epilepsy. *Epilepsia* **16,** 457-461.

Gastaut, H. (1982*a*): A new type of epilepsy: benign partial epilepsy of childhood with occipital spike-waves. *Clin. Electroencephalogr.* **13,** 13-22.

Gastaut, H. (1982*b*): L'épilepsie bénigne de l'enfant à pointe-ondes occipitales. *Rev. EEG Neurophysiol.* **12,** 179-201.

Gibbs, E.L., Gibbs, F.A. (1960): Good prognosis of mid-temporal epilepsy. *Epilepsia* **1,** 448-453.

Glaser, G.H., Dixon, M.S. (1956): Psychomotor seizures in childhood. Clinical study. *Neurology* **6,** 646-655.

Heijbel, J. Blom, S., Bergfors, P.G. (1975): Benign epilepsy of children with centro temporal EEG foci. A study of incidence rate in outpatient care. *Epilepsia* **16,** 657-664.

Holowach, J., Renda, Y.A., Wagner, I. (1961): Psychomotor seizures in childhood. *J. Pediatr.* **59,** 339-345.

Holowach, J., Thurston, D.L., O'Leary, J. (1972): Prognosis in childhood epilepsy: Follow-up study of 148 cases in which therapy has been suspended after prolonged anticonvulsivant control. *New Engl. J. Med.* **286,** 169-174.

Joshi, V., Katiyar, B.C., Mohan, P.K., Misra, S., Shukla, G.D. (1977): Profile of epilepsy in a developing country: a study of 1000 patients based on the International Classification. *Epilepsia* **18,** 549-554.

Kellerman, K. (1978): Recurrent aphasia with subclinical bioelectric status epilepticus during sleep. *Eur. J. Pediatr.* **128,** 207-212.

Laplane, R., Salbreux, R., Tuloup, A.M., Deniaud, J.M. (1977): 149 cas de convulsions dans les 18 premiers mois de la vie: analyse statistique et corrélations électrocliniques. *Ann. Pédiatr.* **24,** 467-473.

Lerman, P. (1975): Benign focal epilepsy of childhood. A follow-up study of 100 recovered patients. *Archs Neurol.* **23,** 261-264.

Lindsay, J., Ounsted, C., Richards, P. (1979): Long-term outcome in children with temporal lobe seizures: social outcome and childhood factors. *Develop. Med. Child Neurol.* **21,** 285-298.

Lombroso, C.T. (1967): Sylvian seizures and midtemporal spike foci in children. *Archs Neurol.* **17,** 52-59.

Morikawa, T., Osawa, T., Higashi, T., Seino, M., Wada, T. (1980): A study of the sylvian seizure by the use of VTR-EEG monitoring system. *Clin. Neurol.* 675-679.

Nayrac, P., Beaussart, M. (1958): Les pointe-ondes pré-rolandiques: expression EEG très particulière. Etude électroclinique de 21 cas. *Rev. Neurol.* **99**, 201-206.

Nishiura, N., Miyazaki, T. (1976): Clinico-EEG study of focal epilepsy with special reference to benign epilepsy of children with centro temporal EEG foci and its age dependency. *Folia Psychiatr. Neurol. Jpn* **30**, 253-261.

Okuma, T., Kumashiro, H. (1981): Natural history and prognosis of epilepsy. Report of a multi-institutional study in Japan. *Epilepsia* **22**, 35-53.

Patry, G., Lyagoubi, S., Tassinari, C.A. (1971): Subclinical 'electrical status epilepticus' induced by sleep in children. A clinical and EEG study of six cases. *Archs Neurol.* **24**, 242-252.

Pazzaglia, P., Frank-Pazzaglia, L. (1976): Record in grade school of pupils with epilepsy: an epidemiological study. *Epilepsia* **17**, 361-366.

Pazzaglia, P., D'Alessandro, R., Lozito, A., Lugaresi, E. (1982): Classification of partial epilepsies according to the symptomatology of seizures: practical value and prognostic implications. *Epilepsia* **23**, 343-350.

Plouin, P., Lerique, A., Dulac, O. (1980): Etude électroclinique et évolution dans 7 observations de crises partielles complexes dominées par un comportement de terreur chez l'enfant. *Boll. Lega. It. Epil.* **29-30**, 139-143.

Rodin, E.A. (1968): *The prognosis of patients with epilepsy.* Charles C. Thomas: Springfield Illinois.

Rodriguez, I., Niedermeyer, E. (1982): The aphasia-epilepsy syndrome in children: electroencephalographic aspects. *Clinical EEG* **13**, 23-35.

Roger, J., Dravet, C., Menendez, P., Bureau, M. (1981): Les épilepsies partielles de l'enfant. Evolution et facteurs de pronostic. *Rev. EEG Neurophysiol.* **11**, 431-437.

Roger, J., Bureau, M. (1983): Facteurs de pronostic et évolution des épilepsies partielles de l'enfant. *Riv. Ital. EEG Neurofisiol. Clin.* (Suppl. 1), 171-174.

Salbreux, R., Laplane, R., Thyl de Lopez, R., Bousquet, J. (1977): Physionomie électroclinique d'une population d'enfants suivis plus de dix ans pour convulsions. *Ann. Pédiatr.* **24**, 475-481.

Sato, S., Dreifuss, F.E., Penry, J.K. (1973): The effect of sleep on spike-wave discharges in absence seizures. *Neurology* **23**, 1335-1345.

Scarpa, P., Carassini, B., (1982): Partial epilepsy in childhood: clinical and EEG study of 261 cases. *Epilepsia* **23**, 333-341.

Shoumaker, M.R., Bennett, D.R., Bray, P.F., Curless, R.G. (1974): Clinical and EEG manifestations of an unusual aphasic syndrome in children. *Neurology* **24**, 10-16.

Smith, I.M.B., Kellaway, P. (1964): Central (rolandic) foci in children: analysis of 200 cases. *EEG Clin. Neurophysiol.* **17**, 460-461.

Tassinari, C.A., Bureau-Paillas, M., Dalla Bernardina, B., Mancia, D., Capizzi, G., Dravet, C., Valladier, C., Roger, J. (1974): Generalized epilepsies and seizures during sleep. A polygraphic study. In *Brain and sleep,* pp 154-166, ed Van Praag and H. Meinardi. De Erven Bohn BV: Amsterdam.

Tassinari, C.A., Dravet, C., Roger, J. (1977): E.S.E.S.: Encephalopathy related to electrical status epilepticus during slow sleep. *EEG Clin. Neurophysiol.* **43**, 529.

Tassinari, C.A., Bureau, M., Dravet, C., Roger, J., Daniele Natale, O. (1982): Electrical status epilepticus during sleep in children (E.S.E.S.) In *Sleep and epilepsy,* pp 465-479, ed M.B. Sterman, M.N. Shouse, P. Passouant. Academic Press: New York and London.

Tassinari, C.A., Daniele Natale, O., Dravet, C., Bureau, M., Dalla Bernardina, B., Michelucci, R., Picornell Darder, I., Vigevano, F., Roger, J. (1984): Sleep polygraphic studies in some epileptic encephalopathies from infancy to adolescence. In *Epilepsy sleep and sleep deprivation,* pp 140-154, ed R. Degen, E. Niedermeyer. Elsevier Science Publ. B.V.: Amsterdam.

*　　　　　*　　　　　*

Discussion pages 213-215

Epileptic syndromes in infancy, child-
hood and adolescence. J. Roger,
C. Dravet, M. Bureau, F.E.
Dreifuss and P. Wolf. John Libbey
Eurotext Ltd ©1985.

Chapter 16
Benign Partial Epilepsy with Centro-Temporal Spikes

Pinchas LERMAN

Pediatric Seizure Unit and EEG Laboratory, Beilinson Medical Center, Petah Tiqva, and the Sackler School of Medicine, Tel Aviv University, Israel

Summary

Benign partial epilepsy of childhood with centro-temporal spikes is an entity that includes characteristic clinical and electroencephalographic manifestations. Clinically, it consists of typical brief,
hemifacial seizures that tend to become generalized when they occur nocturnally. The EEG findings include slow, diphasic, high-voltage, centro-temporal spikes, activated by sleep. These seizures usually appear in the first decade of life and disappear in the second, and, as a rule they
occur in otherwise healthy children who show no evidence of cerebral lesions. The seizures are
mild and variable in frequency and respond well to anticonvulsant therapy. The prognosis is excellent and recovery is the rule. In all patients the EEG normalizes and seizures cease within a
few years without recurrence after discontinuation of medication.

Introduction

It is only during the past 30 years that the interesting features of benign partial epilepsy
with centro-temporal spikes (BECT) have come to be recognized. Gastaut in 1952 was
the first to describe the electroencephalographic features, already noting that these pre-
rolandic discharges had no focal significance. Bancaud *et al.* (1958) and Courjon and
Cotte (1959), who followed these findings into puberty, confirmed their evanescence.
The initial description of the clinical symptoms, made by Nayrac and Beaussart in
1958, was followed by a number of reports, including those of Faure and Loiseau
(1960), Lombroso (1967), Blom *et al.* (1972), Mortureux (1966). Like Gibbs and
Gibbs (1959-1960) all these authors emphasized the good prognosis of BECT. Blom
and Heijbel (1982) followed 37 patients for periods ranging from 13 to 27 years and
found that 36 of these had been seizure-free for 14 to 23 years, all but one of them receiving no medication. Only one 34-year-old patient reported having had two sporadic
grand-mal seizures after alcohol abuse.

Gibbs *et al.* (1954) were the first to note that epileptic foci in the EEG are not
necessarily accompanied by clinical seizures. Since then this phenomenon was also ob-

served by others (Smith and Kellaway, 1964; Blom and Brorson, 1966; Green, 1961; Loiseau *et al.* 1964; Eeg-Olofson *et al.*, 1971; Cavazzuti *et al.*, 1980; Lerman and Kivity, 1981).

Bray and Wiser (1964), even without clear delineation of this syndrome, were the first to note that genetic factors were in evidence and to suggest that it was an idiopathic genetic form of epilepsy. This was confirmed by Loiseau and Beaussart (1969), Heijbel *et al.* (1975), Lerman and Kivity (1981) and others.

Why was this common syndrome not discovered until 1958 despite the characteristic clinical picture and the striking EEG findings? Lombroso (1967) has this to say: 'More surprising is the lack of such description in studies of epilepsies in the child. For example, Losky & Lerique-Koechlin report that facial seizures are quite rare in children . . . What may be rare and difficult is to obtain a full picture of such cases, particularly the key symptoms of sensory and motor interference with the tongue and nearby structures, before rapid propagation, especially in sleep, submerges all into the maelström of a generalized convulsion.' No less surprising is the fact that in the long-term follow-up study of 148 epileptic children reported by Holowach *et al.* (1972, 1982) this syndrome was not mentioned at all. It must be assumed that these cases were lost among the 'major seizures', 'focal seizures' and 'temporal lobe seizures' comprising their classification. Even today BECT is rarely described in English textbooks.

For many years neurologists have been taught to identify partial seizures and focal epilepsy with cortical lesions. Sutherland *et al.* (1974) state that 'It is vital to recognize that partial seizures have an underlying pathology.' However, we are here confronted with partial seizures associated with striking focal EEG discharges in which there is no underlying cerebral pathology and which must be considered as an idiopathic, primary form of epilepsy. This is a concept which is difficult to assimilate and accept.

Clinical data

(based on the studies of Beaussart (1972) and Lerman and Kivity (1975))

This is one of the commonest forms of epilepsy encountered in childhood, being found in approximately 15-20 per cent of young epileptics. The age of onset ranges from 3 to 13 years (a mean of 9.9 years). It may be stated that the seizures usually appear in the first decade of life, to disappear in the second. In 76 per cent they appear between 5 to 10 years, with a peak of 9 years. As in other forms of epilepsy the sex prevalence is 60 per cent males and 40 per cent females.

The frequency of seizures is very variable but is usually low. A single seizure during the entire course is to be expected in 10-13 per cent of cases even without drug therapy. In our material seizures were infrequent in 66 per cent of the cases, recurring once every 2 to 12 months. However, approximately 20 per cent of patients do have frequent fits, sometimes even multiple daily seizures. The occurrence in clusters is common, ie, a series of frequent seizures may be followed by long seizure-free periods. In our experience there is no correlation whatsoever between the severity of the EEG abnormality, the frequency of the seizures, the resistance to drug therapy and the final outcome.

The duration of the seizures is usually quite brief, ranging from several seconds to two minutes, the diurnal fits tending to be shorter, especially the sensory ones.

The temporary distribution of seizures is interesting: most frequently they occur solely during sleep, whether nocturnal or diurnal. In approximately 15 per cent they occur both in sleep and in waking and in 10-20 per cent in the waking state alone. The nocturnal seizures tend to be longer and more severe. The majority of the nocturnal seizures occur in the early morning, sometimes arousing the clinician's suspicion that hypoglycemia is to be blamed.

The past history is usually uneventful. However, 7-9 per cent of patients have a history of febrile convulsions in infancy, 6-10 per cent of neonatal difficulties and 4-5 per cent of mild head injuries. It is doubtful whether any of these factors is causally related to the subsequent epilepsy. Forensic issues may arise. Some children with centro-temporal spikes found after a mild head injury may be labelled as suffering from post-traumatic epilepsy even in the absence of clinical seizures *(vide infra)*.

The somewhat higher incidence of febrile convulsions than in the general population (which is 5 per cent) is probably the reflection of the inborn predisposition to seizures in these children. Most authors dealing with BECT emphasize that these children are neurologically intact and mentally normal. Beaumanoir (1976) states 'The neurological examination must be negative; otherwise the diagnosis of BECT has to be rejected.' Beaussart (1972) and Loiseau and Beaussart (1973) simply excluded from their studies cases with neurological defects. Interestingly, benign epilepsy also may occur, though infrequently, in brain damaged children. Among the 40 patients of Blom *et al.* (1972) three had mild hemiparesis. Three of our 100 cases suffered from cerebral palsy; yet another patient was microcephalic and moderately retarded. Hence partial epilepsy can be benign, even in the presence of brain damage, to which it should not be etiologically attributed. Rather it should be considered as fortuitously superimposed or 'grafted' on an injured brain. The prognosis is as good in these brain-damaged children as in normal children in terms of recovery from the epilepsy.

Description of seizures

The most characteristic features of this type of partial seizures are as follows (Lombroso, 1967): (1) a somatosensory onset with unilateral paresthesias involving the tongue, lips, gums and inner cheeks; (2) unilateral, tonic, clonic or tonic-clonic convulsions involving the face, lips, tongue as well as pharyngeal and laryngeal muscles and causing (3) and (4); (3) speech arrest or anarthria; (4) drooling due to sialorrhea and saliva pooling; (5) preservation of consciousness.

In a typical seizure, occurring either upon waking or out of sleep, the child, usually aged 5 to 10 years, will come to his parents, fully conscious but unable to speak, pointing to his mouth, which is drawn to one side, saliva oozing from one corner, often followed by some hemifacial twitchings. The whole episode lasts for no more than a minute or two and when it is over the child, when questioned, is able to relate that it started with a feeling of numbness, pins and needles, or 'electricity' in his tongue, gums and cheek on one side. We feel that if such a seizure description is obtained this is sufficient for the diagnosis, even before an EEG is performed to definitely confirm the clinical diagnosis.

This typical primordial seizure may spread to the arm ('brachiofacial seizure') and rarely to the leg ('unilateral convulsion'). In some children the partial motor seizure may change sides from time to time. We have never encountered a diurnal generalized major seizure in these children. However, the nocturnal seizures, which are the most frequent variety in this syndrome, often become generalized and since the partial onset is usually missed they tend to be labelled by the family physician as 'grand-mal'.

In a typical case of nocturnal seizures the mother is awakened by vocal noises coming from the child's bed. Rushing to him she finds him unconscious, grunting, gurgling sounds emanating from his mouth, which is drawn to one side and drooling. At this stage the seizure may end or it may develop into a generalized major convulsion.

Thus the nocturnal seizures may be of three types: (1) typical brief hemifacial seizures associated with speech arrest and drooling in a conscious state, ie identical to the diurnal seizures. The child will usually be awakened from sleep by the somatosensory 'aura'; (2) seizures like those above but with a loss of consciousness and usually with gurgling-grunting noises and at times terminating in vomiting; (3) generalized convulsions (so-called *grand-mal*), which are most often secondarily generalized although this is a point which lacks verification since the onset of the seizure is rarely witnessed.

The somatosensory 'aura' is probably quite common (Lombroso, 1967) but often missed since the young child rarely reports these subjective phenomena and when they occur at night they are usually not recalled on the next day. Rarely the diurnal seizure may be purely sensory. In such cases the diagnosis can be delayed for a long time.

The expression of the seizures appears to be age-dependent. In older children pure hemifacial seizures are more common whereas in the younger ones (2-5 years) hemiconvulsions and generalized nocturnal convulsions are more apt to occur. Even when seizures are very frequent in the first decade they tend to die out in adolescence and finally cease altogether, whether treated or not.

EEG findings

Interictal EEG records show centro-temporal spikes, either unifocal or bifocal. Typically, slow, diphasic, high-voltage spikes recur at short intervals, often in clusters (Fig. 1), at times followed by a slow wave. When unilateral they are always synchronous in the central (Rolandic) and midtemporal areas, although they are sometimes of different amplitudes. When bilaterally asynchronous spikes occur, both the rate of firing and amplitude varies from side to side. In a small number of patients the spike discharges are scanty and of low amplitude, tending to become more prominent in sleep. In approximately 60 per cent of patients the spike focus is unilateral. In approximately 40 per cent there are bilateral spike foci either in the initial EEG record or in consecutive ones, the foci tending to shift from side to side. In some patients, occipital spikes are found independently, or replacing centro-temporal spikes. In addition to the centro-temporal focus some of the records show generalized spike-wave discharges, without any concomitant petit mal lapses. In all patients the EEG subsequently normalizes within a period ranging from 6 months to 6 years (Lerman and Kivity, 1975).

No correlation is to be found between the intensity of the spike discharges and the frequency, length and duration of the seizures.

Centro-temporal spikes typically increase in drowsiness and all stages of sleep, then tending to become bilateral. In approximately 30 per cent of children with BECT spikes appear only in sleep (Blom and Heijbel, 1975). Thus a sleep record should be obtained whenever BECT is clinically suspected and the waking tracing is unrevealing. With recovery, normalization is seen first in the waking records and later also during sleep.

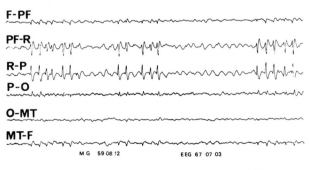

Fig. 1. Interictal EEG. Central (rolandic) diphasic, high voltage slow spikes, in clusters.

Diffuse spike-wave discharges, rarely occurring during waking in these cases, are strongly activated in sleep, appearing in 40 per cent of children with clinical seizures and in 10 per cent of those without seizures (Dalla Bernardina and Beghini, 1976). These authors observed that activation in REM sleep occurred only in children with seizures.

Beaumanoir (1976), who compared cases of petit-mal (with or without grand-mal) with those of BECT, observed the occurrence of diffuse spike-wave discharges in BECT as well as of centro-temporal spikes in petit-mal.

The ictal EEG recorded during a nocturnal seizure in stage II (Dalla Bernardina and Tassinari, 1975) showed an initial discharge beginning in the centro-temporal area on one side, then spreading to the whole ipsilateral hemisphere and finally the contralateral one. The onset of the seizure was marked by low voltage fast activity confined to a limited area.

There is no report in the literature of the EEG correlate during a diurnal seizure. However, in our laboratory such a seizure was recorded: it began with local decremental activity, followed by dense spikes in the centro-temporal area during the tonic phase and 'spike-waves' in the clonic phase, with no spread and no postictal slowing. The whole episode lasted less than one minute.

Various authors have used different terms to describe the EEG findings. American authors (Lombroso, 1967; Gibbs and Gibbs, 1960) have labelled these spike discharges as 'midtemporal' while the French (Gastaut, 1952; Nayrac and Beaussart, 1958; Bancaud et al., (1958) prefer the terms 'Rolandic spikes' or paroxysms. We find that the term 'centro-temporal spikes' proposed by Blom et al. (1972) is the most appropriate, since discharges occur in both areas and the site of origin is probably the lower Rolandic cortex (Lombroso, 1967). Furthermore, it avoids confusion with 'temporal lobe epilepsy', in which spike discharges are recorded in the anterior temporal area and are of different configuration.

In BECT the spikes are typically large, diphasic and blunt. They are often followed by a slow wave and tend to appear in clusters. In contrast, the discharges associated with cortical lesions tend to be smaller, sharper and more uniform.

Pathophysiology

The clinical symptomatology of BECT strongly suggests that the source of disturbance lies in the lower rolandic cortex representing the face and the oro-pharynx. Indeed, Penfield and Rasmussen (1950 — cited by Lombroso, 1967) were able to produce the symptoms suggesting Sylvian epilepsy by stimulating this cortical area. As stated by Lombroso (1967) 'The actual source of such foci projected to the midtemporal region of the scalp is as yet unclear.' From the fact that these spikes tend to be blunt he speculates that their origin might be within the depths of the Sylvian fissure. However, as Aicardi (1979) states, 'Despite its frequency, little is known of the neurophysiological mechanisms which produce such striking localized seizure activity in the face of a structurally normal brain.'

EEG studies demonstrate that quite frequently centro-temporal spikes are associated with bi-synchronous spike-wave discharges.

Both *petit-mal* and BECT are genetically determined. Thus even though we cannot clearly explain the sharp focalization in BECT it is clear that we are dealing with a 'functional' epilepsy, much the same as in *petit-mal*.

The alternation in lateral predominance of the foci in the evolution of BECT, the coexistence or alternance with occipital spike and/or generalized discharges, as well as their evanescence within several years, coupled with the lack of evidence for neurological deficits in these children — all this lends further support to the concept of a primary type of partial epilepsy lacking an anatomical substrate, much in contrast to the majority of the partial epilepsies seen in adults.

Genetic factors

A high percentage (up to 40 per cent) of close relatives (siblings, parents and cousins) have been found to have a history of febrile convulsions, partial or generalized seizures or epileptic discharges in the EEG of a focal or generalized nature, although without clinical seizures.

Bray and Wiser (1964, 1965) were the first to note the importance of genetic factors in this syndrome and came to the conclusion that centro-temporal foci are controlled by a single autosomal dominant gene with age-dependent penetrance, very much the same as in primary epilepsy associated with diffuse spike-wave discharges. This was supported by the findings of Heijbel *et al.* (1975), who conducted a genetic study on 19 probands with BECT. It should be stressed, however, that in the records of a single sibship, and at times of the same proband, one can find independent rolandic, mid-temporal and occipital spike foci as well as spike-wave discharges, so that both centro-temporal and occipital spikes may be the expression of this genetic trait. The number of children who bear the EEG trait exceeds those who have clinical seizures. Obviously those who are seizure-free represent a group of subclinical 'carriers' who have a heightened propensity to seizures.

The pertinent question is, which factors may transform the subclinical state into an active clinical epilepsy? Heijbel *et al.* (1975) postulate the existence of an inhibitory factor capable of preventing seizures which 'can be broken through by external or internal factors.' In illustration they describe three siblings, all with rolandic discharges. In the first there was an initial seizure during an episode of fever at the age of 4 years whereas in the second the first seizure occurred at the age of 10 years while he was watching television and in a state of emotional tension. The third child has had no seizures. In other words, a precipitating factor is needed to convert the inherited trait into the overt disease. Such precipitating factors may include head trauma (found in 4 per cent of our cases), perinatal brain insult (found in 13 per cent of Beaussart's cases (1972)), prematurity, meningitis and probably also emotional factors.

Diagnosis

A correct diagnosis is essential for correct management. Ascertaining the benignity of the condition makes it possible to avoid unnecessary 'invasive diagnostic procedures' (Aicardi, 1979). We feel that even a brain scan is superfluous. In the rare cases in which structural pathology is found (Morikawa *et al.,* 1979) it is not causally related to the seizure disorder and hence is non-contributory to management or prognosis.

BECT should be easy to differentiate from the complex group of 'temporal-lobe epilepsy'. Its symptomatology is elementary and stereotyped. There is no visceral aura, no clouding of consciousness and no automatisms or psychic phenomena. Hence complex partial seizures can easily be ruled out.

In the less common brachiofacial seizures and in the rare unilateral convulsions, it may be difficult to differentiate BECT from Jacksonian epilepsy on clinical grounds alone. The same is true for those cases which seem to present with major generalized nocturnal convulsions without any focal features. Indeed many of our patients were referred with the diagnosis of *'grand-mal'*. In these cases the typical EEG findings help make the correct diagnosis.

Drug therapy

Since the seizures are brief and usually mild there may be no need for medication especially if they are confined to nocturnal seizures of rare occurrence. The drug of choice appears to be phenytoin, which should be administered in a single bed-time dose. Carbamazepine and phenobarbital may also be used. Valproate and clonazepam are of little use. Overmedication (regarding both dose and frequency) and polypharmacy should be avoided. In the past we discontinued medication only after EEG normalization. One current policy is to taper off the anti-convulsant drug after 1-2 years of seizure control, even before the EEG normalizes. Most cases respond well to medication even with low doses. In the relatively few patients appearing to be drug resistant good control is eventually achieved, with the same favourable prognosis as in others.

Prognosis

Long-term clinical and EEG follow-up of BECT in children (Gibbs and Gibbs, 1960; Beaussart and Loiseau, 1973; Lerman and Kivity, 1975; Blom and Heijbel, 1982) has invariably shown that in the course of the years the seizures stopped completely whether they had been treated or not, and whether or not control had been achieved with therapy. In all cases the centro-temporal, as well as the occipital foci, disappeared from the records.

Some authors (Beaussart, 1972; Aicardi, 1979) speak of a 'cure' in BECT. This term implies the use of treatment. 'Recovery' appears more appropriate since it occurs regardless of treatment.

The excellent prognosis can be inferred from the mere fact that neither such partial seizures nor such EEG findings are ever found in adults. The inevitable conclusion would be that all these children recover before adulthood.

No doubt other forms of childhood epilepsy, associated with focal discharges, run a benign course and may end in recovery. This is certainly true for cases associated with occipital spikes and for some cases with multifocal discharges. However, 'Sylvian' seizures have the best prognosis among the benign epilepsies in childhood, as emphasized above. In less than 1 per cent of cases initially classified as BECT, following cessation of the characteristic 'Sylvian' seizures, generalized nocturnal convulsions as well as complex partial seizures may persist or may develop many years later. This may be due to an initial misclassification or simply to the fact that such epilepsy may occur *de novo* in a subject recovered from BECT just as it may occur in previously healthy young adults.

Psychosocial aspects

Our study of two groups of patients (Lerman and Kivity, 1975) both suffering from BECT but managed differently, afforded us a unique opportunity to compare the effect of contrasting attitudes towards the epilepsy on the patient and his family. In the retrospective group the doctors, believing that this was a chronic, disabling, incurable disease, probably due to brain damage, pronounced a grave prognosis and advised that the child be protected and his activities restricted. In the prospective group treated by our team, with awareness of the benignity of the condition, management was utterly different. We conveyed our optimism to the family and encouraged them to consider their epileptic child as a healthy, functioning individual, temporarily under medication to control the seizures, but expected to fully recover in a few years, and therefore not requiring restrictions nor over-protection.

These different attitudes produced quite striking differences in the behaviour and personality of the respective patients. In the retrospective group of patients a wide range of emotional problems was clearly associated with the anxiety and frustrations of the child and family engendered by the grim prognosis and severe restrictions of the child's activities. Behaviour and learning problems were quite common, being attributable to psychosocial factors, or to the adverse effect of barbiturates. Often a clear improvement was evident when the barbiturates had been discontinued. With the approach of adulthood critical problems often arose, particularly for the male patients, who were rejected by the armed forces and refused a driving licence. Many patients suffer from ostracism by peers and the combination of overprotection and rejection which are apt to develop in parents faced with the appalling situation of having an epileptic child, particularly when they have not had proper explanation and guidance as to the nature of this malady and its management. In this case children often develop antisocial attitudes, rebellion and despair, feeling like outcasts and frequently having great difficulty in social adjustment.

It is noteworthy that such problems were hardly ever encountered in the prospective group of patients, who, from the onset, were reassured that their convulsive disorder was benign and curable. In this group hardly any restrictions were imposed and they were encouraged to lead a normal, active life. Indeed out-growing their epilepsy they grew up to become well-balanced productive citizens.

References

Aicardi, J. (1979): Benign epilepsy of childhood with rolandic spikes. *Brain & Development* **1**, 71-73.

Bancaud J., Collomb, J., Dell,M.B. (1958): Les pointes rolandiques: un symptôme EEG propre à l'enfant. *Rev. Neurol.* **99**, 206-209.

Beaumanoir, A. (1976): Les épilepsies infantiles. *Problèmes de diagnostic et de traitement,* pp 54-59. Editions Roche: Bâle.

Beaumanoir, A., Ballis, T., Varfis, G. Ansari, K. (1974): Benign epilepsy of childhood with rolandic spikes. *Epilepsia* **15**, 301-315.

Beaussart, M. (1972): Benign epilepsy of children with rolandic (centro-temporal) paroxysmal foci. *Epilepsia* **13**, 795-811.

Beaussart, M., Loiseau, P. (1973): Evolution et pronostic de l'épilepsie à paroxysmes rolandiques. In *Evolution and prognosis of epilepsies,* ed E. Lugaresi, P. Pazzaglia, C.A. Tassinari, pp 215-228. A. Gaggi: Bologna.

Blom, S. Brorson, L.O. (1966) Central spikes and sharp waves (rolandic spikes) in children's EEG and their clinical significance. *Acta Paediatr. Scand.* **55**, 385-393.

Blom, S., Heijbel, J., Bergfors, P.G. (1972): Benign epilepsy of children with centrotemporal EEG foci - prevalence and follow-up study of 40 patients. *Epilepsia* **13**, 609-619

Blom, S. Heijbel, J. (1975): Benign epilepsy of children with centrotemporal EEG foci — Discharge rate during sleep. *Epilepsia* **16**, 133-140

Blom, S., Heijbel, J. (1982): Benign epilepsy of children with centrotemporal EEG foci: a follow-up study in adulthood of patients initially studied as children. *Epilepsia* **23**, 629-631.

Bray, F. P., Wiser, W.C. (1964): Evidence for a genetic etiology of temporal central abnormalities in focal epilepsy. *New Engl. J. Med.* **271**, 926-933.

Bray, F.P., Wiser, W.C. (1965): Hereditary characteristics of familial temporal central focal epilepsy. *Pediatrics* **30**, 207-211.

Cavazzutti, G.B., Cappella, L., Nalin, A. (1980): Longitudinal study of epileptiform EEG patterns in normal children. *Epilepsia* **21**, 43-55.

Courjon, J., Cotte, M.R. (1959): Les décharges pseudorhythmiques localisées chez l'enfant et leur évolution à la puberté. In *XXIIᵉ Congrès de pédiatrie de Langue Française,* pp 247-250. Dehan: Montpellier, France.

Dalla Bernardina, B., Beghini, G. (1976): Rolandic spikes in children with and without epilepsy (20 subjects polygraphically studied during sleep). *Epilepsia* **17**, 161-167.

Dalla Bernardina, B., Tassinari, C.A. (1975): EEG of a nocturnal seizure in a patient with "benign epilepsy of childhood with rolandic spikes". *Epilepsia* **16**, 497-501.

Eeg-Olofson, O., Petersen, I., Sellden, V. (1971): The development of the EEG in normal children from the age of 1 to 15 years: Paroxysmal activity. *Neuropädiatrie* **4**, 375-404.

Faure, J., Loiseau, P. (1960): Une corrélation clinique particulière des pointe-ondes sans signification focale. *Rev. Neurol.* **102**, 399-406.

Gastaut, Y. (1952): Un élément déroutant de la symptomatologie électroencéphalographique: les pointes prérolandiques sans signification focale. *Rev. Neurol.* **87**, 488-490.

Green, J.B. (1961): Association of behaviour disorders with an EEG focus in children without seizures. *Neurology* **11**, 337-340.

Gibbs, E.L., Gibbs, F.A. (1959-1960): Good prognosis of mid-temporal epilepsy. *Epilepsia* **1**, 448-453.

Gibbs, E.L., Gillen, H.W., Gibbs, F.A. (1954): Disappearance and migration of epileptic foci in children. *Am. J. Dis. Child.* **88**, 596-603.

Heijbel, J., Blom, S., Rasmuson, M. (1975): Benign epilepsy of childhood with centrotemporal EEG foci: A genetic study. *Epilepsia* **16**, 285-293.

Holowach J., Thurston, D.L., O'Leary, J. (1972): Follow-up study of 148 cases in which therapy had been suspended after prolonged anticonvulsant control. *New Engl. J. Med.* **286**, 169-174.

Holowach-Thurston, J., Thurston, D.L., Hixon, B.B., Keller, A.J. (1982): Prognosis in childhood epilepsy. Additional follow-up of 148 children 15 to 23 years after withdrawal of anticonvulsant therapy. *New Engl. J. Med.* **306**, 831-836.

Lerman, P., Kivity, S. (1975): Benign focal epilepsy of childhood - a follow up study of 100 recovered patients. *Archs Neurol.* **32**, 261-264.

Lerman, P., Kivity, S. (1981): Focal epileptic EEG discharges in children not suffering from clinical epilepsy: etiology, clinical significance and management. *Epilepsia* **22**, 551-558.

Loiseau, P., Beaussart, M. (1969): Hereditary factors in partial epilepsy. *Epilepsia* **10**, 23-31.

Loiseau, P., Beaussart, M. (1973): The seizures of benign childhood epilepsy with rolandic paroxysmal discharges. *Epilepsia* **14**, 381-389.

Loiseau, P., Geissmann, P., Cohadon, S., Vincent, D., Faure, J. (1964): Les paroxysmes rolandiques en dehors de l'épilepsie. *Rev. Neurol.* **111**, 374-381.

Lombroso, C.T. (1967): Sylvian seizures and mid-temporal spike foci in children. *Archs Neurol.* **17**, 52-59.

Morikawa, T., Osawa, T., Ishihara, O., Seino, M. (1979): A reappraisal of "benign epilepsy of children with centro-temporal EEG foci". *Brain & Development.* **1**, 253-265.

Mortureux, Y. (1966): Etude électro-clinique de certains paroxysmes d'expression rolandique chez l'enfant. Thèse: Bordeaux.

Nayrac, P., Beaussart, M. (1958): Les pointe-ondes prérolandiques: Expression EEG très particulière. *Rev. Neurol.* **99**, 201-206.

O'Donohoe, N.V. (1979): *Epilepsies in childhood.* Butterworths: London.

Smith, J.M.B., Kellaway, P. (1964): Central (rolandic) foci in children. An analysis of 200 cases. *Electroenceph. Clin. Neurophysiol.* **17**, 460-461.

Sutherland, J.M., Tait, H. Eadie, M.J. (1974): *The epilepsies.* 2nd edn, p 21. Churchill Livingstone: Edinburgh & London.

*   *   *

Discussion pages 213-215

Epileptic syndromes in infancy, childhood and adolescence. J. Roger, C. Dravet, M. Bureau, F.E. Dreifuss and P. Wolf. John Libbey Eurotext Ltd ©1985.

Chapter 17
Benign Epilepsy of Childhood with Occipital Paroxysms

Henri GASTAUT

Institut de Recherches en Neurologie, Centre Collaborateur de l'OMS pour l'Enseignement et la Recherche en Neurologie, Faculté de Médecine, 13385 Marseille Cedex 5, France

Summary

Benign epilepsy of childhood with occipital paroxysms (BEOP) is characterized by seizures which include visual symptoms often followed by motor or psychomotor manifestations and sometimes terminated with post-ictal migrainous headache. The EEG shows distinct repetitive occipital paroxysms appearing only after eye closure. No occipital lesions have been found, the children are neurologically normal and the seizures cease in adult life. This syndrome represents a separate variety of primary partial epilepsy, due at least in part to a constitutional epileptic predisposition similar to that responsible for primary generalized epilepsy. The post-ictal headache may be due to a persistence of the initial vasodilation in the vascular bed of the posterior cerebral and basilar arteries which accompanies the occipital epileptic discharge.

Three decades ago benign epilepsy with occipital paroxysms (BEOP) was proposed by Gastaut (1950) who described an epilepsy with visual ictal symptoms and interictal occipital rhythmic spike waves (SW) appearing only after eye closure in children without occipital cortical lesion, and by Gibbs and Gibbs (1952) who described seizure foci in occipital lobes which tend to disappear with age in young epileptic children. Such a distinct form of epilepsy had not previously been recognized as a separate electroclinical entity — undoubtedly because the following two fundamental characteristics are not always obvious: (1) the visual symptoms, which may be poorly described by younger children; (2) the attenuation of the occipital SW at eye opening, which may not be obvious in a routine EEG recording during which eyes may only be opened once or twice for a few seconds.

BEOP was definitely identified electroclinically two years ago in our department in 35 patients (Gastaut, 1981; 1982 a,b,c,d). Twenty-seven additional cases have been found since this initial differentiation so this study considers a total of 53 patients. The following topics are subsequently discussed: (1) the interseizure patient status; (2) the features of the seizures; (3) the evolution; (4) the diagnosis and finally (5) some theoretical remarks about the etiology of the disorder and the pathophysiology of its seizures. This study concerns 63 cases. Similar cases have been reported by Camfield *et al.,* (1978) and Beaumanoir (1983).

Status of children between seizures

Clinical and neuroradiological symptoms
> *Sex:* 52 per cent males.
> *Age at onset:* 15 months to 17 years (mean age 7 years 5 months).
> *Family history:* of epilepsy in 36.6 per cent of cases; of migraine in 15.9 per cent.
> *Personal history:* 14 per cent febrile convulsions; 6 per cent breath-holding spells; 11 per cent mild perinatal distress.
> *Neuropsychiatric examination:* normal in 90 per cent of cases; developmental re-retardation in 10 per cent, three of these cases with hemiparesis.
> *Ophthalmologic examination:* normal in 100 per cent of cases.
> *Neuroradiologic and CT examination:* normal in 91.7 per cent of cases.

Electroencephalographic features
Normal background activity and very distinct paroxysms outlined as follows (see Figs. 1-10).
> *Morphology:* SW in 80 per cent of cases; sharp waves in 20 per cent.
> *Amplitude:* high (200-300 μV).
> *Topology:* over the occipital as well as postero-temporal regions (electrode positions 01 and/or 02 as well as T5 and/or T6) of one hemisphere, most often the left, or over both hemispheres simultaneously or independently.
> *Chronology:* usually rhythmically repeated from 1 to 3 c/s in bursts or in trains; rarely isolated at irregular intervals.
> *Reactivity:* (i) prompt disappearance with opening of the eyes in 94 per cent of cases; reappearance at closure with a latency of 1-20 s; (ii) no significant effect of hyperventilation, and intermittent photic stimulation; (iii) reinforcement by slow sleep in only 15 per cent of cases.

In 38 per cent of cases, these characteristic occipital paroxysms are associated (i) with generalized bilaterally synchronous SW or polySW, characteristics of primary generalized epilepsy or (ii) with central or mid-temporal spikes characteristic of other types of primary partial epilepsy.

Semiology of seizures

Clinical ictal symptoms: they are ictal (visual and non-visual) as well as post-ictal.

(a) Visual ictal symptoms are represented by: (i) amaurosis, i.e. partial or complete visual loss in the entire visual field, sometimes preceded by initial hemianopsia, in 52 per cent of patients; (ii) elementary visual hallucinations, i.e. phosphenes (moving flashing spots) occupying the entire visual field in two-thirds of cases, in 45 per cent; (iii) complex visual hallucinations in 14 per cent; (iv) visual illusions, including micropsia, metamorphopsia or palinopsia, in 14 per cent. (v) Several of these visual symptoms may be reported by the same patient as part of one or several seizures.

(b) Non-visual symptoms may follow one or more of the visual symptoms and are represented by: (i) hemiclonic seizures in 43 per cent of patients; (ii) complex partial seizures with automatisms, indistinguishable from typical seizures of temporal lobe epilepsy, in 14 per cent; (iii) generalized tonic-clonic seizures in 13 per cent; (iv) other different ictal manifestations, including dysphasia, dysesthesia and adversive seizures, in 25 per cent.

Electroencephalographic ictal features: spontaneous seizures characterized by an occipital self-maintaining discharge over one or both occipital lobes were recorded in six patients (Fig. 4). Similar discharges were seen during sleep in five other patients without any clinical manifestations, probably representing subclinical electrographic seizures.

Post-ictal symptoms are represented by diffuse headache, only rarely hemicranial, in 33 per cent of patients; migraine-like nausea and vomiting were associated in 17 per cent.

Frequency and precipitating factors of seizures: frequency varies in periodic patterns from many attacks daily over several months, to occasional seizures separated by interseizure periods of several years in length.

There are no clear precipitating factors, but seizures were reported by 25 per cent of patients on going from a dark area into a brighter one, or conversely from a well-lit area into a darkened one.

Evolution

Prognosis is usually good, but not as good as in benign epilepsy of childhood with rolandic spikes. Complete seizure control was achieved in 60 per cent of patients with almost all of the classical anticonvulsants, chiefly phenobarbital, valproate, carbamazepine and benzodiazepines. In none of our cases have the typical seizures persisted past adolescence and other types of recurring seizures in adulthood were seen in only 5 per cent of patients.

Diagnosis

Positive diagnosis

In patients with the complete syndrome of BEOP, including ictal visual symptoms and interictal occipital EEG paroxysms (55 per cent of our cases) the diagnosis is clearly evident.

In patients with an incomplete or apparently incomplete syndrome, lacking the ictal visual symptoms or the interictal occipital EEG paroxysms (25 per cent of our cases), diagnosis is more difficult. In fact, many cases of BEOP may be missed if a history of visual manifestation is not carefully sought out, chiefly when the EEG pattern is not well recognized by the electro-encephalographer and the physician is not familiar with seeking such history.

In patients with a complete or incomplete electroclinical syndrome associated with the symptoms of another primary childhood epilepsy, which may be generalized (like *petit mal* absences and/or 3 c/s generalized SW) or partial (like nocturnal hemifacial seizures and/or rolandic spikes) (20 per cent of our cases), diagnosis is more difficult.

Differential diagnosis

Four conditions only must be differentiated from BEOP.

(1) *Secondary (or intermediary) generalized epilepsies* of children suggesting the Lennox-Gastaut syndrome but with occipital SW seen with eyes open as well as closed, in place of the more usual diffuse slow SW.

(2) *Elementary partial epilepsy secondary to occipital lesion,* which is much rarer in childhood than BEOP and differs (a) clinically, by a less complex ictal pattern usually marked by visual symptoms followed by tonic deviation without hemiclonic or psychomotor attacks and (b) EEGraphically, by intermittent spikes unreactive to eye-opening over a single occipital lobe, with abnormal background activity.

161

(3) *Complex partial epilepsy secondary to temporal lesion* which is at least as frequent in children as BEOP. The two may be confused in those rare instances where the psychomotor temporal lobe attacks are preceded by visual illusions or hallucinations, but the EEG is especially useful in the differentiation in showing the typical anterior temporal sharp waves.

(4) *Basilar migraine* (Bickerstaff 1961), which is very exceptional and easy to differentiate from BEOP by the absence of epileptiform occipital activity during and between the attacks of migraine.

Etiology

Normal neurospychiatric status of our patients combined with the finding of epilepsy in 37 per cent of their family histories demonstrate that BEOP, like the benign partial epilepsy with rolandic paroxysms, is a variety of the primary partial epilepsies which depends on an epileptic predisposition and not a cortical lesion. Primary partial epilepsies which have recently been proposed for inclusion in the international classification of epilepsies (Gastaut, 1983) and for the explanation of which Gastaut suggested 34 years ago (1950) and proposed very recently (1984) a thalamo-cortical mechanism comparable to the reticulo-cortical mechanism suggested by Gloor *et al.* (1982) as an explanation for primary generalized epilepsies, but restricted to only an areo-thalamic sector.

Pathophysiology

The pattern of spreading of the occipital ictal discharges has been previously studied in adults with secondary occipital epilepsy by Ajmone-Marsan and Ralston (1957), Bancaud (1969), Olivier *et al.,* (1982) and Gastaut (1958). Such distribution patterns evidently apply to BEOP and explain its four major clinical forms:

- strictly visual seizures, associated with a non-propagated focal occipital discharge;
- visual auras followed by hemisensory and/or hemiconvulsive attacks, related to spread of the occipital discharge to the central region;
- visual auras followed by psychomotor seizures, related to spread of the occipital discharge to the temporal lobe and/or the rhinencephalon;
- seizures without visual auras, corresponding either to the secondary spread of an occipital discharge in which the visual phenomena were not reported, or to the discharge of an independent secondary focus at a distance from the primary occipital focus.

The post-ictal migrainous symptoms of some attacks may be explained by persistance in the vascular bed of the posterior cerebral and basilar arteries of the initial vasodilation which accompanies the occipital ictal activity in children with impaired or labile cerebrovascular autoregulation and who are predisposed to migraines.

APPENDIX

Seven detailed case reports are included here to illustrate the main semiological and evolutive features of BEOP.

Case No. 1 (VB) — 21-year-old female
Seizures began at age 9 years with visual hallucinations sometimes accompanied by right or left hemiclonic convulsions, and disappeared at the age of 18, a few days after the introduction of clobazam. Twenty EEGs performed over nine years consistently showed typical bilaterally synchronous and symmetrical interictal occipitoposterotemporal SW, only on closure of the eyes (Figs 1 and 2).

Case No. 2 (NK) — 14-year-old male
Seizures began at age 4 years with four attacks of complex visual hallucinations, followed by a loss of vision lasting for 4 to 5 minutes and headache with nausea and vomiting. At age 8 years he presented sparkling flashes throughout his visual field for several seconds. Seven EEGs over seven years all showed typical bilaterally synchronous or asynchronous occipito-postero-temporal interictal SW on closure of the eyes (Fig. 3). Several visual seizures were recorded (Fig. 4). He has been free of seizures for the last four years since phenobarbital was prescribed.

Case No. 3 (VK) — 6-year-old male, the brother of case no. 2.
A single seizure occurred at age 6 years. Loss of vision lasting 45 minutes was followed by dysphasia lasting 2 minutes and a major convulsion. An EEG (Fig. 5) showed the same typical occipital SW activity as that of his brother.

Case No. 4 (PL) — 13-year-old male
After a single febrile convulsion at age 3 years, seizures began at age 9 years, heralded by a glowing yellow sphere throughout the visual field, followed by deviation of the head and eyes to the left with twitching of the left side of the mouth. Three EEGs showed posterior sharp wave activity confined to the right hemisphere on closure of the eyes (Fig. 6). A spontaneous seizure was recorded (Fig. 7A, B).

Case No. 5 (LG) — 14-year-old female
Seven generalized convulsions have occurred in early sleep over the last seven years, all followed by severe headache. Two EEGs have shown typical bilateral quasirhythmic occipito-postero-temporal sharp waves on closure of the eyes (Fig. 8). By chance an eighth most recent convulsive seizure occurred on going to bed, before the light was turned out, and was immediately preceded by a one minute loss of vision.
   This case was selected to show that certain instances, which seem to be examples of an incomplete BEOP syndrome, are in fact complete cases in which the history of the initial visual symptoms is not obtained because the patient is amnestic for the aura of the seizures or because the seizures begin during sleep.

Case No. 6. (YG) — 12-year-old female
This was the first case of BEOP recorded in Marseille, on 23 November 1949, published one year later (Gastaut, 1950). Seizures began at age 7 years with sparkling flashes throughout her visual field for several seconds, sometimes followed by a typical petit mal absence. An EEG (Fig. 9) showed: (a) interictal rhythmic SW confined to the right occipital lobe on closure of the eyes; (b) ictal 3 c/s generalized SW associated with petit mal absence induced by hyperventilation.
   Such a case was selected to show that a primary partial epilepsy like BEOP may be associated with a primary generalized epilepsy like petit mal.

Case No. 7(SP) — 7-year-old male, a paternal uncle with primary generalized epilepsy
A first seizure occurred at age 4 years. He awakened around midnight and had an adversive seizure to the right, followed by nausea, vomiting and diarrhoea, before losing consciousness for over one hour. Since then numerous other nocturnal attacks of right hemifacial twitching, salivation and anarthria have occurred. Two EEGs showed typical left occipital SW, attenuated by eye opening, and left-sided rolandic spikes (Fig. 10).
   Such a case was selected to show that two types of primary partial epilepsies (BEOP and benign partial epilepsy with rolandic spikes) may be associated.

Case no. 1

Fig. 1

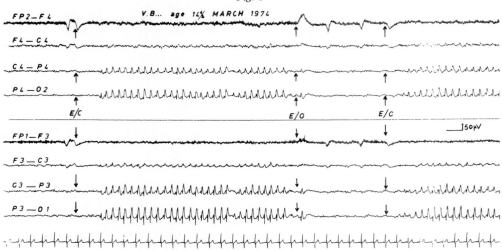

Fig. 2

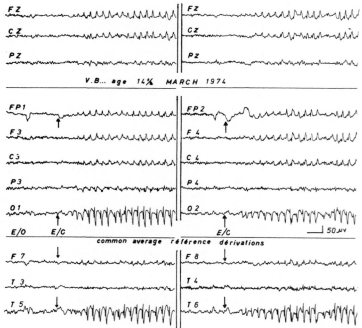

Figs. 1 and 2 (case No. 1). The typical interictal activity of BEOP: bilateral, synchronous, symmetric, surface-negative high amplitude SW, repeated at 3 c/s, localized to the occipital and posterior temporal regions. They appear within only 2 s of eye closure.

Case no. 2

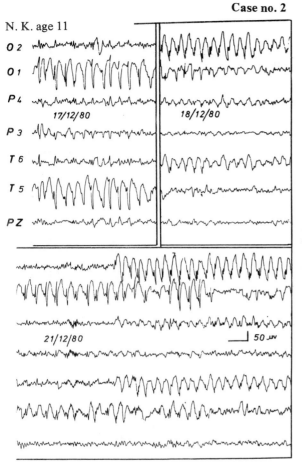

Fig. 3 (case No. 2). Characteristic morphology of the interictal epileptic activity of BEOP, but seen over each hemisphere or both, independently or synchronously.

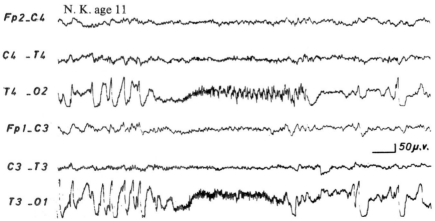

Fig. 4 (case No. 2). Ictal 16-18 c/s activity over both posterior regions. The child describes seeing stars.

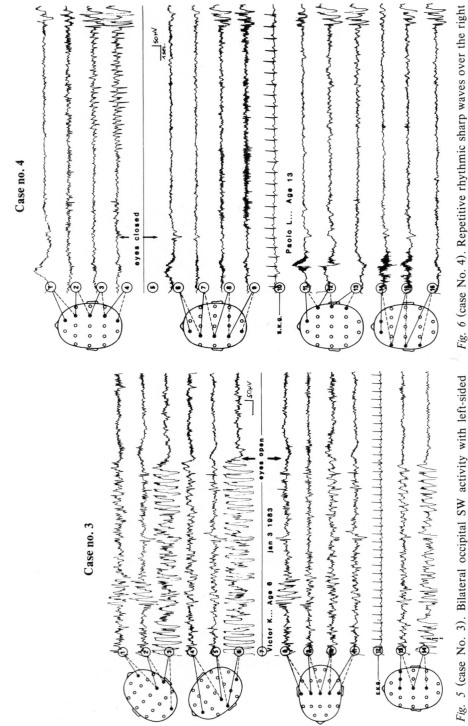

Case no. 4

Paolo L... Age 13

Fig. 6 (case No. 4). Repetitive rhythmic sharp waves over the right posterior quadrant, beginning 6s after eye closure. Note the spread to homologous areas of the left side after the sudden increase in amplitude of the right-sided discharge. Alpha activity is also reduced on the right side.

Case no. 3

Victor K... Age 6   Jan 3 1983

Fig. 5 (case No. 3). Bilateral occipital SW activity with left-sided predominance, suppressed by opening of the eyes. Note the occasional centro-temporal spikes over each hemisphere.

Case no. 4

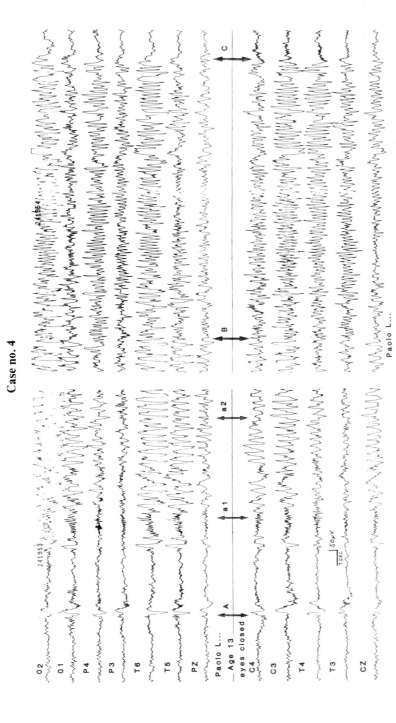

Fig. 7 (case No. 4). Occipital and postero-temporal ictal discharge with right-sided predominance. At A, the child said, 'Here it comes! I see yellow'. At a1 and a2 he is asked what he sees and described 'the lights of a car at night'. At B, he turned his head and eyes to the left and did not respond. At C, he suddenly asked 'Where am I?'.

167

Case no. 5

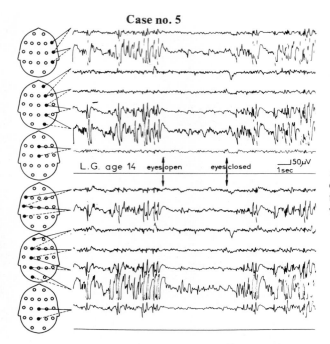

L.G. age 14   eyes open   eyes closed   50µV 1sec

Fig. 8 (case No. 5). Typical activity of BEOP. The visual symptoms of this patient's nocturnal seizures were not apparent for 6 years.

Case no. 6

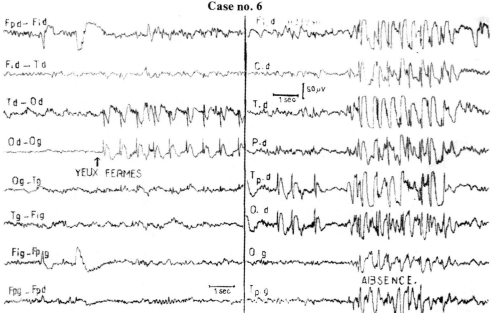

Fig. 9 (case No. 6). Left (bipolar derivations), occipital interictal rhythmic SW occurring after eye closure on the right occipital lobe. Right (common average reference derivation), note the precise occipital and postero-temporal localization of the interictal SW, and the generalized 3 c/s SW during an absence induced by hyperpnea and heralded by phosphenes during one or two seconds. Fpd = Fp2; Fid = F8; Cd = C4; Td = T4; Tpd = T6; Pd = P4; Od = O2; Ppg = Fp1; Fig = F7; Yeux fermés = eyes closed.

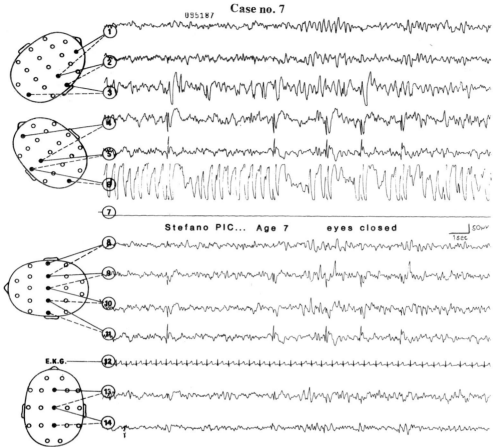

Fig. 10 (case No. 7). Left-sided quasi-rhythmic occipital SW activity with eyes closed. Note the associated left rolandic spikes, seen with the highest-amplitude occipital spikes. In this patient, clinical attacks were typical of epilepsy with rolandic spikes.

References

Ajmone-Marsan, C., Ralston, B. (1957): *The epileptic seizure: its functional morphology,* pp. 211-215. Charles C. Thomas: Springfield, Ill.

Bancaud, J. (1969): Les crises épileptiques d'origine occipitale. *Rev. Oto-Neuro-Ophtal.* **41,** 299-311.

Beaumanoir, A. (1983): Infantile epilepsy with occipital focus and good prognosis. *Eur. Neurol.* **22,** 43-52.

Bickerstaff, E. (1961): Basilar artery migraine. *Lancet* **1,** 5.

Camfield, P.R., Metrakos, K., Andermann, F. (1978): Basilar migraine, seizures and severe epileptiform E.E.G. abnormalities. *Neurology* **28,** 584-588.

Gastaut, H. (1950): Evidences électrographiques d'un mécanisme sous-cortical dans certaines épilepsies partielles. La signification clinique des "secteurs aréo-thalamiques". *Rev. Neurol.* **83,** 396-401.

Gastaut, H. (1958): A propos des décharges neuroniques développées à distance d'une lésion épileptogène. *Bases physiologiques de l'épilepsie,* ed T. Alajouanine. 163-183. Masson: Paris.

Gastaut, H. (1981): L'épilepsie bénigne de l'enfant à pointes-ondes occipitales. *Bull. Acad. Roy. Méd. Belgique* **136,** 540-555.

Gastaut, H. (1982*a*): L'épilepsie bénigne de l'enfant à pointe-ondes occipitales. *Rev. EEG Neurophysiol. Clin.* **12,** 179-201.

Gastaut, H. (1982*b*): Die benigne Epilepsie des Kindesalters mit okzipitalen Spike-wave. *EEG — EMG* **13,** 3-8.

Gastaut, H. (1982*c*): A new type of epilepsy : benign partial epilepsy of childhood with occipital spike-waves. *Clin. Electroencephalogr.* **13,** 13-22.

Gastaut, H. (1982*d*): A new type of epilepsy: benign partial epilepsy of childhood with occipital spike-waves. In *Advances in epileptology,* pp. 19-25. XIIIth Epilepsy International Symposium. Raven Press: New York.

Gastaut, H. (1983): A proposed completion of the current international classification of the epilepsies. In *Progress in epilepsy,* ed F.C. Rose, pp. 8-13. Pitman: London.

Gastaut, H. (1984): Classification des épilepsies. In Encyclopédie Médico-Chirurgicale (Paris), *Neurologie* 17044K[10].

Gastaut, H., Zifkin, B. (In press): Benign epilepsy of childhood with occipital paroxysms. In *Migraine and epilepsy.* Butterworths: Guildford.

Gibbs, F., Gibbs, E. (1952): *Atlas of Electroencephalography Vol. II. Epilepsy,* pp. 222-224. Addison-Wesley Press: Cambridge.

Gloor, P., Metrakos, S., Metrakos, K., Van Guelder, N. (1982): Neurophysiological, genetic and biochemical nature of the epileptic diathesis. In R. Broughton: H. Gastaut and the Marseille School's contribution to the neurosciences. *Electroenceph. Clin. Neuro-Physiol.* (Suppl.) **35,** 45-56.

Olivier, A., Gloor, P., Andermann, F. (1982): Occipito-temporal epilepsy studied with stereotaxically implanted depth electrodes. *Ann. Neurol.* **11,** 428-432.

*　　　　　*　　　　　*

Discussion pages 213-215

Epileptic syndromes in infancy, childhood and adolescence. J. Roger, C. Dravet, M. Bureau, F.E. Dreifuss and P. Wolf. John Libbey Eurotext Ltd ©1985.

Chapter 18
Benign Partial Epilepsy with Affective Symptoms ('Benign Psychomotor Epilepsy')

Bernardo DALLA BERNARDINA, Claudio CHIAMENTI, Giuseppe CAPOVILLA, Emanuela TREVISAN, Carlo Alberto TASSINARI*

*Neuropsichiatria Infantile, Università di Verona, Borgo Roma, 37100 — Verona, and *Clinica Neurologica, Università di Bologna, Italy*

Summary

The authors present the result of an electroclinical study of 26 children (14 girls and 12 boys) having epileptic attacks with affective symptoms. In 38.3 per cent of cases there was a previous familial history of epilepsy. The age of onset was between 2 to 9.4 years. The seizures occurred several times during the 24 hours, both day and night, but were controlled rapidly and permanently. Neurological and intellectual development was normal. This benign progression is correlated with an homogeneous ictal and interictal electroclinical picture enabling an early prognosis to be made. The nosology of this type of epilepsy and its analogy with epilepsy with rolandic spikes are discussed.

Introduction

Epileptic seizures with predominant affective symptoms, particularly an expression of terror, are complex partial seizures usually attributed to temporal lobe epilepsies (Cavazzuti, 1978; Beaumanoir, 1976). The onset of a partial complex epilepsy in a child generally suggests a poor prognosis: mental retardation and behavioural disturbances are said to be common in this form of epilepsy (Ounsted *et al.*, 1966; Stevens, 1975). A lesional aetiology is suspected in most cases and refractoriness to drug therapy is considered a frequent event (Ounsted *et al.*, 1966; Lindsay *et al.*, 1979; Glaser and Dixon, 1956). Some authors however, have reported a few cases with favourable outcome and even with disappearance of all interictal EEG abnormalities (Holowach *et al.*, 1961; Chao *et al.*, 1962; Cappella *et al.*, 1971; Lindsay *et al.*, 1979). The elements of good prognosis are: the single-typed seizures (Rodin,1968), their early onset (Cappella *et al.*, 1971), their affective expression (Cavazzuti, 1978) the existence of familial epileptic antecedents (Holowach *et al.*, 1961) and the lack of any recognizable aetiology (Lindsay *et al.*, 1979). More recently, under the definition of benign partial epilepsy with affective symptomatology or 'Benign Psychomotor Epilepsy', Dalla Bernardina *et al.*, (1980*a*,*b*; 1984), Plouin *et al.*, (1980), Dulac and Arthuis, (1980) have reported some observations characterized by a favourable evolution, probably representing a particular form of Benign Partial Epilepsy of Childhood. The aim of this paper is to describe the electroclinical features of this type of childhood epilepsy on the basis of a brief analysis of some personal observations.

Personal observations

Clinical data

This report describes 26 subjects with a mean age of 11 years 6 months (range 7 years-16 years 9 months) not showing any neurological and/or intellectual deficit.

The group comprised 14 girls and 12 boys. Familial antecedents of epilepsy were present in 38.3 per cent of cases. Between the ages of 9 and 24 months, five children had suffered from febrile convulsions which were either generalized (three patients) or unilateral (two patients), brief in duration and with no residual post-ictal defect. All subjects had normal CT scans.

The age of onset of afebrile fits ranged from 2 years to 9 years 4 months and was unevenly distributed with two peaks: the first between 2 and 5 years and the second between 6 and 9 years of life.

The predominant feature of the seizures was in all cases sudden fright or terror. This terror was expressed by the child starting to scream, to yell or to call his mother (12 cases); he clung to her or to anyone nearby (14 cases) or went to a corner of the room hiding his face in his hands (three cases). This terrorized expression was sometimes associated with either chewing or swallowing movements (six cases), distressed laugh (four cases), arrest of speech with glottal noises, moans and salivation (six cases) or some kind of autonomic manifestation such as pallor, sweating or abdominal pain, that the child expressed by bringing his hands on to his abdomen and saying 'it hurts me, it hurts me' (seven cases). These phenomena were associated with changes in awareness (loss of contact) that did not amount to complete unconsciousness. The mean duration of the fits was between 1 and 2 minutes (maximum 10 minutes). No post-ictal deficit was ever observed but the child could be temporarily sleepy or tired. In four cases the child had, at the same period, a few brief nocturnal orofacial clonic fits. But no child suffered from tonic, clonic, tonic-clonic or atonic fits during the evolution. For many children the seizures became frequent soon after onset, happening several times a day in 50 per cent of cases. From onset, in the great majority of the cases, the fits appeared both during waking and sleep with the similar semiology. In no cases were polymorphous seizures observed in the same child.

EEG data

The background activity was normal in all cases and the organization of sleep was also normal in all cases, even during the periods with frequent seizures. The more frequent interictal abnormalities (73 per cent) were characterized by ample slow spike/slow waves (looking like the rolandic spikes of benign epilepsy with rolandic spikes — BERS) involving the fronto-temporal or parieto-temporal areas of one or both hemispheres. These abnormalities had a great tendency to appear and disappear throughout the course and were always activated by sleep, without changing in morphology.

In the 57.6 per cent of cases the only paroxysmal abnormalities, at least during the first months of evolution, were characterized by rhythmic sharp waves in the fronto-temporal or in the parieto-temporal areas of one hemisphere.

In 57.6 per cent of cases, we observed the appearance of brief bursts of generalized spike waves, alone or in association with one of the two types of focal abnormalities described above. These generalized spike waves could appear during drowsiness but never increased in frequency during slow sleep.

In 19 cases one or several seizures were recorded during waking and/or sleep.

In 15 instances the seizure discharges were clearly localized in the fronto-temporal, the centro-temporal or the parietal areas whereas in four instances they were more diffuse and it was often difficult to recognize a localized onset. The polygraphic records showed that the attacks were associated with various movements but never of a tonic or clonic type. Furthermore they showed that in the same child the ictal pattern was relatively stereotyped both during the awake state and during sleep.

Evolution

Three subjects never received treatment because of their relatively low frequency of seizures. In all but two of treated cases, the treatment was effective even for those patients where treatment was started 6 to 18 months after onset because of misdiagnosis — these children having initially been considered as having psychological problems. In two cases, infrequent attacks persisted for some months or years despite treatment but ultimately disappeared. The most efficient therapy was monotherapy with carbamazepine or phenobarbital. Nine cases, aged more than 13 years and now treatment free for one or more years, did not have any more seizures.

At the time of frequent seizures, some children had major behavioural troubles, associated in three cases with retarded intellectual efficiency. When last seen, the patients had neither intellectual nor motor sequelae, nor social or significant school adaptation difficulties.

Discussion

The diagnosis of this type of seizures may present some difficulties to the clinician. They may first be misdiagnosed as non-epileptic attacks (fear attacks or *pavor nocturnus*), since many features at onset may be misleading: the lack of personal antecedents and of neurological abnormalities; the ictal symptoms and the coincidence of their appearance with behavioural disorders and/or with acute psychological problems and, in some cases, the absence of EEG abnormalities.

However the diagnosis is fairly easy if the following features are taken into account: in the majority of the cases the episodes appeared both during waking and sleep with similar symptomatology; they were very frequent; the nocturnal seizures were most frequent on falling asleep, whereas *pavor nocturnus* appears especially during slow sleep (Gastaut *et al.*, 1965). It is however important to emphasize that the nature of the attacks we report is different from that of *pavor nocturnus* which are not epileptic, even when they appear in epileptic patients (Tassinari *et al.*, 1972). If a precise description of the seizures is not available, or if they are absent or rare during waking, the EEG recording of a seizure may be required to obtain an accurate diagnosis even if EEG interictal abnormalities are observed.

The second and most difficult problem is that once the proper diagnosis of epilepsy has been made, the clinician generally suspects a cerebral lesion and therefore a poor prognosis when faced with frequent complex partial seizures with localized EEG interictal abnormalities. Indeed some patients with a cerebral lesion are known to suffer from attacks of the kind we report. In such cases, however, these either are associated with other kinds of seizures or constitute the aura of longer attacks having a major motor component (Penfield and Jasper, 1954; Williams, 1956; Mullan and Penfield, 1959; Weil 1959).

The evolution of our cases shows that these patients suffer from a benign kind of epilepsy. It is interesting to notice that the epilepsy we report is similar in many respects to BERS which has a well-established favourable outcome (Beaussart and Faou, 1978). The analogies are: the age at onset (Dalla Bernardina *et al.*, 1981), with two peaks of frequency; the frequent familial epileptic antecedents (Heijbel *et al.*, 1975); the brievity of fits (Loiseau and Beaussart, 1973); the good response to treatment (Lerman and Kivity-Ephraim, 1974); the morphology of focal paroxysmal abnormalities and their activation during sleep (Dalla Bernardina *et al.*, 1982); the frequency of associated generalized spike waves discharges, not increasing in frequency during slow sleep (Dalla Bernardina *et al.*, 1982, 1984). Such similarities are a further element in favour of the genetic nature of this epilepsy and consequently of its benignity. From the nosological point of view it is possible to discuss whether this epilepsy does or does not represent a separate form of partial benign epilepsy. In fact, as outlined by Aicardi (1983), the predominance of fear over other ictal manifestations probably has not in itself an independent predictive value which is greater than that of any other ictal symptom occurring in a similar clinical context. From the practical point of view we consider that the homogeneous electroclinical pattern above described may lead the clinician to the proper diagnosis and therefore permits an early favourable prognosis to be set.

As previously recommended (Dalla Bernardina *et al.*, 1980*a, b*, 1984; Dulac and Arthuis, 1980) we propose to call this form of epilepsy Benign Partial Epilepsy with Affective Symptoms or Benign Psychomotor Epilepsy.

References

Aicardi, J. (1983): Complex partial seizures in childhood. In *Advances in epileptology:* XIVth Epilepsy International Symposium, pp. 237-242, ed M. Parsonage. Raven Press: New York.

Beaumanoir, A. (1976): *Les épilepsies infantiles. Problèmes de diagnostic et de traitement.* Roche: Bâle.

Beaussart, M., Faou, R. (1978): Evolution of epilepsy with rolandic paroxysmal foci: a study of 324 cases. *Epilepsia* **19**, 337-342.

Cappella, L., Cavazzuti, G.B., Nalin, A. (1971): Casi di epilessia psicomotoria insorti nel primo triennio. *Minerva Pediatrica* **23**, 1359-1366.

Cavazzuti, G.B. (1978): Nosologia delle convulsioni della prima infanzia. *Boll. Lega It. Epil.* **22-23**, 127-135.

Chao, D., Sexton, J.A., Sautos Pardo, L. (1962): Temporal lobe epilepsy in children. *J. Pediatr.* **60**, 686-693.

Dalla Bernardina, B., Bureau, M., Dravet, C., Dulac, O., Tassinari, C.A., Roger, J. (1980*a*): Epilepsie bénigne de l'enfant avec crises à séméiologie affective. *Rev. EEG Neurophysiol.* **10**, 8-18.

Dalla Bernardina, B., Colamaria, V., Bondavalli, S., Tassinari, C.A., Dulac, O., Dravet, C., Roger, J., Bureau, M. (1980*b*): Epilepsie partielle bénigne de l'enfant à séméiologie affective. *Boll. Lega It. Epil.* **29-30**, 131-137.

Dalla Bernardina, B., Beghini, G., Bondavalli, S., Colamaria, V. (1981): L'epilessia parziale benigna dell'infanzia a parossismi rolandici e/o mediotemporali (EPR). In *Le epilessie infantili benigne,* atti del convegno di Verona, Sigma-Tau 23-35.

Dalla Bernardina, B., Bondavalli, S., Colamaria, V. (1982): Benign epilepsy of childhood with rolandic spikes (BERS) during sleep. In *Sleep and epilepsy,* pp 495-506. ed M.B. Sterman, M.N. Shouse, P. Passouant. Academic Press: London & New York.

Dalla Bernardina, B., Colamaria, V., Capovilla, G., Bondavalli, S. (1984): Sleep and benign partial epilepsies of childhood. In *Epilepsy sleep and sleep deprivation,* pp 119-133, ed R. Degen, E. Niedermeyer. Elsevier Science Publishers B.V.: Amsterdam.

Dulac, O., Arthuis, M. (1980): Epilepsie psychomotrice bénigne de l'enfant. In *Journées parisiennes de Péd.,* pp 211-220. Flammarion: Paris.

Gastaut, H., Batini, C., Broughton, R., Fressy, J., Tassinari, C.A. (1965): Etude EEG des phénomènes épisodiques non épileptiques au cours du sommeil. In *Le sommeil de nuit normal et pathologique,* pp 215-236. Masson: Paris.

Glaser, G.H., Dixon, M.S. (1956): Psychomotor seizures in childhood. Clinical study. *Neurology* **6,** 646-655.

Heijbel, J., Blom, S., Rasmuson, M. (1975): Benign epilepsy of children with centro-temporal EEG foci. A genetic study. *Epilepsia* **16,** 285-293.

Holowach, J., Renda, Y.A., Wagner, I. (1961): Psychomotor seizures in childhood. *J. Pediatr.* **59,** 339-345.

Lerman, P., Kivity-Ephraim, S. (1974): Carbamazepine sole anticonvulsivant for focal epilepsy of childhood. *Epilepsia* **15,** 229-234.

Lindsay, J., Ounsted, C., Richards, P. (1979): Long term outcome in children with temporal lobe seizures: Social outcome and childhood factors. *Develop. Med. Child. Neurol.* **21,** 285-298.

Loiseau, P., Beaussart, M. (1973): The seizures of benign childhood epilepsy with rolandic paroxysmal discharge. *Epilepsia* **14,** 381-389.

Mullan, S., Penfield, W. (1959): Illusions of comparative interpretation and emotion. *Arch. Neurol. Psychiatry* **81,** 269-284.

Ounsted, C., Lindsay, J., Norman, R. (1966): *Biological factors in temporal lobe epilepsy.* Heinemann: London.

Penfield, W., Jasper, H.H. (1954): *Epilepsy and the functional anatomy of the human brain.* Little Brown: Boston.

Plouin, P., Lerique, A., Dulac, O. (1980): Etude électroclinique et évolution dans 7 observations des crises partielles complexes dominées par un comportement de terreur chez l'enfant. *Boll. Lega It. Epil.* **29-30,** 139-143.

Rodin, E.A. (1968): *The prognosis of patients with epilepsy.* Charles C. Thomas: Springfield, Illinois.

Stevens, J.R. (1975): Interictal clinical manifestations of complex partial seizures. In *Complex partial seizures and their treatment.* Advances in Neurology, Vol. 11, pp. 85-107, ed J.K. Penry, D.D. Daly, Raven Press: New York.

Tassinari, C.A., Mancia, D., Dalla Bernardina, B., Gastaut, H. (1972): Pavor nocturnus of non epileptic nature in epileptic children. *EEG Clin. Neurophysiol.* **33,** 603-607.

Weil, A.A. (1959): Ictal emotions occurring in temporal lobe dysfunction. *Archs Neurol.* **1,** 87-111.

Williams, D. (1956): The structure of emotions reflected by epileptic experience. *Brain* **79,** 29-67.

*　　　　*　　　　*

Discussion pages 213-215

Epileptic syndromes in infancy, child-
hood and adolescence. J. Roger,
C. Dravet, M. Bureau, F.E.
Dreifuss and P. Wolf. John Libbey
Eurotext Ltd ©1985.

Chapter 19
Benign Partial Epilepsy
with Extreme Somato-Sensory
Evoked Potentials

Carlo Alberto TASSINARI* and Pasquale DE MARCO‡

* Istituto di Clinica Neurologica, Bologna, Italy
‡ Divisione di Neuropsichiatria Infantile Ospedali Riuniti, Trento, Italy.

Summary

In a population of 15 000 children, it was found that tactile stimulation, mainly tapping on the
soles or heels of the feet, could elicit high-voltage evoked potentials in the EEGs of 1 per cent of
them. A longitudinal study of 16 of these subjects showed a stereotyped electroclinical evolution
in four stages. Seizures began (fourth period) within five months to two years after the appearance of the focal abnormalities. Such seizures were rare, but in some cases they were grouped in
status epilepticus. They were usually of the partial motor type, with version of the head. They
occurred mainly during the daytime. The fits were short-lived, however, and after a year had
mostly disappeared, while the ESEPs and spontaneous interictal focal abnormalities sometimes
persisted for several years before disappearing too. The subjects were otherwise neurologically
and psychologically normal throughout the observation and follow-up period.

Definition and prevalence

This short review is based on the De Marco and Tassinari work in 1981. Since the De
Marco and Negrin report (1973), it was found that in 1 per cent of children without
overt neurological pathology, tapping of the feet could elicit high-voltage evoked
potentials. Such extreme somatosensory evoked potentials (ESEPs) were evident on
the EEG as high-voltage spikes, up to 400 μV of amplitude, involving the parietal and
parasagittal regions. It was found that 155 children (out of 15 000 who have had tapping
of the feet during EEG records), mainly males (105), showed ESEPs at an age ranging
from 1 to 13 years with a peak between four to six years (80 cases) of age. Thirty of
these 155 patients had epileptic seizures when ESEPs were discovered; of the remaining 125, 16 later developed epileptic seizures.

ESEPs and epilepsy

The electroclinical evolution of this syndrome in the 16 patients who developed epileptic seizures progressed through four distinct periods.

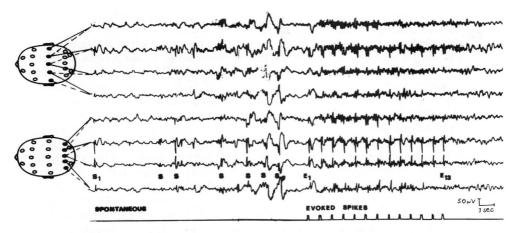

Fig. 1. Subject during the second period of the evolution, showing both spontaneous focal spikes (S1-S8) and ESEPs (E1-E13) evoked by tapping the left heel, both involving the same region and with phase reversal around Pz. Last bottom trace is a mechanical signal for the stimulus.

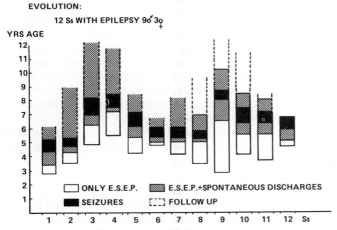

Fig. 2. Electroclinical evolution of 12 subjects first having ESEPs on an otherwise normal EEG record (white area, first period). Second and third period (hatched areas) are characterized by the presence of both ESEPs and interictal spontaneous focal discharges on the EEG (see Fig. 1). Seizures occur in the fourth period (black areas), last approximately 1 year, and then subside. ESEPs and focal discharges may persist after the seizures have stopped (hatched areas as in second period) and then disappear, as in cases 8-11 (follow-up showed normal EEGs and no ESEPs).

In the *first period* (Fig. 2), which occurred between the ages of 2.5 and 5.5 years, the only abnormal EEG feature was the presence of ESEPs evoked by tapping of one or both feet or, less frequently, other parts of the body. Such ESEPs constituted the only EEG findings (in some cases, until their disappearance) in the absence of other spontaneous paroxysmal EEG abnormalities in patients without seizures or other neurological impairment. The subjects had previously had a normal EEG record (at rest as well as during hyperventilation and photic stimulation).

177

The *second period* was marked by the appearance of spontaneous focal EEG abnormalities during sleep (for further details, see Negrin and De Marco, 1977).

In the *third period,* spontaneous focal abnormalities appeared when the subjects were awake. This period was characterized by the occurrence of spontaneous discharges, usually focal spikes, involving the same regions where the ESEPs were first observed. The morphology and topography of the spontaneous focal abnormalities and the ESEPs were strikingly similar (Fig. 1). The time interval between the onset of the ESEPs and the occurrence of the spontaneous focal discharges is not precisely known, since we do not know in each case when the ESEPs originally appeared; they were presumably present for an unknown period before the first EEG investigation. However, the latency between the discovery of the ESEPs and the appearance of the spontaneous focal spikes varied from nine months to four years (mean, 21 months).

The *fourth period* was characterized by the appearance of electroclinical seizures. Following the spontaneous focal discharges, seizures occurred with a delay varying from five months (Fig. 2, case 7) to two years (Fig. 2, case 9), with a mean interval of about one year. The mean age at onset of seizures was six years (range, 4.5-8 years).

Types of seizures

According to the clinical description, most seizures in each patient were of the same type and consisted of motor seizures with head and body version (12 subjects). Two patients had generalized tonic-clonic seizures, apparently without focal onset, while in another patient seizures were mainly of the tonic type. One patient had primarily somatosensory seizures with a slight impairment of consciousness, if any at all.

In one subject, repeated seizures were clinically characterized by version of the head to the right, and hyperextension of the right arm, followed by a few jerks, without motor manifestations of the legs, during the seizures the EEG showed an abrupt disappearance of the preexisting background rhythmic activity, with flattening of the activity lasting 10-15s, followed by a short period of some slow theta and delta waves disturbed by numerous artifacts. Interictal abnormalities consisted of spikes in the left parietal and central regions, where ESEPs could also be evoked by tapping the sole of the right foot. A probable focal onset could be presumed from clinical and interictal findings but was not documented during the ictal recordings.

Frequency of seizures

Seizures were rare, occurring two to six times a year. They always occurred during the day in 14 subjects, but were present during both day and night in two subjects. Their repeated occurrence in two patients, however, amounted to partial motor status epilepticus lasting several hours. In one patient, seizures were extremely frequent, ranging from 200-800 daily for 15 days. Consciousness was slightly impaired during the ictal state but was normal during the interictal period. The seizures were controled only temporarily by various treatments. They were finally stopped by corticotropin (ACTH) therapy. On the occasion of a second status in this same patient, both ACTH and antiepileptic drug therapy failed. The seizures eventually diminished and then stopped spontaneously after several days.

The seizures usually persisted for about one year and then subsided. As shown in Fig. 2, the attacks disappeared before nine years of age and did not recur during the follow-up period, which lasted an average of eight years. The spontaneous interictal focal discharges, as well as the ESEPs, sometimes persisted for years after the seizures had stopped (hatched areas between the dotted lines in Fig. 2), while in some patients (e.g., cases 8-10), they disappeared within 1-3 years after cessation of the seizures, and the ESEPs were no longer observed.

Neurological and psychological appraisal

Neurological and neuroradiological assessment (arteriography or CT scans) of the patients who had epileptic seizures that later subsided showed no evidence of neurological damage. Noteworthy, however, is the history of simple febrile convulsions in seven (43.8 per cent) of the 16 subjects who developed epileptic seizures. The IQ, assessed by a standard group of tests, showed normal values throughout the electroclinical evolution, suggesting that the seizures did not lead to psychological impairment (De Marco and Burighel, 1979).

Antiepileptic therapy

Antiepileptic drugs, mainly barbiturates, phenytoin, or carbamazepine, in various dosages, were given to the 16 patients who developed seizures. The effectiveness of the treatment was difficult to assess, however.

Discussion

It seems appropriate to discuss both the similarities and the differences in the benign focal epilepsy described here, characterized by the ESEPs, and the benign epilepsy of children with rolandic or mid-temporal foci (Lombroso, 1967; Loiseau and Beaussart, 1973). Clinical features common to both forms of epilepsy are the absence of organic brain lesions, seizures of the partial motor type, the rarity of the seizures, and the tendency of the fits to regress with age. Both syndromes share an increased incidence of febrile convulsions, which were eight times more prevalent in our patients than in the general population.

A common EEG trait is the presence of focal or multifocal spikes, which tend to disappear with age. The two syndromes are distinguished however, by the following clinical aspects:

(1) Although the seizures of both syndromes are chiefly of the motor type, the seizures in patients with ESEPs usually do not affect the facial muscles, and they occur predominantly during the daytime.

(2) Seizures accompanied by ESEPs persist for about one year, whereas the fits of benign epilepsy with rolandic foci may persist for several years.

(3) A male predominance (3 : 1) seems evident in the ESEP cases, and it is not due to a preponderance of males (49 per cent) in our population; a sex difference was not observed in the syndrome of benign epilepsy with rolandic foci (Loiseau and Beaussart, 1973).

(4) Electroencephalographically, the topography of the spikes in the latter syndrome is mainly rolandic or mid-temporal, while in the case of the ESEPs the spikes are mostly parietal and parasagittal.

(5) Finally, and most important, ESEPs have been observed in only one case of benign epilepsy with rolandic foci out of more than 100 such cases examined by one of us (De Marco, 1980).

Conclusion

Thus, it seems that we are dealing with a particular form of benign epilepsy, which is expressed primarily as partial motor seizures preceded by ESEPs and associated with interictal focal EEG abnormalities involving mainly the parietal regions. The appearance of ESEPs before the possible occurrence of seizures constitutes an interesting and important EEG sign, which should be searched for systematically in children. In the absence of cerebral organic lesions, the ESEPs suggest that we are dealing with a functional phenomenon, which is likely to be age-related, having a maximum expression around four years of age and greater prevalence in boys.

References

De Marco, P. (1980): Possibilities of a temporal relationship between the morphology and frequency of parietal somato-sensory evoked spikes and the occurrence of epileptic manifestations. *Clin. EEG* **11**, 132-135.

De Marco, P., Burighel, F. (1979): Correlazioni fra le punte evocate parietali e alcune comuni turbe neuropsichiatriche infantili. *Riv. Ital. EEG Neurofisiol. Clin.* **2**, 683-688.

De Marco, P., Negrin, P. (1973): Parietal focal spikes evoked by contralateral tactile somatotopic stimulations in four non-epileptic subjects. *Electroenceph. Clin. Neurophysiol.* **34**, 308-312.

De Marco, P., Tassinari, C.A. (1981): Extreme Somatosensory Evoked Potential (ESEP): an EEG sign forecasting the possible occurrence of seizures in children. *Epilepsia* **22**, 569-575.

Loiseau, P., Beaussart, M. (1973): The seizures of benign childhood epilepsy with rolandic paroxysmal discharges. *Epilepsia* **14**, 381-389.

Lombroso, C.T. (1967): Sylvian seizures and mid-temporal spike foci in children. *Archs. Neurol* **17**, 52-59.

Negrin, P., De Marco, P. (1977): Parietal focal spikes evoked by tactile somatotopic stimulation in 60 non-epileptic children: The nocturnal sleep and clinical and EEG evolution. *Electroenceph. Clin. Neurophysiol.* **43**, 312-316.

*   *   *

Discussion pages 213-215

Epileptic syndromes in infancy, childhood and adolescence. J. Roger, C. Dravet, M. Bureau, F.E. Dreifuss and P. Wolf. John Libbey Eurotext Ltd ©1985.

Chapter 20
The Landau-Kleffner Syndrome

Anne BEAUMANOIR

Division de Neurophysiologie Clinique, Hôpital Cantonal Universitaire, Genève, Switzerland

Summary

The Landau-Kleffner syndrome is a childhood disorder associating an acquired aphasia and multifocal spikes and spike and wave discharges, which are not stable in the course of the evolution. Two other symptoms are also observed: epileptic seizures (67.6 per cent) and behavioural and psychomotor disturbances (71.4 per cent). From the neuropsychological point of view, there is a verbal auditory agnosia with rapid reduction of spontaneous oral expression. Epileptic seizures are generally rare and various, more often generalized convulsive or partial motor. They always disappear before the age of 15, as well as the EEG abnormalities in the cases which had been studied for that. It is suggested to consider only cases with clinical seizures as an epileptic syndrome. The two following names could be used: Landau-Kleffner syndrome with epilepsy or acquired aphasia of childhood with epilepsy.

Introduction

A review of the literature to get the most complete features of the Landau-Kleffner syndrome (LKS) suggests the following main characteristics. It is a disease of the child associating two major symptoms: an acquired aphasia and a paroxysmal electroencephalographic (EEG) recording with spikes and spikes and waves, mostly multifocal and unstable in the course of evolution, and two accessory symptoms: a psychomotor or behavioural disturbances and an epilepsy of favourable outcome.

Although most usable observations (about two-thirds of the 130 cases published since the original work of Landau and Kleffner in 1957) are suitable to evaluate only one, at the most two criteria, the association of acquired aphasia with paroxysmal EEG recording is constantly mentioned.

Epidemiology

The prevalence cannot yet be ascertained. However only 61 observations have been published between 1957 and 1978, while 70 new cases have been added in the last 5 years. Dugas *et al.* (1982), in a Parisian psycho-pathological clinic, see one new patient per year.

Sex ratio shows a clear male predominance with about two affected boys to each girl. Familiar and personal medical history are irrelevant and there are no associated neurological signs.

Hemispheric dominance has been thoroughly reported in only a few cases. It does not seem to influence the outbreak or evolution of the LKS.

Semiological study

Aphasia

Aphasia commonly starts (except in less than 1/10 of cases) with an auditory verbal agnosia sometimes extending to familiar noises. Patients are then incapable of attributing a semantic value to acoustic signals and their consequent indifference makes them often appear as hypoacousic or autistic children. Their history can reveal pre-existing difficulties in language acquisition; it then could be a congenital deaf-mutism revealed at the moment of emerging speech (Cavazzuti, 1979; Dugas et al., 1976; Lou et al., 1977; McKinney and McGreal, 1974). Spontaneous verbal expression is always reduced early (with stereotypies, perseverations, paraphasias) or even abolished. Recovery of language essentially depends on the age of onset of the syndrome (most often before 7 years of age) and on the logopedic re-education, with a better prognosis when started early. Operational and intellectual capacities are usually preserved during the complete course of evolution.

When aphasia starts after the child has acquired writing, and if the child retains this capability, re-eduction is facilitated.

Psychomotor disturbances

Psychomotor disturbances, especially hyperkinesia, are mentioned in about half of the observations. Personality disturbances are also frequently noted but seldomly analysed. Development disturbances other than those linked to language problems are frequent. However, search for a primitive personality disorder has been advocated by certain authors, especially when the character of afferential disorganization of LKS has led to confusion with a psychotic syndrome of psychogenic origin.

Electroencephalogram

EEG is non-specific and can be seen in affections other than LKS. Fundamental awake activities when mentioned are normal. However in some cases, dysrhythmia is noted. It is probably due, although only one author mentions this possibility, to the frequent heavy medication with three, sometimes four antiepileptic drugs. The typical EEG findings are repetitive spikes and spikes and waves of great amplitude, organized in foci variable in time and space. These multiple foci express themselves either constantly, or during certain periods of the evolution. They are preferentially located in the temporal regions (Fig. 2) (1/2 of cases), in parieto-occipital regions (1/3 of cases), without clear hemispheric predominence. Anterior and mid-temporal foci are more seldom found. Data in the literature are scarce to figure out the influence of age on the topographical distribution of foci. In 90 per cent of the observations available for this specific point, focus was already present on the first EEG recorded, that is between the ages of 3 to 9 years. The peak of appearance seems to be around 3 to 5 years of age. Age at the moment of last recording is seldomly mentioned. Recordings made after the age of 15 did not show spikes. According to the very few authors having studied this point, recordings show little sensitivity to hyperpnea or photic stimulation. Sleep, especially slow sleep, activates the record with diffusion of the paroxysmal discharges. Despite good agreement between various authors about this point, the number of nocturnal recordings (25 as a whole) is however not sufficient to definitely define the sleep pattern of LKS. The pattern seems quite similar to sleep epileptic status. In a state of low vigilance, short bursts of diffuse slow spikes and waves may arise. These abnormalities have been interpreted variously. The existence of such slow spike and waves has suggested to some that the LKS and the Lennox-Gastaut syndrome (LGS) were identical. This is however contradicted by favourable electroclinical evolution, by the constantly normal fundamental trace and by the absence of diurnal or nocturnal tonic seizures in LKS. Results of neuroradiological examinations (pneumoencephalography, arteriography, CT-scan) have failed to demonstrate any morphological abnormalities. In the cases where investigations were performed in order to search a specific encephalopathy or a subacute encephalitis (cerebral biopsy, serological examination), the findings are heterogeneous. (Lou *et al.*, 1977, McKinney and McGreal, 1974; Pouplard and Pasquier, 1978).

Thus the paroxysmal discharges recorded during wakefulness and sleep do not seem to be promoted by a detectable structural epileptogenic lesion. The EEG in LKS is characterized by a normal recording but adding multiple functional foci of the type already described by numerous authors since 1951 in various situations which suggest an immaturity of afferent systems or a sectorial disorganization consecutive to deafferentation.

Epilepsy

As Landau and Kleffner already noted, not all patients present epileptic fits. Seizures occur in about 70 per cent of patients. In one-third of cases, there is a single seizure or status epilepticus, mostly at the beginning of evolution. Isolated seizures appear between 5 and 10 years. In cases of recurrent fits, the first ones mostly occur between 4 and 6 years. After the age of 10 only 20 per cent of patients still present seizures and there is none noted after the age of 15. Repetitive seizures are rare, mainly nocturnal and usually well controlled by therapy. Therapy is however often heavy, probably an attempt to abolish all electrical paroxysmal events. Ictal semiology has been poorly studied, is heterogeneous and includes convulsive and non convulsive seizures. However, the infrequency of complex partial seizures with psychomotor automatisms is striking. Tonic seizures have been described in only one patient, but never recorded.

A familial history of epilepsy is noted in 12 per cent of cases when it has been looked for. This proportion falls down to 5 per cent in non-epileptic cases.

Discussion

Pathogenesis of the syndrome remains hypothetical. We propose to consider the LKS as a rupture in the loop: hearing — verbal integration - spoken language. Aphasia usually begins during the crucial period of language acquisition and of functional lateralization of the hemispheres. When it takes place, it corresponds to an auditive agnosia in almost all cases. These data are taken as evidence (for example by Kellerman, 1978, or Dugas *et al.*, 1982) to localize the interruption at the level of subcortical connexions which are responsible for the activation of the temporal regions. Other authors, and among them Njiokitgien (1983), suggest that a delayed or halted maturation of the functional structures and of the interhemispheric pathways (particularly corpus callosum) could be the cause of the LKS.

The aphasia disturbs the apprehension of the patient's sensory, cognitive and affective environment, leading to behavioural disturbances. However some authors eg, Revol *et al.* (1982) note that if interest in communication is lacking, due to social relational difficulties or to an affective shock, LKS could be related to pre-existing personality disorders, being in this case an aspect of the afferential disorganization of a psychotic syndrome.

The EEG non-specific foci of the LKS can result from de-afferentation which can occur at various levels of the corticopetal pathways, thalamic connexions of the cortical receptive and integrative areas or interhemispheric pathways. In accordance with the results of electrophysiological and neurochemical experients on disuse supersensitivity of the isolated and epileptic cortex (Sharpless, 1969) the presence of functional spike foci as well as the occurrence of seizures in certain patients finds an explanation.

Whatever their place in the chain of events, the EEG foci, most often bi-temporal or bi-temporo-occipital, reflect a local bi-hemispheric dysfunction. The diffusion into multiple foci in the course of evolution may be due to remodelling of speech areas or to dysfunction of one or more areas of integration consecutive to a new mode of organization needed by aphasia. The EEG anomalies are moreover not specific of the LKS. Similar foci have been described in various clinical situations and in particular in cases of disturbed language acquisition not related with the LKS. They constitute the EEG interictal sign of the benign epilepsy of childhood.

Therefore can the LKS be considered as an epileptic syndrome and, in this case, how should it be classified? In 30 per cent of the affected subjects, a seizure (a brief episode starting and ending abruptly) does not occur. Consequently, to consider the LKS as an epileptic syndrome attaches undue relevance to the EEG findings in the absence of electroclinical correlation. Nevertheless, taking into account the fact that a simultaneous improvement in EEG and in aphasia can occasionally be observed, which may sometimes be attributed to antiepileptic therapeutics, certain authors believe that the LKS is a kind of epilepsy. This seems hazardous; on the one hand because it is based on the observation of only few cases followed during many years, and on the other hand because it gives way to the persisting but erroneous opinion which identifies spikes and spikes and waves with epilepsy.

A common pathogenesis has been suggested for the spikes originating from the immature isolated cortex, de-afferented by an adjacent lesion, as well as from the epileptic cortex. These data could suggest the possibility of a place for 'bio-electric epilepsy' among the epileptic syndromes of childhood; this entity would be characterized by an EEG overloaded with localized or diffuse spikes and spike and waves, adding an aphasia in the case of the LKS.

Should the classification of the epilepsies include such a 'bio-electric epilepsy', the LKS could belong to it. But if one takes into account the definition of the epilepsies - diseases or syndromes characterized by recurring epileptic seizures - only two out of three cases of LKS could be classified among epilepsies.

For the moment, the LKS must be considered as a pathologic entity of childhood whose EEG reflect bihemispheric dysfunctioning. It is probably responsible for (or secondary to) de-afferentation, leading (or consecutive to) an auditory agnosia which constitutes an aphasic syndrome very similar to the deaf-mutism with complex perceptive problems as described by De Ajuriaguerra et al. (1962). In certain cases, seizures took place, the clinical and evolution characteristics of which are those of the benign epilepsy of childhood or primary partial epilepsy.

If LKS must be retained among the epileptic syndromes, then a special mention should notify the presence of seizures, such as 'LKS with epilepsy' (LKSE) or childhood-acquired aphasia with epilepsy (AAE).

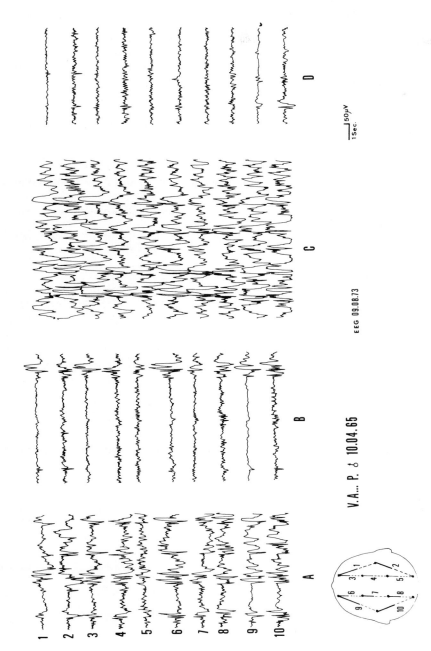

Fig. 1. Telemetric record during one day. A = 9.30a.m. B = 11a.m. C = 3p.m. (sleep); D = 5p.m.

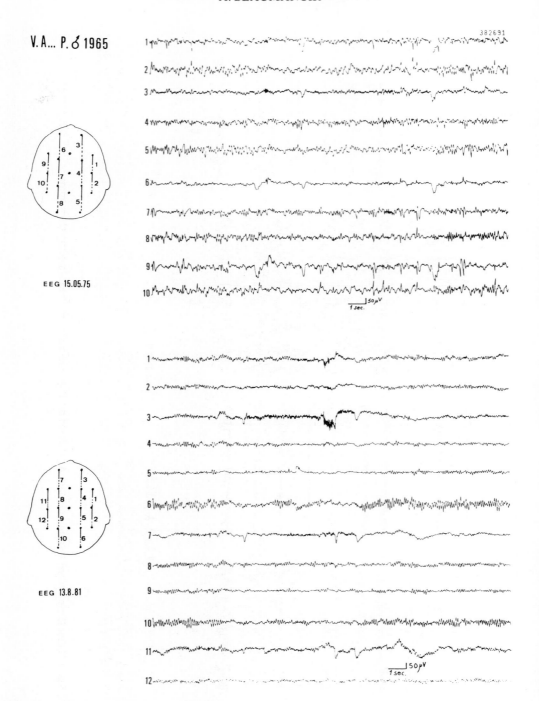

Fig. 2. Follow-up. EEG at 10 years and at 16 years.

Case report

Pascal V.A. was born in 1965. He is ambidextrous and free of any relevant family medical history. He developed febrile convulsions at age 17 months. EEG recording was then normal. Following this episode, parents noted during a couple of weeks a slowing in his — so far normal — psychomotor development, especially in speech-acquisition. A second EEG was done because of appearance of hyperkinetic behaviour with sudden bursts of anger. It showed left occipital spike and wave focus. At age 5 and for no obvious reason, the child developed difficulties in understanding with phonemic distortions and started to be unresponsive to familiar noises. These difficulties increased over 2 or 3 weeks; they progressively led to diminished oral expression finally reduced to a couple of words. EEG recordings showed paroxysmal abnormalities, either focal, multifocal or diffuse, depending on the state of vigilance and the moment of recording. Epileptic seizures appeared at the same time and were characterized by 'absences' mostly astatic, sometimes preserving the started movement. They were easily controlled by treatment and stopped at age 6.5 years. The whole follow-up period has been 18 years. Complete aphasia has lasted 3.5 years. At age 7, verbal score at WISC test was 0 and performance score 96. At age 9, verbal score improved to 62 with performance at 107. He then underwent re-education in a school for the deaf for 2 years. At age 10.5, there was a light persisting dysphasia and dysgraphia. On control in 1983, while 17 years old, there was still some degree of dyslexia and dysorthographia. Mnesic records remained below normal on verbal testing but were normal on spatial testing. Scores at Wechsler intelligence scale were quite heterogeneous; verbal scale was subnormal while performance was above average. Operational capacities were preserved. There was slight abruptness in behaviour.

As a whole, 19 EEGs have been recorded, and among them five nocturnal recordings and three 24-h telemetries. Paroxysmal diurnal focal or multifocal abnormalities have been present for 5.5 years and were discovered before the occurrence of aphasia. 'Absences' have lasted 1.5 year. Figures 1 and 2 illustrate the EEG evolution.

Summary of the published data
(Based on the references cited in the bibliography)

	Number of cases reconsidered	
	n	%
Sex (124 cases)		
Female	48	38.7
Male	76	61.3
Handedness (42 cases)		
right-handed	24	57
left-handed	10	23.5
ambidextrous	8	19
Semiology (102 cases)		
acquired aphasia	102	100
EEG abnormalities	102	100
epilepsy	69	67.6
Behavioural anomalies (95 cases)		
80 percent with		
hyperkinetic syndrome	68	71.4

Semiology at onset

	n	*%*
Age at first symptoms (94 cases)		
2-3 years	12	
3-5	50	53.6
6-8	24	25.8
9-11	7	
older than 11	1	
Mode of onset (68 cases):		
aphasia	31	45.5
epilepsy	11	16.1
epilepsy and aphasia	12	17.6
others	2	2.9
Total aphasia	43	63
Total epilepsy	23	33.8
Age at first EEG (69 cases)		
3 years-5 years	10	
with spikes and waves	3	
without spike and wave	7	
5-7 years	40	
with spikes and waves	38	
without spike and wave	2	
6-8 years	16	
with spikes and waves	15	
without spike and wave	1	
9-11 years	3	
with spikes and waves	2	
without spike and wave	1	

Aphasia (92 cases)		
Onset semiology		
Auditory agnosia	75	81.5
Pre-existing disturbance of language acquisition	9	9.8
Aphasia installation by stage	17	18.4
Relapses	7	7.6

EEG data
(**SW** = spikes and waves)

	n	%
A single record	23	
EEG followed for:		
2 years	15	16.3
2-5 years	19	20.6
2 EEG	15	
>2 EEG	4	
5 years	25	27.7
2-4 EEGs	14	
>4 EEG	11	11.9
Sleep EEGs	17	
Age at last record:		
Between 8 and 9 years	26	
Persistent SW	8	30
Between 10 and 12 years	19	
Persistent SW	5	26
Between 13 and 15 years	11	
Persistent SW	2	18
15 years or more	13	
Persistent SW	0	0

Epileptic seizures symptomatology

Frequent seizures (39 cases)
    Several types of seizures   17   43.5

Seizures described:
    GM   9
    Partial, evocative of BERS   14
    Hemiclonic   5
    Partial complex   3
    Absence PM?   4
    Astatic   5
    Convulsive (not identified)   3
    Motor Jacksonian   1

Rare seizures (19 cases)

    GM   3
    Partial, evocative of BERS   6
    Hemiclonic   2
    Partial complex   1
    Absence PM?   4
    Astatic   2
    Convulsive (not identified)   5

Epileptic seizures symptomatology	*n*

Single seizure (7 cases)

GM	2
Partial, evocative of BERS	1
Hemiclonic	1
Partial complex	1
Convulsive (not identified)	2

Unique episode of status epileptcus (7 cases)

Status epilepticus during follow-up (3 cases)

References

Ajuriaguerra, J. D., Borel-Maisonny, D., Diatkine, R., Narlian, S., Stambak, M. (1962): Le groupe des audimutités. *Psychiat. de l'Enfant* **1**, 7-62.

Beaumanoir, A. (1984): Epilepsies partielles primaires. In Encycl. Med. Chir. (Paris) *Neurologie* 17044 N10.

Billard, C., Autret, A., Laffont, F., de Giovanni, D., Luca, B., Santini, J.J., Dulac, O., Plouin, P.(1981): Aphasie acquise de l'enfant avec épilepsie: à propos de 4 observations avec état de mal électrique infraclinique du sommeil. *Rev. E.E.G. Neurophysiol.* **11**, 457-467.

Billard, C., Santini, J.J., Dulac, O., Autret, A., de Giovanni, E. (1981): Surdité verbale acquise de l'enfant. A propos de 5 observations (syndrome aphasie-épilepsie). *Rev. Oto-neuro-ophtalmol.* **53**, 331-336.

Brissaud, H.E., Richardet, J.M. (1974): Le syndrome "désintégration du langage et comitialité". *Journées parisiennes de Péd.*, 441-445. Flammarion: Paris.

Büchsenschutz, E. (1979): Troubles sévères de la compréhension du langage associés à une épilepsie. *Neuropsychiatr. de l'Enfant* **7-8**, 361-373.

Cavazzuti, G.B. (1979): Afasia acquisita con crise epilettiche. Descrizione di un caso a esordio precocissimo. *Rivista Pediatrica Siciliana,* Anno XXXII Fasc. 4, 313-321.

Cooper, J.A., Ferry, P.C. (1978): Acquired auditory verbal agnosia and seizures in childhood. *J. Speech Dis.* **43**, 176-184.

Deonna, T., Beaumanoir, A., Gaillard, F., Assal, G. (1977): Acquired aphasia in childhood with seizure disorder: a heterogeneous syndrome. *Neuropädiatrie* **8**, 263-273.

Deonna, T., Fletcher, P., Voumard, C. (1982): Temporary regression during language acquisition: a linguistic analysis of a 2 1/2 year old child with epileptic aphasia. *Develop. Med. Child Neurol.* **24** 156-163.

Deuel, R.K., Lenn, N.J. (1977): Treatment of acquired epileptic aphasia. *J. Pediatr.* **90**, 959-961.

Dugas, M., Grenet, P., Masson, M., Mialet, J.P., Jaquet, J. (1976): Aphasie de l'enfant avec épilepsie. Evolution régressive sous traitement antiépileptique. *Rev. Neurol.* **132**, 489-493.

Dugas, M., Masson, M., Le Heuzey, M.F., Regnier, N. (1982): Aphasie "acquise" de l'enfant avec épilepsie (syndrome de Landau et Kleffner). *Rev. Neurol.* **138**, 755-780.

Forster, G. (1977): Aphasia and seizure disorders in childhood. In *Epilepsy: the Eighth International Symposium,* pp 305-306, ed J.K. Penry. Raven Press: New York.

Gascon, G., Victor, D., Lombroso, C.T., Goodglass, H. (1973): Language disorder, convulsive disorder and electroencephalographic abnormalities. Acquired syndrome in children. *Archs Neurol.* **28**, 156-162.

Harms, D. (1972): Die Sprachstörungen bie Kindern mit cerebralen Krampfanfällen. *Klinische Pädiatr.* **184**, 41-46.

Humphrey, I.L., Knipstein, R., Bumpass, E.R. (1975): Gradually developing aphasia in children. A diagnostic problem. *J. Am. Acad. Child Psychiatr.* **14**, 625-665

Huskisson, J.A. (1973): Acquired receptive language difficulties in childhood. *Br. J. Disord. Communic.* **8**, 53-54.

Julien, J., Lagueny, A., Darriet, D., Boulat, M. (1978): Syndrome aphasie acquise de l'enfant-épilepsie idiopathique. *Bordeaux Médical* **11**, 965-967.

Kellerman, K. (1978): Recurrent aphasia with subclinical bioelectric status epilepticus during sleep. *Eur. J. Pediatr.* **128**, 207-212.

Koepp, P., Lagenstein, I. (1978): Acquired epileptic aphasia. *J. Pediatr.* **92**, 164-166.

Landau, W.M., Kleffner, F.R. (1957): Syndrome of acquired aphasia with convulsive disorder in children. *Neurology* **7**, 523-530.

Lou, H.C., Brandt, S., Bruhn, P. (1977): Aphasia and epilepsy in childhood. *Acta Neurol. Scand.* **56**, 46-54.

Mantovani, J.F., Landau, W.M. (1980): Acquired aphasia with convulsive disorder: course and prognosis. *Neurology.* **30**, 524-529.

McKinney, W., McGreal, D.A. (1974): An aphasic syndrome in children. *Canad. Med. Ass. J.* **16**, 636-639.

Mialet, J.P. (1977): Le syndrome d'aphasie acquise de l'enfant avec épilepsie. Revue de la littérature à propos de deux nouveaux cas. Thèse Paris.

Njiokiktjien, Ch. (1983): Callosal dysfunction as a possible pathogenetic factor in developmental dysphasia. *Neuropediatrics* **14**, 123.

Noël, /A. (1980): Le syndrome de Landau et Kleffner (aphasie acquise de l'enfant et épilepsie). Revue de la littérature à propos de quatre observations personnelles. Thèse Lyon.

Pateiski, K., Presslich, O. (1968): Electro-encephalographisch-experimentelle Untersuchungen bei einem Fall von errvorrenen Sensorischer Aphasie mit Epilepsie in Kindesalter. *Wien Klin. Wsch.* **80**, 851-855.

Petersen, U., Koepp, P., Solmsen, M., Villez, TH.V. (1978): Aphasie im Kindesalter mit E.E.G. veranderungen. *Neuropädiatrie* **9**, 84-96.

Pouplard, F., Pasquier, C. (1978): Le syndrome d'aphasie acquise avec épilepsie est-il une complication du Mycoplasma pneumoniae? *La Nouvelle Presse Médicale* **7**, 33, 2970.

Rapin, I., Mattis, S., Rowan, A.J., Golden, G.G. (1977): Verbal auditory agnosia in children. *Develop Med. Child. Neurol.* **19**, 192-207.

Revol, M., Bourdelon, G. et Brochard, E. (1982): Syndrome Aphasie acquise de l'enfant avec épilepsie et psychose infantile. In *Epilepsies et psychoses. Aspects médicaux.* Ligue française contre l'épilepsie, pp 65-80. Labaz: Paris.

Rodriguez, I., Niedermeyer, E. (1982): The aphasia-epilepsy syndrome in children: electroencephalographic aspects. *Clin. Electroencephal.* **13**, 23-35.

Sharpless, S.K. (1969): Isolated and deafferented neurons: disuse supersensitivity. In *Basic mechanisms of the epilepsies,* Jasper, Ward and Pope, pp. 329-348. Churchill: London.

Shoumaker, M.D., Bennett, D.R., Bray, P.F., Carless, R.G. (1974): Clinical and E.E.G. manifestations of an unusual aphasic syndrome in children. *Neurology* **24**, 10-16.

Toso, V., Moschini, M., Gagnin, G., Antoni, D. (1981): Aphasie acquise de l'enfant avec épilepsie. Trois observations et revue de littérature. *Rev. Neurol.* **137**, 425-434.

Van Harskamp, F., Van Dongen, H.R., Loonen, M.C.B. (1978): Acquired aphasia with convulsive disorders in children. A case study with a seven-year follow-up. *Brain and Language* **6**, 141-148.

Worster-Drought, C. (1971): An unusual form of acquired aphasia in children. *Develop. Med. Child Neurol.* **13**, 563-571.

*   *   *

Discussion pages 213-215

Epileptic syndromes in infancy, childhood and adolescence. J. Roger, C. Dravet, M. Bureau, F.E. Dreifuss and P. Wolf. John Libbey Eurotext Ltd ©1985.

Chapter 21
A Case of Landau-Kleffner Syndrome: Effect of Intravenous Diazepam

Igor RAVNIK

Department of Child Neurology and Psychiatry, Laboratory for Functional Neurological Diagnostics, University Children's Hospital, Vrazov trg 1, 61000 Ljubljana, Yugoslavia

The following clinical observation allows a discussion on the relations between the seizure-discharges and the aphasia in the Landau-Kleffner syndrome.

The patient was in good health until the age of $8^1/_2$ years when he had his first generalized convulsion. His paternal uncle had suffered from primary epilepsy, and his father had had a single seizure in early childhood. The boy had some difficulties with grammar prior to the convulsion; these were attributed to his multilingual environment.

After the seizure his speech and understanding deteriorated. He had difficulties in understanding spoken language and his speech became low-pitched and garbled. Speech therapy was started. In one lesson a questionable absence was observed. Another convulsion occurred in sleep, with clonic jerks of the jaws. EEG showed bitemporal synchronous or independent spikes and generalized spike discharges, with a normal background. There was no evidence of absence seizures. Subsequently the child stopped talking altogether. Later there was some improvement following therapy with carbamazepine to which sodium valproate was added. The child's behaviour got worse and he became rather aggressive. The father had to shift to night work so that he could tend to the boy's needs. The pediatricians considered his behaviour as psychotic.

Following a further deterioration the child was hospitalized. On examination he had impairment of auditory discrimination of expression and of understanding. He was able to understand only short questions pronounced slowly and clearly, to which he gave short and stereotyped answers. In addition to the aphasic problem he also displayed dyspraxia and impaired spatial orientation and body image. Also minor seizures, of which the family was ignorant, were observed. They consisted of fine myoclonic jerks of the upper limbs, disturbing writing, and brief absence seizures associated with eyelid myoclonus, which could be provoked by hyperventilation.

The EEG at that time showed bitemporal asynchronous spikes as well as generalized discharges. During sleep continuous discharges were recorded. Intravenous diazepam (0.3 mg/kg) was given; the EEG normalized and the child, after sleeping for 2 min, could speak much better than before. Nonetheless, the qualitative language impairment persisted. He spoke mainly of bodily needs expressing desire to be checked by a dentist because of toothache, and by an optician to fix glasses for him. He read aloud what was written on the wrapping of a bar of chocolate, apparently wanting to show his capacities. A reading test, 1 hour after the injection, confirmed the improvement.

When clonazepam was added to his medication, the EEG normalized and verbal communication improved, though remained imperfect. He was placed in a special school. He is still dyspractic, but his behaviour is considered to be normal. Incontestably, improvement was faster since the EEG normalization. It seems to us that the spectacular effect of the diazepam injection demonstrates the existence of a correlation between EEG abnormalities and the speech impairment.

To the best of my knowledge, this observation is unique. I believe that in all such cases this therapeutic test should be conducted, and that medication should be adjusted with the aim of obtaining EEG normalization and control of seizures, even when 'the seizures do not seem to cause trouble'. This does not exclude the need for psychiatric help which is valuable in the management of problems resulting from the language impairment.

*   *   *

Discussion pages 213-215

Epileptic syndromes in infancy, childhood and adolescence. J. Roger, C. Dravet, M. Bureau, F.E. Dreifuss and P. Wolf. John Libbey Eurotext Ltd ©1985.

Chapter 22
Epilepsy with Continuous Spikes and Waves during Slow Sleep

— otherwise described as ESES (epilepsy with electrical status epilepticus during slow sleep)

Carlo Alberto TASSINARI*, Michelle BUREAU**, Charlotte DRAVET**, Bernardo DALLA BERNARDINA‡ and Joseph ROGER.

*Institute of Clinical Neurology, University of Bologna, Via Ugo Foscolo 7, Bologna, Italy; **Centre Saint-Paul, Marseille, France; and ‡Department of Childhood Neuropsychiatry, University of Verona, Verona, Italy*

Summary

From their 19 personal cases and from the literature, the authors describe the clinical and EEG features of epilepsy with electrical status epilepticus during slow sleep (ESES). They outline the variable onset and the constantly favourable (when known) evolution of seizures and emphasize the need of a SW index superior to 85 per cent to affirm the diagnosis. They discuss the relationships between ESES and benign epilepsy with rolandic spikes (BERS), Lennox-Gastaut syndrome, Landau-Kleffner syndrome and atypical benign epilepsy in childhood. From the terminological point of view they consider that the term 'ESES' might be used as well as the term 'Epilepsy with continuous spikes and waves during slow sleep' (CSWS).

Definition

A condition characterized by continuous spikes and waves occurring during sleep was described by one of us in collaboration with Patry and Lyagoubi in 1971 under the title *Subclinical electrical status epilepticus induced by sleep in children* and later under the title of *Electrical status epilepticus during sleep* (ESES) (Tassinari *et al*, 1977). The original description stressed the importance for the definition of the syndrome of the fact that the spikes and waves should occupy no less than 85 per cent of the time of slow sleep. These conditions were observed in five patients with epileptic seizures while one other patient was 'mute'. We will consider here only the cases with epileptic seizures and an electrical status epilepticus during slow sleep (ESES syndrome), while retaining for the diagnosis and nosographic discussion the cases of ESES without seizures.

Incidence

Exact figures cannot be given since the data in the literature are still inadequate. However, the condition must be rare. Since 1972, despite a worldwide interest in sleep studies in epileptic patients, we can find 18 personal cases in the St-Paul Center (Tassinari *et al,* 1982), and 25 additional cases in literature were described as having ESES (Laurette and Arfel, 1976; Giovanardi-Rossi and Sineti, 1976; Dalla Bernardina *et al.,* 1978; Calvet, 1978; Kellerman, 1978; Ohtahara *et al.,* 1979; Aicardi and Chevrie, 1982; Billard *et al.,* 1982; Ohtsuka *et al.,* 1983). Additional observations are presented by Morikawa *et al.* in chapter 23. However, as we will discuss later, the parameters used for the definition of ESES were not the same for all the authors, with a consequent variability of incidence and of prognosis (see below).

In addition, the review of literature is difficult because the various parameters are not consistently adhered to by the various authors.

Sex-ratio
Sex is not recorded in all reports. When mentioned (26 cases) we find a probably not significant preponderance of males (15 cases).

Genetic Factors

- Genetic factors for ESES are impossible to establish. No sleep study has been made in siblings and parents. Moreover, since this condition has only been recognized in 1971 and since it exists in childhood only, no information is yet available concerning the offsprings of the patients.
- Genetic factors for epilepsy: there is no evidence of significant genetic factors in the relatives of the patients with ESES.

Epilepsy in patients with ESES

1. *The seizures*

(a) *Before ESES:* Epileptic seizures appeared in our series of 18 patients (Tassinari *et al.,* 1982) at a mean age of 4 years 6 months (range: 8 months-11.5 years). A similar age of onset is reported by Aicardi and Chevrie (1982), Billard *et al.* (1982), and Morikawa *et al.* (chapter 23). In our series the seizures at the onset consisted of unilateral seizures in five patients (as unilateral clonic status in one case), generalized motor seizures in eight patients (six of mainly clonic type, two not sufficiently described) motor manifestation involving the facial muscles with a mandibular contraction and a loss of consciousness in four patients, and myoclonic absences in one patient. In nine of these 18 patients the first seizure occurred during sleep. Partial motor seizures are similarly described by Morikawa *et al.* (chapter 23), including one case with unilateral status, and by Billard *et al.* (1982).

(b) *At the time of the discovery of ESES:* We can distinguish, based on the evolution of the seizures, three groups of patients

Group I: patients having only *motor seizures* throughout their evolution. It consists of 4 patients in our series (indicated as class I in Tassinari *et al.,* 1982), some patients in groups II of Calvet (1978) and Billard *et al.* (1982). Usually the seizures are rare, nocturnal, and they tend to disappear in the early adolescence.

Group II: patients with initially unilateral partial motor seizures, or generalized tonic clonic seizures (mainly occurring during sleep), in whom *'absences'*, similar to typical petit mal absences in some cases, appear at the time of the discovery of ESES. There are seven cases of our series (indicated as class II in Tassinari *et al.,* 1982) and four cases reported by Dalla Bernardina *et al.,* (1978), of whom three are also included in our series.

The evolution of the epilepsy was favourable, with the disappearance of the seizures between 10 and 16 years (usually before 13 years, as in five out of our seven cases).

Group III: patients in whom the *rare nocturnal seizures* become associated, at the time of ESES, with *'atypical absences'*, frequently with *atonic and clonic components.*

Such was the case in seven of our patients (class III in Tassinari *et al.,* 1982), of the seven patients described by Aicardi and Chevrie (1982) under the heading of Atypical Benign Epilepsy of Childhood, of five patients of group III of Billard *et al.* (1982) and of five patients of Morikawa *et al.* (chapter 23).

The *absence of tonic seizures* during sleep was accurately pointed out by us and as well by Morikawa *et al.* (chapter 23), and tonic seizures are not noted by Billard *et al.* (1982) and by other workers who did complete polygraphic sleep studies. Thus, it can be assured that tonic seizures were absent in all cases.

(c) *The evolution of epilepsy:* All the authors agree that seizures are *per se* self-limited, rare and disappear around 10 to 15 years of age.

2 *Electroencephalographic findings*

(a) *Before ESES;* During wakefulness, in our series of 18 patients, three cases had more or less generalized spikes and waves (SW), sometimes in bursts, clinically accompanied by a consciousness impairment with twitching of the eyelids. Fifteen cases had focal interictal spikes, or slow spikes, with or without associated slow waves, involving the fronto-temporal or the centro-temporal region. Among these 15 cases with focal abnormalities, nine also had associated diffuse interictal SW discharges. Similar findings are reported by Morikawa *et al.* (chapter 23). Sleep recordings, performed in five patients of our series, showed an increase of the interictal abnormalities without the features of ESES.

(b) *During ESES:* During wakefulness, the interictal abnormalities, with the same focal distribution as previously reported, and the diffuse abnormalities tend to increase in comparison with the previous periods. The EEG abnormalities reported by other authors are rather focal, with spikes in the frontal and centro-temporal regions, at times associated with diffuse SW (Aicardi and Chevrie, 1982; Billard *et al.,* 1982; Morikawa *et al.,* chapter 23).

As soon as the patient falls asleep continuous bilateral and diffuse slow SW appear, persisting through all the slow sleep stages in our series (Figs 1 and 2). As we have already stressed it is not a matter of an 'important' or 'almost subcontinuous activation'.

See next page

Fig. 1. Awake recording (left), showing focal spikes. Drowsiness (middle) provokes the appearance of spike and wave discharges, which become continuous during NREM or slow sleep (right).

Fig. 2. Top: at 6 years 6 months, sleep recording showing an important activation of abnormalities which are bilateral but of higher voltage on the left hemisphere and which are discontinuous. Bottom: at 9 years, in the same child, occurrence of continuous diffuse spikes and waves during slow sleep, realizing an ESES. Note the extremely high voltage of these discharges (1 cm = 200 μV).

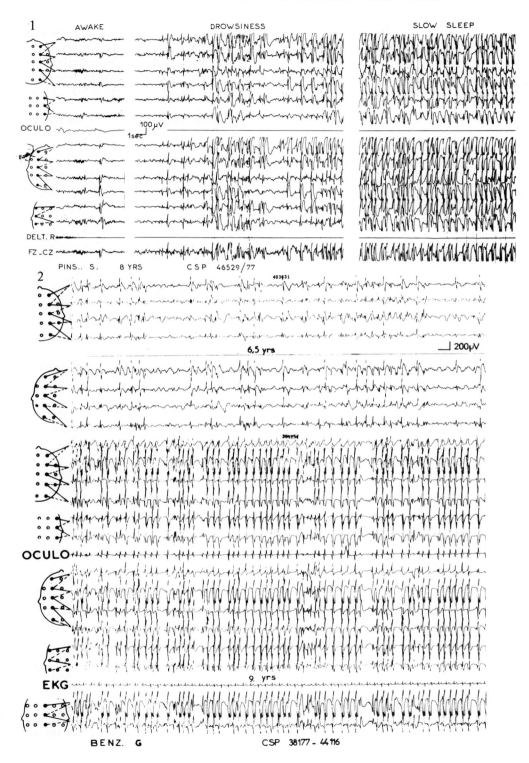

Indeed, the discharges are continuous and the SW index ranges from 85 to 100 per cent. The same parameter was used by Morikawa *et al.* (chapter 23). However, other authors (Calvet, 1978; Billard *et al.,* (1982) also included cases with a SW index higher than 50 per cent. Thus, they considerably widen the definition of ESES, from a continuous status of SW, as in our own definition, to a considerable amount of SW during slow sleep.

In some cases, focal abnormalities, with frontal predominance, can be observed during the rare short periods (seconds) of fragmented diffuse SW discharges in non REM sleep.

During REM sleep the electrical status disappears and the paroxysmal abnormalities consist of rare bursts of diffuse SW, or of focal, predominantly frontal, discharges (Fig. 3). In three patients (also described by Dalla Bernardina *et al.,* 1978) focal, fronto-central rhythmic discharges organized as a subclinical seizure were observed at the end of REM sleep (Fig. 4).

The SW were so continuous that spindles, K-complexes or vertex sharp waves were seldom distinguishable. This rendered impossible the differentiation of NREM sleep stages. The proportion of NREM and REM sleep was approximatively 80 versus 20 per cent. The cyclic organization of sleep was grossly preserved, and these children appeared not to present any obvious sleep disorders, although a number of children had some difficulty awakening in the morning. On awakening, EEG abnormalities were similar to those of the wakefulness prior to sleep.

(c) *Onset of ESES:* In our group, the average age of diagnosis of ESES was 8 years 3 months (range: 4.5-14 years). However these data should be considered with an obvious reservation, since only five children had an EEG during sleep prior to the tracing

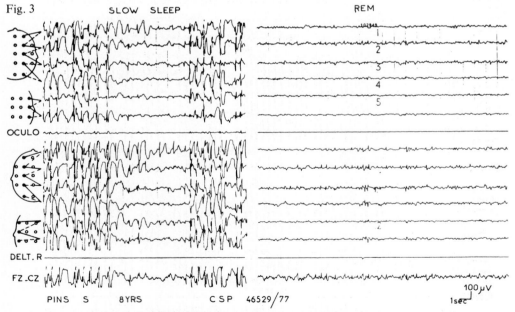

Fig. 3. Left: A short period of fragmentation of generalized spike-waves discharge with left frontal spikes during NREM or slow sleep. Right: during REM, continuous generalized spike and wave discharge disappears, and only localized spike bursts are seen, predominating over the left hemisphere.

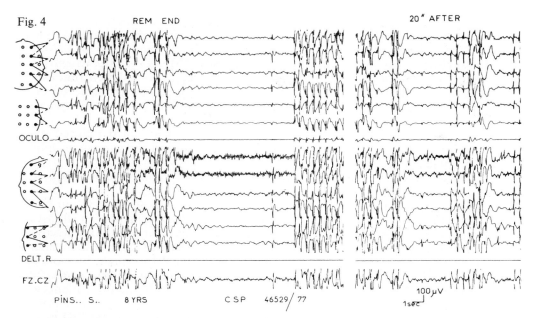

Fig. 4. Left: at the end of a REM stage, when the generalized spikes and waves reappear, occurrence of a subclinical ictal discharge in the left fronto-central area. Right: After 20 sec another shorter and smaller ictal discharge.

indicating ESES. In addition the sleep EEG without ESES was performed less than 1 year before the first sleep recording with ESES in only two patients.

Overall, from our data and from the literature, ESES seems to start 1 to 2 years after the appearance of the seizures.

(d) *End of the ESES:* The average age at the time of the last EEG with ESES was 10 years (range: 5-15 years). In nine patients, tracings obtained showing the disappearance of the ESES pattern allowed the determination of approximate duration of the condition. In these patients, the end of ESES occurred at an average age of 12.5 years (range: 8-13 years). The exact duration of the ESES could be determined with accuracy in only two patients. In one patient, the ESES lasted from 8.5 to 12.5 years with a six-month remission. In the other patient, the ESES lasted from 9 to 11.5 years. In cases for which it was impossible to know the time of onset or termination of ESES, status was recorded over periods ranging from 6 months to 5.5 years.

Neuropsychological and psychic disorders related to ESES

As we have suggested since 1971 there is now an increasing evidence that *the long lasting (years) persistence of continuous SW during sleep characterizing the ESES* is responsible for the appearance of complex and severe neurological impairment, mainly concerning language function, with mental impairment and psychiatric disturbances (Tassinari *et al.,* 1982; Billard *et al.,* 1982; Morikawa *et al.,* chapter 23).

We can distinguish two groups of patients.

Group A

Patients with a *normal psychomotor development* prior to the occurrence of ESES. In our series it consists of 11 children who were normal and attended school before the onset

of ESES and who presented, in relation to ESES, the following disturbances:
- all had *a severe decrease* in IQ, ranging from a score of 78 in the best case to one of 45 in the worst case, as measured by the Wechsler Intelligence Scale for Children. Similar clear cut findings characterize also the cases of Morikawa *et al.* (chapter 23)
- *a very marked reduction of language* function occurred in six children (but two of them presented an isolated speech retardation prior to the probable onset of ESES), associated with a severe impairment of *memory* and *of temporo-spatial orientation*
- in 10 cases disturbances also involved the behavioural sphere, with reduced attention span, hyperkinesis, aggresiveness, difficulty in contact and sometimes inhibition manifestation
- psychotic states were observed in two of our cases and in one case of Billard *et al.* (1982).

After ESES, psychological problems were evaluated in only seven children in our group, since the other four still evidenced ESES on the last examination. In all cases, a global improvement was noted in performance and/or behaviour after ESES. Recovery was always slow, returning to a normal level in only two patients. In the other patients there was a slight degree of recovery, which corresponded to a slight or moderate mental deficiency. It was only after training in a specialized institution that some children were able to achieve satisfactory psychosocial adjustment. In the two patients who presented retardation of speech, one recovered his former level and the other maintained an increased discrepancy between verbal and performance scores (PIQ = 103, VIQ = 57). Billard *et al.* (1982) and Morikawa *et al.* (chapter 23) confirmed the variable degree of improvement after the end of ESES, supporting the hypothesis that ESES is responsible for the intellectual, language and psychiatric disturbances.

Group B

Patients with an *abnormal psychomotor development* prior to the occurrence of ESES. In our series seven patients came into this category. During ESES a worsening of mental deficiency was observed in these seven patients. In one patient who had a previous homogeneous IQ of 75, the VIQ collapsed. But, in this case, loss of speech was part of a picture of massive regression, with loss of interest in all activities except those related to alimentary function. This child also presented recurrent episodes of absence status.

After ESES, the intellectual evolution was appraised in three patients only. Their level of mental activity was not very different from previous performance during ESES. However, psychiatric disturbances were always considerably improved.

Neurological conditions

Eight patients out of 18 of our series presented an evidence of encephalopathy prior to the onset of ESES: congenital hemiparesis in two cases, hemiplegia observed at 5.5 years in one case and spastic tetraparesis in one case.

There is no evidence of previous neurological disorders in the patients reported in literature, except one case of Billard *et al.* (1982) who had a diffuse hypotonia and a static ataxia.

Response to treatment

We can distinguish the effectiveness of treatment with regard to seizure control and electrical status during sleep.

Various drugs have been employed (benzodiazepines, sodium valproate, carbamazepine...) in chronic oral treatment. On the whole no drug seems effective in abolishing the continuous SW during sleep. ACTH therapy (Kellerman, 1978; Billard *et al.*, 1982; Morikawa *et al.*, chapter 23; Inokuma *et al.*, 1983; Dalla Bernardina, unpublished observation) can be effective in suppressing the ESES and can occasionally improve the language function. However the amelioration is limited to the duration of treatment.

In two personal cases an IV injection of benzodiazepine during slow sleep (the vein was canulated prior to the sleep onset in order to not awake the patient) arrested the continuous SW for approximately one hour, after which it reappeared as before.

Diagnosis of Atypical form

Two considerations should be made. The first concerns the diagnosis of *electrical status* itself: we consider that the cases with a SW index below 85 per cent should not be considered as ESES. In this context it is significant that when we consider the cases with a SW index superior to 85 per cent the overall electroclinical condition is quite homogeneous, with a quite constant behavioural, psychiatric and intellectual impairment, as in our cases and in those of Morikawa *et al.* (chapter 23).

The second consideration concerns the *duration of the ESES:* we consider that it is a long lasting condition, with the characteristic features of continuous SW appearing and persisting every time the child sleeps for a considerable length of time (months and usually more than one year).

If there is only a 'considerable amount' of SW during sleep limited to a few days, it is unlikely that we are dealing with the ESES syndrome. It is probably the long duration of ESES which is related to the appearance of the intellectual, language and behavioural disturbances observed in ESES.

Differential diagnosis and nosology of ESES

Four syndromes must be considered in the differential diagnosis.

(1) *Benign epilepsy of childhood with rolandic spikes (BERS)*

In some cases of ESES the ictal symptomatology and the evolution of epilepsy are identical to those observed in BERS (Group I in our series). Moreover, in some other cases (Group II in our series) seizures recalling those of BERS are associated with more or less typical absences. Such an association has been described in BERS by Beaumanoir *et al.* (1974) and by Dalla Bernardina *et al.* (1982).

It should be noted that in the case of patients with ESES interictal abnormalities usually are in the fronto-central regions, while in the case of BERS the spikes have a more centro-temporal distribution. However this is a minor point in the distinction between ESES and BERS. They are two major points of differentiation.

(a) While the sleep of patients with BERS activates discharges, this activation exceptionally reaches the degree observed in ESES with a SW index greater than 85 per cent. Ambrosetto (personal communication) never found such a high degree of activation in a polygraphic nocturnal study of 60 patients with BERS.

(b) When such extreme activation occurs, indicating a true ESES, patients considered as having BERS indeed get a different evolution, because of the appearance of behavioural, intellectual and eventually language disturbances, as in our Group I. In these cases we have the choice of saying that they have an atypical BERS or a typical ESES, and it does not really matter what we call them. What is important is that the occurrence of subclinical status epilepticus makes the prognosis less favourable. In addition, some children with ESES have an evidence of various degrees of organic encephalopathy, which is usually absent in patients with BERS.

(2) *The Lennox-Gastaut syndrome (LGS)*

The patients with ESES having, in addition to nocturnal seizures, frequent daily atypical absences, with atonic or myoclonic components, certainly call for a differential diagnosis with the LGS. This need for such a differential diagnosis between ESES and LGS, first pointed out by Dalla Bernardina *et al.* (1978), becomes even more evident when intellectual performances decline and behavioural and language difficulties appear. This is the case of patients with ESES described in our Group III (class III in Tassinari *et al.,* 1982), of the patients of the Group III of Billard et al. (1982) and of those described by Morikawa *et al.* (chapter 23). A need for a differential diagnosis with the LGS was also felt by Aicardi and Chevrie when they described 7 patients who had atypical absences, atonic and clonic seizures, and who presented a sleep condition identical or similar to the ESES. Despite that, in their cases there was no intellectual impairment.

The benign evolution of the seizures, the absence of tonic seizures and the other features analyzed in details by Morikawa et al constitute the main element of differential diagnosis between the ESES (or 'atypical benign childhood epilepsy' so called by Aicardi and Chevrie (1982)) and the LGS.

(3) *The Landau-Kleffner syndrome (LKS)*

The nosological situation and the electroclinical features of the acquired aphasia with paroxysmal discharges with or without epilepsy are reviewed by Beaumanoir (chapter 20).

Here we will only discuss the cases in whom sleep studies allow us to compare the LKS and the ESES. We have already reported that one patient in our first work on ESES (Patry *et al.,* 1971) was mute but not epileptic.

Kellerman (1978, see also Shoumaker *et al.,* 1974) suggested a close relationship between ESES and acquired aphasia. Since then, additional cases of acquired aphasia, or of 'developmental dysphasia', have been reported, occurring concomitantly with ESES: one case by Maccario *et al.,* 1982 (case 4), three cases by Billard *et al.,* 1982 (one case with seizures and two without, Group I), and other cases have been observed by Dalla Bernardina and Vigevano (1983, personal communication).

In this context, Morikawa *et al.* (chapter 23) quoted the papers of Inokuma *et al.* (1983) and of Ohtsuka *et al.* (1983) which are not available to us.

In our material of 19 patients with ESES, speech functions were impaired in eight cases, representing the major clinical problem in two.

The relationship between ESES and language disturbances was clearly evident in the cases of Billard *et al.* (1982), particularly in the case 1, where 'a marked improvement in language, accompanied by a complete remission of PA (ESES) occurred under hydrocortisone therapy'.

In this context, Billard *et al.* (1982) concluded: 'if one is to accept the hypothesis of a causal relationship between nocturnal paroxysmal activities and language disorders, the question arises as to a possible relationship between sleep and the acquisition of the language'.

Dulac *et al.* (1983), in a review of 66 cases from literature and 10 personal cases, furtherly supported the hypothesis that the language disturbance and the degree of paroxysmal activities are in a strict relationship.

(4) *ESES in patients without related neuropsychological impairment*

In five cases classified as BERS (Calvet, 1978), in case 5 of Billard *et al.* (1982), as well as in the series of seven patients of Aicardi and Chevrie (1982), the presence of ESES was not related to a neuropsychological impairment. These data are evidently at variance with the other cases with ESES.

Two comments can be made:

(a) the development of neuropsychological impairment may depend on the degree of activation of SW during sleep, as well as their duration in time. Thus, it would be important:
(i) to have the SW index during sleep in the cases without neuropsychological impairment, and
(ii) to know how long the ESES persisted: weeks, months, years?
Such factors could understandably account for the differences between cases with a normal neuropsychological evolution and the others.
(b) concerning the Calvet findings, Billard *et al.* (1982) appropriately commented that 'even in these cases (five cases of BERS) one suspects that a thorough neuropsychological evaluation would have uncovered discrete deterioration'.

Terminological discussion

The term 'electrical status epilepticus during sleep' can be criticized for two reasons: because it is difficult to accept that continuous SW during sleep without detectable simultaneous clinical signs can be considered a status, and because ESES can be found in non-epileptic patients. Consequently one could refer to this condition with the term 'continuous spikes and waves during sleep' (CSWS) as did Morikawa *et al.* (chapter 23).

However if we accept the importance of continuous SW during sleep in the determination of neuropsychological disturbances described above, the condition is really a status with clinical correlates and the term ESES can be used to indicate both epileptic patients and patients without clinical seizures. For example, could we consider the aphasia as the epileptic condition resulting from the continuous SW during sleep? Indeed we now treat the aphasic patients with antiepileptic drugs to suppress the discharges presumably responsible for this aphasia.

Alternatively, and more conservatively, we could suggest to use *ESES* as a term to indicate the condition in epileptic patients and to use *CSWS* when the condition occurs in non-epileptic patients. Broughton (1983) suggested the term 'non convulsive status epilepticus' as an alternative to ESES.

Beside any terminological discussion we strongly feel that the condition of having continuous SW during sleep deserves an individual categorization because it exists and it has practical and theoretical implications.

References

Aicardi, J. Chevrie, J.J. (1982): Atypical benign partial epilepsy of childhood. *Devlop. Med. Child. Neurol.* **24**, 281-292.

Beaumanoir, A., Ballis, T., Varfis, G., Ansari, K. (1974): Benign epilepsy of childhood with rolandic spikes : a clinical, EEG, and tele. EEG study. *Epilepsia* **15**, 301-315.

Billard, C., Autret, A., Laffont, F., Lucas, B., Degiovanni, E. (1982): Electrical status epilepticus during sleep in children: a reappraisal from eight new cases. In *Sleep and epilepsy,* pp 481-494, ed M.B. Sterman, M.N. Shouse, P. Passouant, Academic Press: London and New York.

Broughton, R.J. (1983): Epilepsy and sleep. In *Epilepsy, sleep and sleep deprivation,* pp 317-356 ed R. Degen, E. Niedermeyer. Elsevier: Amsterdam.

Calvet, U. (1978): Epilepsies nocturnes de l'enfant. Thèse, Toulouse.

Dalla Bernardina, B., Tassinari, C.A., Dravet, C., Bureau, M., Beghini, G., Roger J. (1978): Epilepsie partielle bénigne et état de mal électroencéphalographique pendant le sommeil. *Rev. EEG Neurophysiol.* **8**, 350-353.

Dalla Bernardina, B., Bondavalli, S., Colamaria, V. (1982): Benign epilepsy of childhood with rolandic spikes during sleep. In *Sleep and epilepsy,* pp 495-506, ed M.B. Sterman, M.N. Shouse, P. Passouant, Academic Press; London and New York.

Dulac O., Billard, C., Arthuis, M. (1983): Aspects électrocliniques et évolutifs de l'épilepsie dans le syndrome aphasie-épilepsie. *Archs Fr. Pédiatr.* **40**, 299-308.

Giovanardi-Rossi, P., Sineti, F. (1976): La sindrome 'afasia-epilessia' di Landau-Kleffner. In *Le Disfasie dell'età evolutiva,* pp 93-109, ed Oppici, Parma.

Inokuma, K., Watanabe, K., Negoro, T., Sigiura, M., Matsumoto, A., Takaesu, E. (1983): Acquired expressive dysphasia with paroxysmal EEG abnormalities treated with ACTH-Z. Report of two cases. *J. Jpn Epil. Soc.* **1**, 153-158.

Kellerman, K. (1978): Recurrent aphasia with subclinical bioelectric status epilepticus during sleep. *Eur. J. Pediatr.* **128**, 207-212.

Laurette, G., Arfel, G. (1976): "Etat de Mal" électrographique dans le sommeil d'après-midi. *Rev. EEG. Neurophysiol.* **6**, 137-139.

Maccario, M., Hefferen, S.J., Kebluser, S.J., Lipinski, K.A. (1982): Developmental dysphasia and electroencephalographic abnormalities. *Develop. Med. Child Neurol.* **24**, 141-155.

Ohtahara, S., Oka, E., Yamatogi, Y., Ohtsuka, Y., Ishida, T., Ichiba, N., Ishida, S., Miyake, S. (1979): Non convulsive status epilepticus in childhood. *Folia Psychiatr. Neurol. Jpn* **33**, 345-351.

Ohtsuka, Y., Yoshida, H., Matsuda, M., Terasaki, T., Iyoda, K., Yamatogi, Y., Oka, E., Ohtahara, S. (1983): A peculiar type of non-convulsive status epilepticus in childhood : a clinical and electroencephalographic study. *J. Jpn Epil. Soc.* **1**, 107-115.

Patry, G., Lyagoubi, S., Tassinari, C.A. (1971): Subclinical 'electrical status epilepticus' induced by sleep in children. *Archs Neurol.* **24**, 242-252.

Shoumaker, M., Bennet, D.R., Bray, P.F., Carless, R.G. (1974): Clinical and EEG manifestations of an unusual aphasic syndrome in children. *Neurology* **24**, 10-16.

Tassinari, C.A., Terzano, G., Capocchi, G., Dalla Bernardina, B., Vigevano, F., Daniele, O., Valladier, C., Dravet, C., Roger, J. (1977): Epileptic seizures during sleep in children. In *Epilepsy. The 8th International Symposium,* pp 345-354, ed J.K. Penry. Raven Press: New York.

Tassinari, C.A., Bureau, M., Dravet, C., Roger, J., Daniele-Natale, O. (1982): Electrical status epilepticus during sleep in children (ESES). In *Sleep and epilepsy,* pp 465-479, ed M.B. Sterman, M.N. Shouse, P. Passouant. Academic Press: London and New York.

*　　　　*　　　　*

Discussion pages 213-215

Epileptic syndromes in infancy, child-hood and adolescence. J. Roger, C. Dravet, M. Bureau, F.E. Dreifuss and P. Wolf. John Libbey Eurotext Ltd ©1985.

Chapter 23
Five Children with Continuous Spike-Wave Discharges during Sleep

Tateki MORIKAWA, Mazakazu SEINO, Takeshi OSAWA and Kazuichi YAGI

National Epilepsy Center, Shizuoka Higashi Hospital, 886 Urushiyama, Shizuoka (MZ 420), Japan

Summary

A comparative study of clinical characteristics between two relevant epileptic syndromes was carried out; five patients with 'continuous spike-and-wave discharges during sleep' (CSWS) and seven patients with 'Lennox-Gastaut syndrome (L-G)'.

(1) In the CSWS group, there was a period of co-existence of atypical absences and partial motor seizures which was not found in the L-G group. Tonic seizure manifestations in both clinical and EEG expressions during sleep were characteristic of the L-G group whereas none was found in the CSWS group.

(2) A quantitative comparison of the occurrence of spike-and-wave discharges using spike-and-wave index of non-REM sleep revealed a striking difference; more than 95 per cent in the CSWS group against less than 51 per cent in the L-G group in all-night EEG recordings.

(3) The significance of age-dependency to this epileptic encephalopathy was emphasized by the combination of generalized and partial seizures, development of behavioral aberrations, and occurrence of continuous spike-and-waves all manifesting between the ages of five and seven.

Introduction

The term 'electrical status epilepticus induced by sleep' was first proposed by Patry *et al.* (1971) and resumed later by Tassinari *et al.* (1982). Since a status epilepticus originally implied clinical manifestations, an alternative nomenclature such as 'continuous spike-wave discharges during sleep' (CSWS) would be a better choice. In this study, we attempted to investigate clinical and electroencephalographic characteristics of the CSWS to compare them with those of the Lennox-Gastaut syndrome (L-G) (Gastaut *et al.*, 1966; Doose and Völzke, 1979).

Patients

The age at the first examination of CSWS group was matched with that of L-G. They were 4 to 9 years of age (mean, 7 years 6 months), and follow-up observation period ranged from 4 to 8 years (mean, 5 years 10 months).

EEG examination was repeatedly carried out with the aid of simultaneous video recording, that is 8 to 46 recordings, average 20, for one patient. All-night polygraphic EEG recording was also conducted in all patients.

Results

1. Individual cases
Case 1. Female, 7 years 7 months, right-handed. No convulsive disorders in family history. Six days after birth she suffered from pyogenic meningitis which did not, however, result in convulsion. At age 2 years 8 months, a left-sided unilateral convulsive status epilepticus occurred and recurred about twice a year until 5 years of age. The status epilepticus was then replaced by partial motor seizures accentuated on the left side. At age 6 years 1 month, atypical absence seizures were noticed, the mental state deteriorated obviously and presence of CSWS became evident (Fig. 1). She was hospitalized in our clinic at age 7 years 7 months, because of disturbed coordination, clumsiness, hyperactive behavior and inattentiveness. Her IQ scores decreased markedly from 97 (5 years 5 months, tested by Tanaka-Binet) down to 40. Her habitual seizures mentioned above were eventually controlled at age 8, but the hyperkinetic behavior and the CSWS persisted until 10 years (Fig. 4). At age 11 years 11 months, it was noted in all-night recordings that the EEG abnormalities diminished strikingly until no CSWS were observed in any EEG recordings at all. As the EEG expressions improved, her hyperkinetic tendency disappeared completely, but her mental deficit still remained with an IQ at 52 (Fig. 4).

Case 2. male, 7 years 8 months, right-handed. No family history of convulsive disorders. Partial motor seizures, occasionally evolving to generalized convulsions beginning at age 3 years, and atypical absences occurred at 6 years 6 months when his mental deterioration became increasingly obvious.

At age 7 years 8 months, he experienced an episode of absence status epilepticus lasting for two weeks (Fig. 2), following which he developed various behavioral problems; a tendency toward apathy, loss of contact with the surroundings,

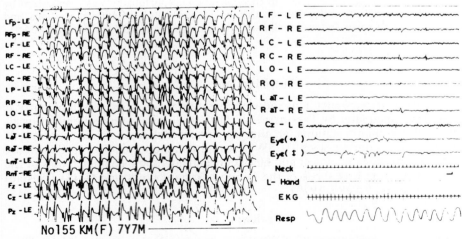

No155 KM(F) 7Y7M

Fig. 1. Case 1. Pseudorhythmic and continuous burst of slow spike-and-wave discharges without showing any clinical manifestations during non-REM sleep (left) were completely suppressed during REM sleep (right).

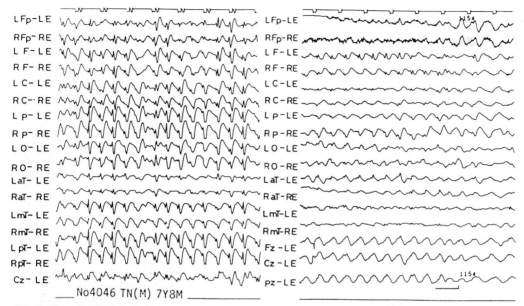

Fig. 2. Case 2. EEG during atypical absence status lasting for two weeks. Continuous 2 c/sec diffuse slow spike-and-wave complexes are maximum in the posterior parts (left). Following intravenous injection of 5 mg diazepam, diffuse 2 c/sec slow activity with residual small spikes in the left frontal region were observed. The patient became responsive (right).

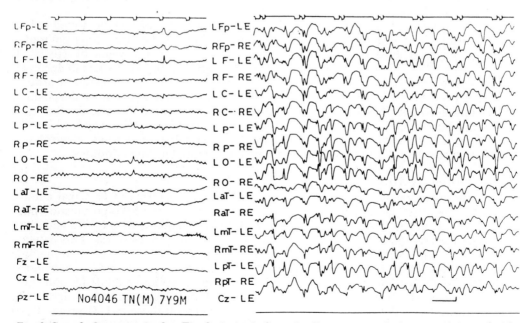

Fig. 3. Case 2. One month after Fig. 2. A single frontal spike was seen during wakefulness (left); continuous 1.5-2 c/sec diffuse slow spike-and-waves and high voltage slow waves continued during non-REM sleep (right).

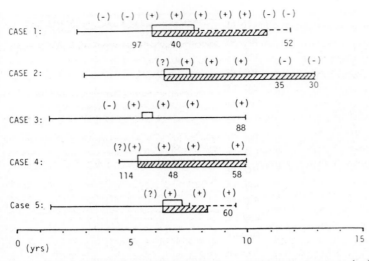

Fig. 4. Clinical course of each patient with CSWS. The symbols (+) and (−) are for existence and absence of CSWS, respectively, white columns for absence seizures, solid lines for partial motor seizures or for predominantly unilateral convulsions, dotted lines for seizure free periods, hatched columns for behavioral problems and numbers for IQ scores tested by Tanaka-Binet.

restlessness, and a short attention span. During this period there was no voluntary speech but he was able to reiterate heard words and his ability to read was unimpaired. CSWS was noted during this period and persisted for more than two years (Figs 3 and 4). After age 11 years, in spite of gradual improvement of CSWS on EEGs, his behavioral abnormalities still continued.

A summary of the clinical course of the five patients with CSWS is illustrated in Fig. 4. The onset of atypical absence seizures was always preceded by that of partial motor seizures. Atypical absence seizures occurred between 5 and 7 years of age in all patients. An EEG expression specified as CSWS developed before 7 years of age in all five children. Progressive intellectual and behavioral difficulties appeared at around the same time except in case 3. There was one patient (case 1) who showed a positive correlation between CSWS and hyperkinetic behavior but there was also another case (case 2) whose CSWS diminished earlier and the hyperkinetic tendency tapered off. Laboratory examinations of blood cells, measles titer, hepatic functions, electrolytes, urine amino acids and cerebrospinal fluid were all without abnormal findings.

2. Comparison of CSWS with L-G

Comparison was made between CSWS and L-G group in terms of principal clinical features. The onset age of epilepsy was under 4 years of age in CSWS group and under 2 years in L-G group. Medical histories showed that two patients with CSWS had acute pyogenic meningitis and two patients with L-G were born in asphyxia. Two patients with CSWS and other two patients with L-G had hemiplegia, and the remaining eight patients from both groups showed some minor motor and/or behavioral disorders, such as clumsiness, disturbed coordination, hyperactive tendency and short attention span. The IQ scores evaluated by Tanaka-Binet Test were rather high in the CSWS group (with the exception of case 2) compared with those in L-G group. Positive CT findings were found in nine patients (four out of five in CSWS group, five out of seven in L-G group), all of which were slight to moderate uni- or bi-lateral atrophic features.

Clinical seizure manifestations

In the course of epilepsy, atypical absence seizures were observed in all patients. Generalized tonic seizures were never seen in the patients with CSWS throughout the observation period whilst those in the L-G group, without exception, inevitably had tonic seizures of various degrees.

It was noteworthy that all patients with the CSWS developed partial motor seizures which occasionally evolved to generalized convulsions. These seizures of the patients with CSWS either ceased or decreased in frequency to a few per year. In contrast, all patients with L-G continued to have generalized tonic and/or atypical absence seizures as frequently as several times a day.

As described above, all five patients with CSWS displayed a peculiar period of a coexistence of absence seizures and partial motor seizures. In the seven patients with L-G, however, the combination of generalized nonconvulsive seizures and partial convulsive seizures was never found. The majority of partial motor seizures seen in the patients with CSWS occurred during sleep and the seizure types confirmed by witnesses were: versive seizure to the left (case 1), right hemifacial spasms accompanying clonic convulsions of the right arm (case 2), right mouth-corner retraction with hemifacial twitchings (case 3), clonic convulsions of the left arm (case 4) and of the right arm (case 5).

Interictal EEG findings

Three patients out of the five with CSWS showed almost normal EEG background activities, whereas none with L-G. By definition, slow spike-and-waves were observed during sleep in all patients with CSWS and also in the patients with L-G. However, bursts of generalized rapid spike rhythm were never observed in patients with CSWS throughout the repeatedly examined EEGs including all-night recordings. The occur-

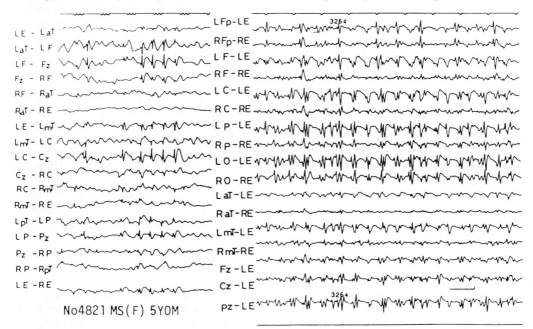

Fig. 5. Case 3. An atypical case (see text). Note that the less generalized and rather focal spike-and-wave activities were found during both waking (left) and non-REM sleep (right).

Table 1. Comparison of the all-night recordings

Case	Total sleep (min)	sp-w/non-REM (min)	sp-w/REM (min)	sp-w indices % non-REM	REM
1*	499	389/401	12/98	97	12
2	580	482/507	47/73	95	64
3	473	365/376	5/97	97	5
4	661	536/547	36/114	98	32
5	494	345/363	1/131	95	1
6**	397	185/362	15/35	51	43
7	522	43/434	4/88	10	5
8	582	105/550	2/32	19	6
9	497	129/431	1/66	30	2
10	497	50/455	1/42	11	2
11	501	54/414	2/87	13	2
12	502	123/441	7/61	28	11

*Cases 1-5; patients with CSWS. **Cases 6-12; patients with L-G.

rence of runs of rapid spike rhythm seemed almost diagnostic to the patients with L-G. In the CSWS group, the occurrence of spike-and-wave discharges appeared suddenly on falling asleep, disappearing abruptly on awakening. This is in sharp contrast to the pattern observed in the L-G group in which the appearance and disappearance of spike-and-wave discharges were more insidious.

In addition to the above-mentioned generalized seizure discharges, focal epileptic EEG abnormalities were randomly observed during waking and drowsy state in the CSWS patients (Figs 2, 3 and 5). The persistent focal findings were: spikes or spike-and-waves in frontal regions (three out of five patients) and centro-frontal region (case 3), and the laterality of the EEG foci, so far demonstrated, was anatomically concordant with that of the clinical partial seizures.

Spike-and-wave index
The spike-and-wave indices were calculated and comparisons drawn between the CSWS and the L-G groups during the period when their seizure activities were greatest between 6 and 9 years in both groups. According to Patry *et al.* (1971), the spike-and-wave index was calculated from a 30-min uninterrupted EEG recording, whereas ours were taken from all-night EEG recordings (Table 1), namely, spike-and-wave index (per cent) of non-REM sleep = total sum of spike-and-wave (min) x 100/total non-REM duration (min).

The spike-wave indices of non-REM sleep in the five patients with CSWS were more than 95 per cent whereas those of the seven patients with L-G were less than 51 per cent. As was expected, the spike-wave indices in REM stages decreased significantly compared with those in non-REM stages (Table 1).

Discussion

The similarity and dissimilarity between two epileptic syndromes: 'electrical status epilepticus induced by sleep' or 'continuous spike-and-waves during sleep' and the Lennox-Gastaut syndrome were pointed out first by Patry *et al.* (1971) and later by Tassinari *et al.* (1982). In order to clarify the framework of the symptomatology of CSWS, making a precise comparison with the L-G appeared to be meaningful. It is needless to say that all-night EEG recording should be carried out on the patients under study.

Tonic seizures during sleep, accompanying particular runs of spike rhythm on EEG, were commonly observed in, and therefore almost diagnostic of, the Lennox-Gastaut syndrome, whereas tonic seizures were, without exception, absent in the CSWS group in terms of both clinical and EEG expressions. A modulating or inducing effect of antiepileptic drugs, especially of benzodiazepines, on the occurrence of the tonic state was suggested first by Tassinari *et al.* (1972). In this study, all the patients of both groups were receiving a combination of valproate and benzodiazepines as a part of the medication. Nonetheless, only the patients with CSWS failed to develop tonic seizures. A possibility of drug-induced effect was thus eliminated.

Although the presence of slow spike-and-wave discharges during sleep is a hallmark of the Lennox-Gastaut syndrome, they can be easily differentiated from the CSWS by the continuity of bursting. This was unequivocally shown by the spike-and-wave indices: more than 95 per cent in the CSWS group versus less than 51 per cent in the L-G group. This fact may reflect different pathophysiological mechanisms underlying these two epileptic syndromes.

The most characteristic features of the CSWS seen in our five patients were a peculiar coexistence of partial motor seizures with atypical absences, that was observed in all five patients, and the occurrence of absence seizures, roughly coincident with the onset of CSWS, inevitably accompanied by behavioural problems which seemed progressive at least at the beginning of CSWS (Landau and Kleffner, 1957; Kellermann, 1978; Inokuma *et al.* 1983; Ohtsuka, 1983). The triad, a combination of generalized and partial seizures, development of behavioural and intellectual impairments, and the occurrence of continuous spike-and-wave discharges during sleep, was observed between 5 and 7 years of age. All these clinical features support Patry's opinion that 'the condition is a form of encephalopathy secondary to a focal or multifocal brain lesion', if the term 'age-dependent' was added before 'encephalopathy'. Secondary bilateral synchronization (Lombroso and Erba, 1970) is a possible explanation of the unique EEG expression of the CSWS.

Among the five patients with CSWS, case 3 had different features from those of the remaining four cases as she displayed the partial, Sylvian seizure often seen in benign epilepsy of children with centro-temporal EEG foci (Lombroso, 1967). The spike-wave discharges were less generalized and with centro-frontal spike focus. Lastly, there were practically no behavioral impairments in association with the CSWS. It is most possible that this case is not identical with the typical cases presented by Patry and Tassinari, and may belong to the cases grouped as 'atypical benign partial epilepsy of childhood' by Aicardi and Chevrie (1982). These facts tempt us to hypothesize the CSWS may situate between generalized and partial epilepsies.

References

Aicardi, J., Chevrie, J.J. (1982): Atypical benign partial epilepsy of childhood. *Develop. Med. Child Neurol.* **24,** 281-292.

Doose, H., Völzke, E. (1979): Petit mal status in early childhood and dementia. *Neuropädiatrie* **10,** 10-14.

Gastaut, H., Roger, J., Soulayrol, R., Tassinari, C.A., Régis, H., Dravet, C., Bernard, R., Pinsard, N., Saint-Jean, M. (1966): Childhood epileptic encephalopathy with diffuse slow spike-waves (otherwise known as 'petit mal variant') or Lennox syndrome. *Epilepsia* **7,** 139-179.

Inokuma, K. Watanabe, K., Negoro, T., Sugiura, M., Matsumoto, A., Takaesu, E. (1983): Acquired expressive dysphasia with paroxysmal EEG abnormalities treated with ACTH-Z.

Report of two cases. *J. Jpn. Epil. Soc.* **1,** 153-158.

Kellermann, K. (1978): Recurrent aphasia with subclinical bioelectric status epilepticus during sleep. *Eur. J. Pediatr.* **128,** 207-212.

Landau, W.M., Kleffner, F.R. (1957): Syndrome of acquired aphasia with convulsive disorder in children. *Neurology* 7, 523-530.

Lombroso, C.T. (1967): Sylvian seizures and midtemporal spike foci in children. *Archs Neurol.* **17,** 52-59.

Lombroso, C.T., Erba, G. (1970): Primary and secondary bilateral synchrony in epilepsy. *Archs Neurol.* **22,** 321-334.

Ohtsuka, Y., Yoshida, H., Matsuda, M., Terasaki, T., Iyoda, K., Yamatogi, Y., Oka, E., Ohtahara, S. (1983): A peculiar type of non-convulsive status epilepticus in childhood: A clinical and electroencephalographic study. *J. Jpn. Epil. Soc.* **1,** 107-115.

Patry, G., Lyagoubi, S., Tassinari, C.A. (1971): Subclinical 'electrical status epilepticus' induced by sleep in children *Archs Neurol.* **24,** 242-252.

Tassinari, C.A., Dravet, C., Roger, J., Cano, J.P., Gastaut, H. (1972): Tonic status epilepticus precipitated by intravenous benzodiazepine in five patients with Lennox-Gastaut syndrome. *Epilepsia* **13,** 421-435.

Tassinari, C.A., Bureau, M., Dravet, C., Roger, J., Daniele Natale, O. (1982): Electrical status epilepticus during sleep in children (ESES). In *Sleep and epilepsy,* ed M.B. Sterman, Margaret N. Shouse, P. Passouant, pp. 465-479. Academic Press: New York.

*　　　*　　　*

Discussion pages 213-215

Epileptic syndromes in infancy, childhood and adolescence. J. Roger, C. Dravet, M. Bureau, F.E. Dreifuss and P. Wolf. John Libbey Eurotext Ltd ©1985.

Discussion of
Benign Partial Epilepsies
(Chapters 15-23)

Summarized by Pinchas LERMAN

Benign partial epilepsy with centro-temporal spikes (BPCT)

O'Donohoe and Lerman emphasize how difficult it is to make parents and doctors realize that the prognosis is always good, even when the seizures are frequent.

O'Donohoe thinks that parents would be more convinced if you give them a precise description of the seizures, immediately after a brief interview.

Lerman estimates that even cases with frequent seizures can be fully controlled by the administration of a higher dose of phenytoin at bedtime.

Benign partial epilepsy with occipital spikes (BPO)

Lerman: What is the relationship between BPO as described by Gastaut and basilar migraine with occipital spiking?

Gastaut replies that the article of the Canadian authors (Camfield *et al.*) entitled *Basilar migraine, seizures and marked epileptiform EEG anomalies* is wrong. The cases described by these authors are identical to his. In true basilar migraine there are no occipital spikes and no occipital seizures.

O'Donohoe wonders if this syndrome is not more common but being confused with migraine no EEG is performed and consequently it is underdiagnosed.

Benign partial epilepsy with exaggerated somatosensitive evoked potentials

Plouin asks whether such evoked potentials may be observed also in lesional epilepsies.

Tassinari replies that by definition the population studied by De Marco did not show evidence of brain damage nor neurological signs. However, one can find such responses also in patients with cerebral lesions (such as hemiplegia) or a degenerative disease.

The Landau-Kleffner syndrome (LKS)

Dulac: Should the LKS always be considered as an epileptic syndrome, since generally there is no strict correlation between the aphasia and the EEG discharges? It is difficult to be sure about this point since in most cases it is impossible to eradicate the EEG abnormalities by the anticonvulsant therapy. However, in one clinical observation the aphasia disappeared during the period when the EEG discharges were suppressed by clobazam therapy, to reappear concomitantly with the reappearance of spike discharges in spite of therapy (cf, with case reported by Ravnik in this meeting).

In his cases he always observed a temporal predominance, mainly on the left side, in the waking records. In the eight cases in which sleep tracings were performed during the active periods of aphasia, CSWS was observed. The earlier the onset of aphasia, the poorer is its prognosis, contrary to other aphasias of childhood.

Lerman: Hormonotherapy with steroids suppresses the EEG discharges and consequently aphasia is resolved. Hence, I believe that aphasia is clearly related to the EEG dysrhythmia. However, in long standing cases recovery from aphasia occurs several months after the EEG normalizes.

Revol: Behaviour problems are rather frequent in LKS; being observed in 49 out of 82 cases reviewed in the literature.

As to the aphasia certain authors have speculated that it is not a true aphasia, but rather a psychogenic mutism. However, the prevalent opinion is that aphasia, though true, may appear as a psychogenic mutism; similarly the behaviour problems may take a psychotic aspect even though, in effect, they are secondary to the communication difficulties and the seizures.

He considers this differentiation between psychogenic and organic symptoms, unjustified. Indeed, in four out of his six observations there was an early disturbance of the organization of the personality. Subsequently, the psychological problems, the language disability and the seizure disorder became so entangled that each one turned out to be one of the modes of expression of the global disturbance regardless of the cause.

At any single instant it becomes impossible to distinguish between what is psychogenic and what is somatic and then an open mind is necessary.

Epilepsy with continuous spike-wave discharges during sleep (CSWS)

Dalla Bernardina: (1) In the benign partial epilepsies there is often a marked increase in the focal abnormalities during sleep, becoming almost continuous but remaining focal all the same. These should not be confused with the picture of CSWS. These cases have an overall good prognosis.

(2) In his opinion there is a relationship between the CSWS and the BPE since this condition can occur in the course of the evolution of the BPE, both with CT spikes as well as with occipital discharges. These CSWS are seen concomitantly with the occurrence of behaviour problems, the diffusion of anomalies in waking and the appearance of absence seizures. Personally he thinks that, while the morphological aspects are hard to distinguish, the generalized spike-wave discharges and the absences are not due to a primary generalized discharge but are the result of a secondary generalization.

General discussion

Problems of terminology
Gastaut proposes to call them primary partial epilepsies for two reasons:

214

(1) because the term 'primary' enables one to distinguish them from those which are secondary to brain lesions; (2) because the terms 'primary' and 'secondary' have already been used in the proposal for an international classification of the generalized epilepsies.

Munari to Gastaut: In your proposition of the classification of the partial organic epilepsies you distinguish between elementary partial seizures and complex partial seizures. Why not adopt the same attitude with regard to the BPE?

Gastaut: It is feasible, but often in the BPE the same patient may have both elementary and complex seizures; eg in the BPO, it depends on the propagation of the discharges.

Genetic problems and relations between BPE and primary generalized epilepsy (PGE)
Roger and Lerman: In the same family cases of various types of BPE may coexist as well as cases of PGE, mainly of the absence type.

Doose: Since the predisposition to absences and to other PGE are genetically determined traits, we may think it a coincidence when the two types are found in the same family. However, since the studies are based on a collection of epileptics, and the combination of many factors lowers the convulsive threshold even further, these combinations are overrepresented in a collection of epileptics.

Beaumanoir: Long-term follow-up of patients with BPE shows the disappearance of both seizures and EEG abnormalities in all cases. However, the seizures may reappear later, generalized in nature, associated with spike-wave discharges. Hence, there must be two genetic factors in those patients expressing themselves in different ages.

Cavazzuti: In his epidemiological study he found that the prevalence of BECT was 1 : 1000 in school age, corresponding to 20 per cent of the epilepsies in this age. In a population of 3000 normal children, 30 had CT spike discharges without clinical seizures. They were followed throughout the school period, and only one developed BPE.

BPE and cerebral lesions
Doose: It is possible for BPE to occur also in brain damaged children. Indeed, if BPE depends on a special genetic predisposition (found in 3 per cent of healthy children) one should expect to find this predisposition also in children afflicted with brain damage. Moreover, since such lesions lower the convulsive threshold, it is expected that in such a population patients with brain damage will be overrepresented. Hence a cerebral lesion can co-exist with a BPE with a good prognosis.

Lerman and *Roger* emphasize that many physicians would not accept the diagnosis of BPE in patients suffering from brain damage.

Roger presents an example of BECT in a child with congenital toxoplasmosis and residual cerebral lesions.

Sorel indicates that one of the elements of distinction between lesional foci and the foci of BPE is the polarity of the spikes. In the former the spikes are cortex-negative. In the BPE the polarity field is different. The polarity is negative in the rolandic and temporal regions and positive in the prefrontal area. The spikes should be studied using referential electrodes.

Epileptic syndromes in infancy, childhood and adolescence. J. Roger, C. Dravet, M. Bureau, F.E. Dreifuss and P. Wolf. John Libbey Eurotext Ltd ©1985.

Chapter 24
Is There an Epilepsy with Unilateral Seizures?

Luis OLLER-DAURELLA

Escuelas Pias, 89, Barcelona - 17, Spain.

Introduction

The concept of a unilateral epileptic seizure is defined in the *Dictionary of epilepsy* (Gastaut, 1973) as 'an epileptic seizure which presents all the clinical characteristics of a generalized epileptic seizure, but with motor manifestations predominant on one side of the body or only on this same side'. A series of varieties are described: (1) unilateral tonic-clonic epileptic seizures; (2) unilateral tonic epileptic seizures; (3) unilateral clonic epileptic seizures; (4) unilateral atonic epileptic seizures; (5) complex absences with unilateral motor symptoms, for example the atonic or myoclonic absences which affect only one side of the body. From the EEG point of view, the unilateral epileptic seizures are accompained by generalized epileptic discharges which correspond to each clinical variety but whose amplitude appears to be greater in the contralateral half of the scalp. It is pointed out that they are specific of infancy and childhood. In the same way the *Dictionary* defines 'unilateral epilepsy' as 'an expression sometimes used to name the epilepsy of those people suffering mainly or exclusively from unilateral epileptic seizures. Synonym: Asymmetric Epilepsy'.

A short time later Gastaut *et al.*, (1974) published an extensive chapter in the *Handbook of clinical neurology,* in which they described the different types of unilateral seizures (USs), adding to those mentioned in the *Dictionary* unilateral infantile spasms, unilateral massive myoclonias, and including within the complex absences with unilateral motor manifestations, the adversive, hypertonic, myoclonic or unilateral atonic seizures. They emphasized the difference between the unilateral atonic seizures and Todd's paralysis. We have described all these varieties of unilateral epileptic seizures and the corresponding ictal tracings (Oller-Daurella and Oller-F-V., 1977-1981).

The best known of the epilepsies with USs is the Hemiconvulsion Hemiplegia-Epilepsy (HHE) syndrome, in which the US usually appears as a status in an infant during a febrile illness. The hemiplegia can be transient or definitive. Later, a partial temporal lobe epilepsy (Gastaut *et al.,* 1959) is often observed.

However, the USs may be seen in many other conditions, usually corresponding to an organic etiology, (Aicardi *et al.*, 1969; Beaumanoir, 1976). They can also be seen in patients with an evident organic etiology but with a favourable evolution (Beaussart *et al.,* 1978).

We thought it interesting to revise our cases of USs in 3000 epileptics, whose characteristics were stored in a data bank, and, from the results, to discuss the possible existence of a unilateral epilepsy or specific epileptic syndromes in patients with USs.

Methods and Material

Our data bank of 3000 epileptics is composed of non-selected patients, first seen between 1966 and 1976. These patients belonged to a neurological service of a general hospital, to an epilepsy centre or to our own private practice. Without previous selection, the data concerning the patients were stored until 3000 had been observed. The patients having only febrile seizures, a single seizure, or with seizure or status due to an acute cerebral insult and not followed by other seizures were excluded (Oller-Daurella *et al.,* 1978, 1981).

All patients with USs were revised statistically, excluding those cases in which the USs constituted an epiphenomenon of the epileptic disease. Thus we only kept the 151 patients in whom epilepsy started with clonic USs (hemiclonic seizures) and who were followed up for more than one year. As a matter of fact the other types of USs are rare and already belong to well definite syndromes (myoclonic absences, for example).

Results and Discussions

These 151 patients can be separated into four groups:
Group 1: 39 patients whose further epilepsy consisted of partial complex seizures belonging to a temporal lobe epilepsy (Temp. E.).
Group 2: 32 patients with a Lennox-Gastaut syndrome (LGS).
Group 3: 6 patients with a primary generalized epilepsy (PGE)
Group 4: 74 patients in whom seizures remain USs.

In each group we studied: sex, age at the first seizure, circumstances and duration of the first seizure, interval between the first seizure and the others, different types of seizures during the evolution and their frequency, EEG data (background activity, localized and generalized paroxysms, localized slow waves and depression) neurological signs, psychic symptoms, aetiological acquired and genetic factors, evolution (Tables 1,2,3,4 and 5).

In group 1: with Temp. E, we noted a slight prevalence of females, a variable age at the first seizure, later than in the other groups, the frequency of initial status (as in group 2), a long interval between the first seizure and the others, the frequency of neurological and psychiatric signs, the severity of the subsequent epilepsy, as we never succeded in suppressing seizures in these patients.

The complex partial seizures (CPS) could be isolated (12 cases) or associated with simple partial seizures (SPS) (six cases), with secondarily generalized seizures (sec. gen.s.) simple (seven cases), with SPS and sec.gen.s (five cases), with USs (one case). Eight patients did not have CPS but they had a temporal focus on the EEG (three with USs, three with SPS and sec.gen.s., one with SPS and one with sec.gen.s). In half of the cases only, epilepsy was controlled by treatment for a time. Only eight patients were seizure-free during 5 years and all the attempts to stop drugs led to a relapse.

In group 2: with LGS, we noted a prevalence of males, as is usual in epilepsy, the earliness of the first seizure, and frequency of initial status. In five cases this status was symptomatic (one encephalitis, two neonatal asphyxias, one cerebral hemorrhage, one kernicterus). On the contrary, there was no interval between the first seizure and the

Table 1. Age at the 1st seizure (in years)

	n	< 1 y n	%	1-5 y n	%	6-10 y n	%	> 10 y n	%
Group 1 (Temp. E.)	: 39	5	12.7	17	43.5	12	31	5	12.7
Group 2 (LGS)	: 32	24	75	7	21.8	1			
Group 3 (PGE)	: 6	3	50	1		2			
Group 4A (US)	: 48	15	31.2	22	45.8	8	16.6	3	6.2
Group 4B (US)	: 26	7	26.9	9	34.6	7	26.9	3	11.5
Total	: 151	54	35.7	55	36.4	30	19.8	11	7.2

Table 2. Data on the first seizures

	Sex M F	Age at the 1st seizure (years)	Circumstances of the 1st seizure (s = seizure)	Duration of the 1st seizure Brief	Status	Interval between the 1st seizure and others (years)
Group 1 (n = 39; Temp. E)	18 21	1-20 y (m = 5.4)	7 febrile s. 1 meningo. enceph. 1 cranial trauma 1 neonatal asphyxia	22	17	11 cases :0 18 cas : 1-18 (m = 4.8)
Group 2 (n = 32;LGS)	18 14	< 1-8 y (m = 1)	0 febrile s 1 encephalitis 2 neonatal asphyxias 1 cereb. hem. 1 kernicterus	16	16	30 cases :< 1 1 case : 1.5 1 case : 5
Group 3 (n = 6; PGE)	1 5	< 1-9 y	1 febrile s.	4	2	4 cases :0 2 cases :3-9
Group 4A (n = 48; US)	27 21	< 1-17 y (m = 3.5)	11 febrile s.	36	12	36 cases :0 12 cases :< 1-9 (m = 1.8)
Group 4B (n = 26;US)	14 12	< 1-14 y (m = 4.3)	1 febrile s.	24	2	2 cases :< 1

Table 3. Seizures during evolution

	Type		Frequency	Recorded	
Group 1 (*n* = 39; Temp. E.)	CPS	31	Always frequent	CPS	13
	US only	3	Status: 28 cases		
	SPS	4			
	sec. gen. s.	1			
Group 2 (*n* = 32;LGS)	LGS s.		Always very frequent	LGS s.	16
	± US		Status: many	hemiclon s.	2
	partial s. rare				
	GMs + Myocl. (very rare)				
Group 3 (*n* = 6;PGE)	Absences	3		Absences	3
	Myocl.	2		Myocl.	2
	GMs	1			
Group 4A (*n* = 48; US)	hemiclon. s.	46	± frequent	hemiclon. s.	3
	hemiton. s.	1	Status: 19 cases	US	1
	hemi. GMs	1		SPS	1
	+ SPS	1			
Group 4B (*n* = 26; US)	hemiclon. s.	26	Rare	hemiclon. s.	4
	+ SPS	5	Status: 4 cases	hemi.GM s.	1
	+ Myocl.	1			

Table 4. EEG characteristics

	Slow background activity		Localized paroxysms		Generalized paroxysms		Localized slow waves		Localized depressions	
	n	*%*	*n*	*%*	*n*	*%*	*n*	*%*	*n*	*%*
Group 1 (*n* = 39; Temp. E.)	9	23.1	37	94.9	10	25.6	12	30.8	1	2.5
Group 2 (*n* = 32; LGS)	25	78	15	46.8	31	96.8			6	18.9%
Group 3 (*n* = 6; PGE)		-	4	66.6	5	83.3				
Group 4A (*n* = 48; US)	13	27.1	32	66.7	15	31.2	13	27.1	6	12.5
Group 4B (*n* = 26; US)	1	3.8	16	61.5	5	19.2	8	30.7	3	11.5

Table 5. Some clinical characteristics of patients: no. of subjects affected (% in parenthesis)

	Neurological signs	Psychological signs	Acquired aetiology		Genetic factor	Evolution 5 yr without seizures
Group 1 (*n* = 39: Temp. E.)	11 (28.2)	17 (43.6)	10 (25.6) perinatal meningo enceph trauma septicemia	4 3 1 1	10 (25.6)	8 (20.5)
Group 2 (*n* = 32; LGS)	23 (71)	30 (93.7)	28 (87.5) perinatal meningo enceph malformation metabolic	10 3 1 1	8 (25)	5 (15.6)
Group 3 (*n* = 6; PGE)	0	0	0		3 (50)	5 (83.3)
Group 4A (*n* = 48; US)	27 (56.2)	33 (68.7)	19 (39.5) perinatal meningo enceph trauma phacomatosis others	11 3 1 2 2	11 (22.9)	23 (47.9)
Group 4B (*n* = 26; US)	0	0	0		5 (19.2)	14 (53.8)

others. As in group 1, permanent neurological signs were very frequent: nine hemiplegias or other hemispheric syndromes, seven diplegias or tetraplegias, seven severe diffuse alterations. Only two patients had an intellectual level in normal limits. Epilepsy was very severe. Seizures persisted in spite of treatment in 75 per cent of cases. Five patients were seizure-free for more than 5 years, but the withdrawal of treatment was followed by a relapse in three cases out of these five.

Group 3: with PGE, is too small to allow any conclusion. However we noted the prevalence of females, as in petit mal absences, the absence of neurological and psychological signs, the good results of treatment. In only one case seizures persisted. Other patients had a good response to treatment which was stopped without relapse in 1 case.

Group 4: patients with only USs — they were divided in two subgroups:
- Group 4A, so called lesional, 48 patients for whom organic damage could be assessed, because of a demonstrated acquired aetiology, permanent neurological signs, or intellectual deficit;
- Group 4B, non-lesional, 26 patients for which no organic lesion could be demonstrated.

In both subgroups we observed a prevalence of males. The age of onset of seizures was more variable than in the three other groups. On the contrary we noted the follow-

ing differences between the two subgroups:
- The onset by a status, often febrile, was much more frequent in subgroup A;
- A free interval was more often observed between the first seizure and the others in the lesional subgroup, and this can be compared to the observations of group 1, with Temp. E.
- Epilepsy was more severe in the lesional subgroup. Seizures were more frequent during evolution and could evolve in status. The seizures were not controlled by treatment in 27 per cent of cases. Twenty-three patients remained seizure-free during 5 years (47.9 per cent) and in eight of them the treatment could be withdrawn without relapses.

Conversely, in the non lesional subgroup B, seizures were rare: 11 patients had less than five seizures throughout the evolution. Only in two cases the treatment was ineffective (7.6 per cent). Fourteen patients were seizure-free during 5 years (53.8 per cent) and in 10 of them the treatment could be withdrawn without relapse.

Conclusion

We think that it is possible to individualize a form of epilepsy in childhood characterized by the unique or greatly predominant presence of hemiclonic USs.

In some cases (groups 1,2, and 3) it is only a phase in the course of the epileptic disease, which probably cannot be regarded as a form of epilepsy. But if one considers the physiopathology, the HHE syndrome remains individualized.

In the other cases (group 4A, B) in whom USs are the main feature during the entire course, it is possible to speak of a unilateral epilepsy, and we propose to divide it into two groups, according to the existence or the absence of an associated lesional symptomatology. This unilateral epilepsy would correspond to group 1: 'epilepsies with both generalized and focal features' included within the undetermined epilepsies in the unpublished draft of classification proposed by the Commission on Classification and Terminology of the ILAE (11 August, 1982).

References

Aicardi, J., Amsili, J., Chevrie, J.J. (1966): Acute hemiplegia in infancy and childhood. *Develop. Med. Child Neurol.* **11**, 162-173.

Beaumanoir, A. (1976): *Les épilepsies infantiles. Problèmes de diagnostic et de traitement.* Edition Roche: Bâle.

Beaussart, M., Faou, R., Grégoire, L.-P. (1978): Devenir des enfants ayant présenté une ou plusieurs crises convulsives unilatérales primitives. *Pédiatrie* **33**, 543-549.

Gastaut, H., Poirier, F., Payan, H., Salamon, G., Toga, M., Vigouroux, M. (1959): H.H.E. Syndrome. *Epilepsia* **1**, 418-447.

Gastaut, H. (1973): *Dictionnaire de l'épilepsie.* OMS: Genève.

Gastaut, H., Broughton, R., Tassinari, C.A., Roger, J. (1974): Unilateral epileptic seizures. In *Handbook of clinical neurology. Vol. XV. The Epilepsies,* pp. 235-245, ed P.J. Vinken, G.W. Bruyn. Elsevier: Amsterdam and New York.

Oller-Daurella, L. and Oller-F.V.,L. (1977): *Atlas de crisis epilépticas.* Geigy Division Farmacéutica: Barcelona.

Oller-Daurella, L. and Oller-F.V.,L. (1978): Banco de datos de epilepsia: analisis computarizado de 3.000 enfermos epilépticos. *Bol. Lega It. Epil.* **17**, 15-21.

Oller-Daurella, L. and Oller-F.V.,L. (1981): *Atlas de crisis epilépticas,* 2nd editn, apéndice 1 pp. 319-343. Geigy Division Farmacéutica: Barcelona.

*   *   *

Discussion pages 228-229

Epileptic syndromes in infancy, childhood and adolescence. J. Roger, C. Dravet, M. Bureau, F.E. Dreifuss and P. Wolf. John Libbey Eurotext Ltd ©1985.

Chapter 25
Comments on an Epileptic Syndrome with Unilateral Seizures

Charlotte DRAVET

Centre Saint-Paul, 300 Boulevard Sainte-Marguerite, 13009 Marseille, France

Symptomatology

A hemiclonic seizure is rarely observed from its onset. The onset can be either a unilateral deviation of head and eyes, associated with horizontal clonic jerks of eyeballs, sometimes with head jerks, or with pallor, nausea, vomiting, abdominal pain, or a fall and generalized clonic jerks then lateralized during the seizure. Usually the patient cannot speak but there is not always an early diminution of consciousness.

Whatever the onset may be, the hemiclonic seizure is characterized by clonic jerks involving one side of the body. These jerks can be rhythmic and stable in their site. But, often, there are unceasing variations of their amplitude, their frequency and their distribution which give an anarchic aspect: they can disappear in the face and persist in the arm, then in the leg, or the contrary, involve only the hand or the foot for some seconds, yet they never have an orderly jacksonian propagation. Some seizures principally consist of a lateral deviation of eyes and head and of very small twitchings involving a small part of the body only (eyeballs, hemilip, frontalis).

The loss of consciousness can be the initial event or the process may be gradual. Automatic phenomena, like pallor, perspiration, hypersalivation, are usual.

In some cases the clonic jerks can cease in the side affected and suddenly appear in a part of the other side or involve this whole side of the body (alternating seizure), or they can become generalized.

The onset of the seizure is sudden. In spite of the existence of a homolateral hemiparesis the child rapidly returns to a normal consciousness if the seizure is brief.

During the seizure, the EEG shows a continuous, bilateral, synchronous discharge of slow waves at 2-3 c/s, higher in the hemisphere opposite to the clinical seizure and in this hemisphere only mixed with a 10 c/s rhythm, sometimes more evident in the posterior region. (Fig. 1A). This feature gives variable appearances, sometimes like pseudorhythmic spike-waves. The polygraphic recording shows the clonic jerks (Fig. 1B). But the relationship between EEG and muscular phenomena is not always very close. At the end of the seizures, the slow waves and the spikes suddenly cease and are replaced by a brief flattening of the rhythms, followed by very slow waves of higher amplitude in the hemisphere which was the site of the ictal discharge. After an intrave-

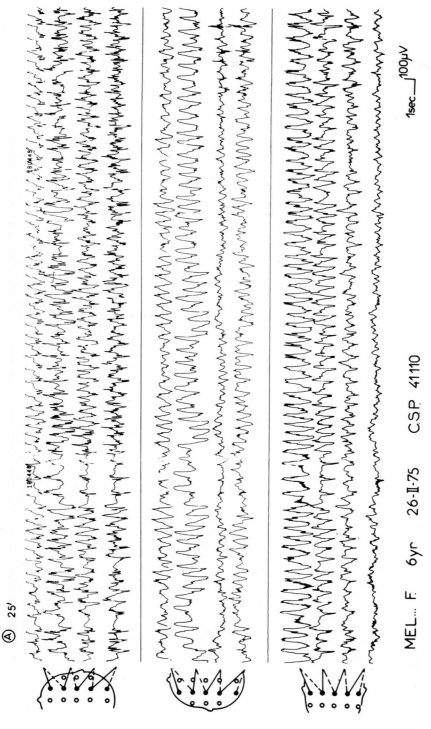

Fig. 1A. A left hemiclonic seizure recorded 25 min. from the onset in a 6-year-old boy with a left hemiplegia.

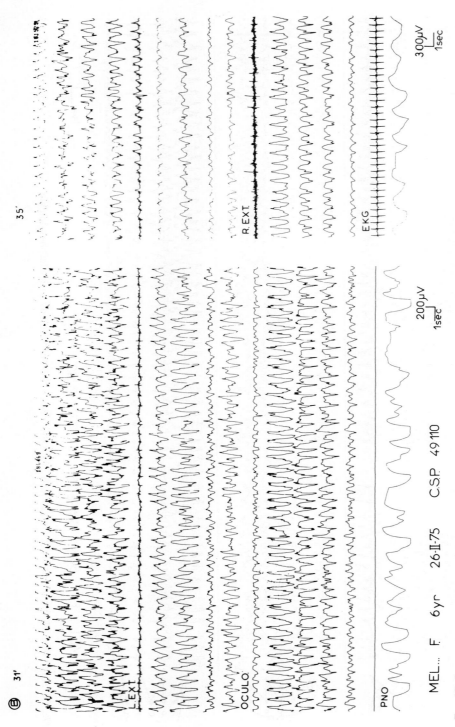

Fig. 1B. Polygraphic recording of the seizure 31 min. later. Left: extensor of the left hand, oculogram, pneumogram. Right: extensor of the left and of the right hands, electrocardiogram and pneumogram. Amplitude of record has been progressively reduced.

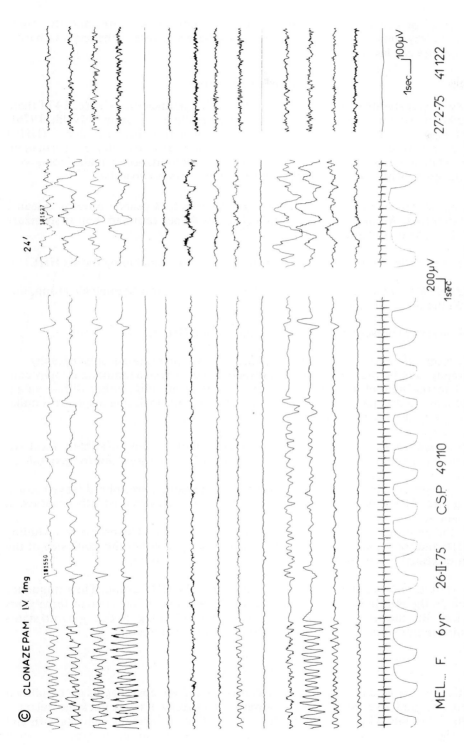

Fig. 1C. Left: end of the seizure after an intravenous injection of 1 mg of clonazepam. Centre: 24 min. after the end of the seizure. Right: 24 h after the end of the seizure (normal record amplitude).

225

nous injection of benzodiazepine the post-ictal asymmetry is clearer and the drug-induced rapid rhythms are seen only in the hemisphere opposite to the ictal discharge. This asymmetry can last several days (Fig. 1C).

Study of 14 patients

In a study of 95 patients whose epilepsy started with a hemiclonic seizure, 14 of them continued to present only seizures of this type all along their evolution (Vivaldi, 1976).

Out of these 14 patients, six had a Hemiconvulsion-Hemiplegia-Epilepsy (HHE) syndrome and were hemiplegic, eight did not present any neurological permanent disorder. They are eight boys and six girls, with a predominance of males being very clear in the group without neurological signs (six boys versus two girls).

The age of onset of seizures is variable: from 8 months to 8 years 7 months (mean 2 years 10 months). Among the non-hemiplegic cases 87 per cent had their first seizure between 1 and 5 years of age.

Circumstances of the first seizure: hyperthermia in nine cases (including the six HHE).

Acquired aetiological factors: three neo-natal anoxias in the non-hemiplegic group, one Sturge-Weber disease in the HHE group.

A genetic factor was present in five cases (including one HHE).

Neuroradiological data. Only eight patients had pneumoencephalography or arteriography: among the HHE one was normal, one displayed a temporal atrophy contralateral to the hemiplegia, two displayed a bilateral atrophy, either diffuse or bi-temporal; among the non-hemiplegic cases, three were normal, one displayed a unilateral atrophy on the site opposite to that of the seizures.

Electroencephalographic data. Paroxysmal abnormalities are variable, focal or multifocal, but sometimes associated with hemispheric (five cases) and/or generalized (seven cases) abnormalities.

When the abnormalities are always localized in the same hemisphere (seven cases, including three HHE and four non-hemiplegic) the seizures are constantly observed in the opposite side of the body.

When the abnormalities are localized in both hemispheres (seven cases, including three HHE and four non-hemiplegic) the seizures involve either the same side of the body (three cases) or vary from one side to the other (four cases).

Data concerning the evolution: Seizures are frequent in the HHE group. Their frequency is variable in the non-hemiplegic group and some patients can have two or three years seizure-free. But the seizures always have a tendency to be long, to develop into status and require an intravenous injection of benzodiazepine to end them.

Conclusion

We think there is actually a group of patients whose epilepsy begins in childhood (between one and five years) and is always characterized by hemiclonic seizures during its evolution. This group is heterogeneous since it includes subjects with and without sign of brain damage. It probably represents a particular type of partial epilepsy, either primary or secondary, which must be acknowledged, in our opinion, because its treatment raises specific problems.

References

Vivaldi, J. (1976): Les crises hémicloniques de l'enfant, modalités évolutives. Thèse, Marseille.

*　　　　　*　　　　　*

Discussion pages 228-229

*Epileptic syndromes in infancy, child-
hood and adolescence.* J. Roger,
C. Dravet, M. Bureau, F.E.
Dreifuss and P. Wolf. John Libbey
Eurotext Ltd ©1985.

Discussion of
Unilateral seizures
(Chapters 24 and 25)

Summarized by Joseph ROGER

Since Oller-Daurella had presented a total statistical profile of unilateral seizures (US),
— both of the most frequent variety, hemiclonic seizures and the others (hemitonic,
hemitonic-clonic, absences with unilateral manifestations, myoclonic or atonic) — the
first discussion dealt with the symptomatology of US.

Munari and Loiseau suggested that US could represent a particular form of motor partial epilepsy and that the unilateral nature of the seizure, without Jacksonian
characteristics, might correspond to a special type of organization of the discharge in
the motor cortex.

Oller-Daurella, Roger and *Dravet* presented the electo-clinical data which, in their
opinion, differentiate the US from the other types of partial motor seizures: usual long
duration of the fit, non-Jacksonian motor manifestations, apparent stability of the ictal
EEG discharge with varying clinical symptomatology during the course of the seizure,
presence of rhythmical bilateral slow waves with spikes discharges in one hemisphere
only, possibility of alternating or 'see-saw' seizures.

Oller-Daurella could not suggest any satisfactory explanation for the generalized spike-
waves accompanying some unilateral clinical manifestations.

Munari asked how effective neuroradiology was in locating lesional epilepsies and pin-
pointing the site of the lesions.

Oller-Daurella answered that neuroradiological examinations were positive in one
third of cases. Closely defined localized lesions are rare, while slightly extended lesions
(such as scars of infarcts, porencephalic cysts) or unilateral atrophy are observed more
often.

Dreifuss questionned *Munari* about the use of stereo-encephalograph who answered
that this type of investigation was reserved for cases of hemiplegia.

Oller-Daurella and *Dravet* emphasized the variable significance of US since different
types of successive epilepsy can be observed. In particular some patients will have a

later primary generalized epilepsy with petit mal absences, for example.

Dulac thought that it was necessary to separate the US from the other motor partial seizures because they can be long, even during evolution. They can occur again in status and cause cerebral damage, even in children. One must be very prudent before discontinuing treatment because relapses are frequent, and possibly severe, above all when there is a previous neurological symptomatology.

Roger thought that US might be the only manifestation of some primary partial seizures, but the reasons are still being debated.

IV
Epileptic syndromes in childhood and adolescence

Epileptic syndromes in infancy, childhood and adolescence. J. Roger, C. Dravet, M. Bureau, F.E. Dreifuss and P. Wolf. John Libbey Eurotext Ltd ©1985.

Chapter 26
Photosensitive Epilepsies

Peter M. JEAVONS

Clinical Neurophysiology Unit, Department of Ophthalmic Optics, University of Aston in Birmingham, Woodstock Street, Birmingham, B4 7ET, United Kingdom

Summary

To establish photosensitivity the photostimulator must carry a pattern and the fovea and macula must be stimulated. The basic EEG is often normal. A photoconvulsive response (PCR) commonly consists of a spike and wave or polyspike and wave discharge involving all areas. Photosensitivity is genetically determined, commoner in females and usually manifests itself around puberty. Seizures may occur spontaneously, or in response to flickering light (television, sunlight) or patterns. Rarely seizures are self-induced. Eyelid myoclonia with absences is a form of photosensitive epilepsy. Seizures evoked by flicker are commonly tonic-clonic or myoclonic, absences and partial seizures being rare. In pure photosensitive epilepsy there are no spontaneous seizures and drug therapy may not be needed. Sodium valproate is the most effective drug therapy. The prognosis is uncertain, and photosensitivity often persists beyong the age of 20.

The literature on photosensitive epilepsy is extensive, and references will be found in Jeavons and Harding (1975), Newmark and Penry (1979) and Jeavons (1982).

Photosensitivity and pattern sensitivity are essentially laboratory findings which can only be established by using adequate techniques, as described elsewhere (Jeavons and Harding, 1975; Jeavons, 1982; Darby *et al.,* 1980*b*). For photosensitivity one important factor is the use of a line or grid pattern on the front of the lamp of the photostimulator (Jeavons *et al.,* 1972), since without such a pattern a photoconvulsive response may not be elicited (Fig. 1). It is also essential that the patient looks directly at the centre of the lamp, which must be placed at 30 cm from the eyes. This ensures adequate stimulation of the macula and fovea. The effect of a slight shift of gaze is shown in Fig. 2.

The diagnosis of photosensitive epilepsy depends on the evocation by intermittent photic stimulation (IPS) of a photoconvulsive response (PCR) which consists of a generalized discharge recorded from all areas of the scalp (Fig. 1). This discharge consists most commonly of a spike and wave or polyspike and wave discharge, though a variety of other discharges may be found. Photomyoclonic responses which are confined to the anterior regions, and those confined to the posterior or occipital regions (occipital spikes) are excluded.

Photosensitive epilepsy is genetically determined and quite often familial occurring in 8 per cent of our cases (Jeavons and Harding, 1975). Photosensitivity is more common in females than males in a ratio of 1.7 to 1.

The median age of onset is 14 years suggesting that puberty is a factor.

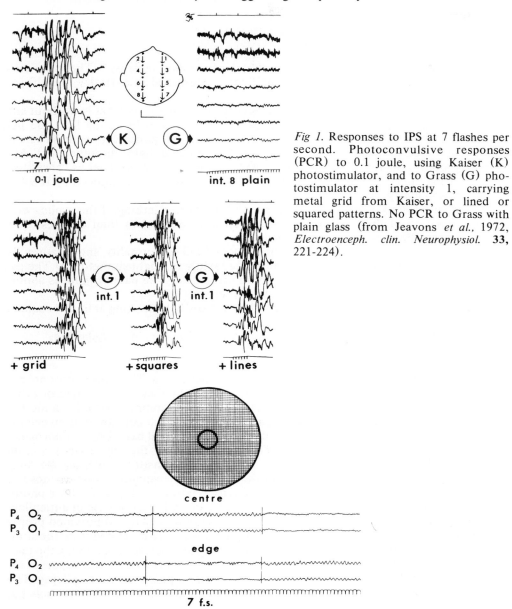

Fig 1. Responses to IPS at 7 flashes per second. Photoconvulsive responses (PCR) to 0.1 joule, using Kaiser (K) photostimulator, and to Grass (G) photostimulator at intensity 1, carrying metal grid from Kaiser, or lined or squared patterns. No PCR to Grass with plain glass (from Jeavons et al., 1972, *Electroenceph. clin. Neurophysiol.* **33**, 221-224).

Fig 2. Photic driving in response to stimulation at 7 flashes per second, seen only when subject looks at centre of Grass photostimulator, and not when subject looks at edge of lamp (distance 30cm from eyes) (from Jeavons, 1982. In *Textbook of epilepsy,* ed. J. Laidlaw, A. Richens, pp 195-211. Churchill Livingstone: Edinburgh).

Subjects who show a photoconvulsive response may or may not have seizures, but if myoclonic jerking is associated with the PCR it is very probable that the subject has epilepsy. Most commonly seizures are generalized tonic-clonic, less commonly absences or myoclonic jerks. Partial seizures may occur, but are uncommon.

Classification

Photosensitive epilepsy is found in 6 main groups.

(1) *Pure photosensitive epilepsy* (television epilepsy, reflex epilepsy). These patients only have seizures provoked by flickering light encountered in everyday life (40 per cent of 454 patients).

(2) *Epilepsy with photosensitivity:* (a) Seizures occur spontaneously (that is, without any evidence of flicker as a precipitant), but they also occur with flickering light (33 per cent of 454 patients). (b) 'Spontaneous' seizures occur, but none occur with flickering light encountered in everyday life (television, flickering sunlight, discotheques). Abnormality occurs on IPS (27 per cent of 454 patients). (c) Spontaneous 'absences' occur, but may not be evoked by everyday flicker. Absences are induced by IPS (31 per cent of 454 patients).

(3) *Eyelid myoclonia with absences* (Jeavons, 1977). Marked jerking of the eyelids with upward deviation of the eyes occurs on eye closure, but not in total darkness. IPS evokes abnormality. Spontaneous absences occur.

(4) *Self-induced epilepsy:* (a) The patient induces EEG abnormality and seizures by waving the hand in front of the eyes or blinking rapidly in bright sunlight. (b) The patient is impulsively attracted to the television screen. (c) The patient induces abnormality by slow blinking in front of the television screen.

(5) *Pattern-sensitive epilepsy.* Seizures are induced, usually by looking at lined or square patterns.

(6) *Seizures are induced by IPS in the laboratory,* but none occurs in everyday life.

1. Pure photosensitive epilepsy

In pure photosensitive epilepsy there are no spontaneous fits. The commonest precipitant is television viewing, though fits may be induced by flickering sunlight or other sources of flickering light or patterns. Seizures are most commonly tonic-clonic (84 per cent), absences occur in 6 per cent, partial seizures in 2.5 per cent and myoclonic seizures in 1.5 per cent. Nearly half the patients have a normal basic EEG, abnormality only occurring when exposed to IPS. The most effective therapy is with sodium valproate, although clonazepam may also control photosensitive epilepsy. We have shown that spike and wave discharges in the basic EEG respond to a lower dose of VPA than is required to abolish all photosensitivity (Harding *et al.,* 1978). Pure photosensitive epilepsy, especially TV epilepsy, can be treated without the use of antiepileptic drugs provided there is no spike and wave in the basic EEG, and provided proper precautions are taken to avoid the stimulus. Most patients are protected from the stimulus if they firmly cover one eye with the palm of the hand before approaching the television set. The recent increase in video games using TV sets has led to the report of so-called 'space-invader' epilepsy, but such cases belong to photosensitive epilepsy. The increasing use of a television set in home computer and in computers in schools has also increased the likelihood of television epilepsy.

2. Epilepsy with photosensitivity

Epilepsy with photosensitivity is not a syndrome, and the subdivision of photosensitive patients on the basis of whether or not they have 'spontaneous' seizures or whether or not they have seizures precipitated by flickering light met in everyday life, must be provisional since follow-up of patients may reveal that 'spontaneous' seizures appear or that flicker induced seizures appear neither having been present in the early years of follow-up. A group of 31 patients who had spontaneous absences differed from other photosensitive patients in that 3 cycles per second spike-wave absence was evoked by a narrow range of flash rates. Seventy per cent of these patients were female and nearly half of them did not have seizures provoked by flicker in everyday life.

3. Eyelid myoclonia with absences
I have previously suggested (Jeavons, 1977), that eyelid myoclonia with absences is a separate entity, on clinical, EEG and therapeutic evidence, and it should be separated from the other types of absence epilepsy. The characteristics are that of very marked myoclonic jerks of the eyelid with upward deviation of the eyes. The EEG shows spike-wave or polyspike-wave discharges on eye closure which are not present in the dark. Abnormalities are invariably provoked by IPS. Spontaneous absences occur associated with spike-wave discharges and there are occasional tonic-clonic seizures. Unlike other photosensitive epilepsies the age of onset is similar to that of simple and complex absences (mean age 6 $\pm$ 2 years). This compares with the later onset of photosensitivity which is usually around puberty. Therapy is more difficult than that of the other types of absence seizure and remission around puberty is less likely. Sodium valproate and ethosuximide alone or in combination may be effective.

4. Self-induced epilepsy
Self-induced epilepsy may occur very rarely following precipitants other than light; it is uncommon and its delineation as a syndrome is unclear from the literature. Most of the cases refer to hand waving in a source of bright light, and mental retardation is said to be quite common. More females are affected than males and the most common type of attack is an absence. Some patients are reported to blink rapidly in bright sunlight. From personal experience and the evidence of Ames both in written papers and cine-film (Ames 1971, 1974), and from the work of other authors, I agree that in many of these patients the hand-movements are part of the seizure and not the precipitating factor. Furthermore, I regard a number of these patients, particularly those who blink rapidly in bright sunlight, as having eyelid myoclonia with absences.

A few patients have been reported as using the television screen to induce seizures (Harley et al., 1967; Andermann, 1971). We have reported 30 patients with impulsive attraction to the television set (Jeavons and Harding, 1975). These patients, unlike other photosensitive patients, show a male predominance and are not usually retarded. Furthermore, the most frequent seizure is tonic-clonic and not an absence. They have a wide sensitivity range evoked by IPS and 80 per cent of them show spike and wave discharges in the basic EEG.

Darby et al. (1980a) reported patients who induced spike and wave discharges by slow eye closure when watching a television set in the laboratory and it is probable that the number of these patients is greater than has previously been reported since it depends on an adequate technique in the laboratory. The patients reported by Darby et al. (1980a) can be separated from the classical self-induced cases and possibly from those impulsively attracted to the TV screen.

5. Pattern-sensitive epilepsy
Pattern-sensitivity is allied to photosensitivity. Patients who present clinically with pattern sensitivity are rare, but it has been shown that pattern-sensitive epilepsy is more common than is generally recognized and the recognition depends on an adequate

technique (Darby *et al.*, 1980*b*). Patients who are pattern-sensitive are photosensitive and patients who are photosensitive are often pattern-sensitive. Pattern-sensitivity should not be separated from photosensitivity.

6. Seizures induced only by IPS in the laboratory
If seizures have only been induced when exposed to IPS in the laboratory, and none have occurred in everyday life, the case should be excluded from photosensitive epilepsy.

Prognosis

We do not yet know the long-term prognosis of photosensitive epilepsy, but photosensitivity tends to appear around puberty and to persist into adult life. Our current follow-up programme, which has continued for 16 years, has shown that a number of patients are still photosensitive after the age of 20.

Impulsive attraction to the television set tends to disappear but occasionally persists. Eyelid myoclonia with absences may well persist into adult life.

If we are to regard photosensitive epilepsy as a syndrome, we must exclude all groups other than pure photosensitive epilepsy and eyelid myoclonia with absences. However, I do not think it is justified to regard photosensitive epilepsies as a syndrome.

References

Ames, F.R. (1971): 'Self-induction' in photosensitive epilepsy. *Brain* **94**, 781-798.
Ames, F.R. (1974): Cinefilm and EEG recording during 'hand-waving' attacks of an epileptic, photosensitive child. *Electroenceph. Clin. Neurophysiol.* **37**, 301-304.
Andermann, F. (1971): Self-induced television epilepsy. *Epilepsia* **12**, 269-275.
Darby, C.E., de Korte, R.A., Binnie, C.D., Wilkins, A.J. (1980*a*): The self-induction of epileptic seizures by eye-closure. *Epilepsia* **21**, 31-42.
Darby, C.E., Wilkins, A.J., Binnie, C.D., de Korte, R. (1980*b*): A method for the routine testing for pattern sensitivity. *J. Electrophysiol. Technol.* **6**, 202-210.
Harding, G.F.A., Herrick, C.E., Jeavons, P.M. (1978): A controlled study of the effect of sodium valproate on photosensitive epilepsy and its prognosis. *Epilepsia* **19**, 555-565.
Harley, R.D., Baird, H.W., Freeman, R.D. (1967): Self-induced photogenic epilepsy. Report of four cases. *Arch. Ophthalmol.* **78**, 730-737.
Jeavons, P.M. (1977): Nosological problems of myoclonic epilepsies in childhood and adolescence. *Develop. Med. Child. Neurol.* **19**, 3-8.
Jeavons, P.M. (1982): Photosensitive epilepsy, Part Two. In *A textbook of epilepsy,* pp 195-211, ed J. Laidlaw, A. Richens, Churchill Livingstone: Edinburgh.
Jeavons, P.M., Harding, G.F.A., Panayiotopoulos, C.P., Drasdo, N. (1972): The effect of geometric patterns combined with intermittent photic stimulation in photosensitive epilepsy. *Electroenceph. Clin. Neurophysiol.* **33**, 221-224.
Jeavons, P.M., Harding, G.F.A. (1975): *Photosensitive epilepsy.* Clinics in Developmental Medicine No. 56. Heinemann: London.
Newmark, M.E., Penry, J.K. (1979): *Photosensitivity and epilepsy: a review.* Raven Press: New York.

*   *   *

Discussion pages 237-241

Epileptic syndromes in infancy, child-hood and adolescence. J. Roger, C. Dravet, M. Bureau, F.E. Dreifuss and P. Wolf. John Libbey Eurotext Ltd ©1985.

Discussion of
Absence and Photosensitive Epilepsies

(Chapters 12,13 and 26)

Summarized by Fritz DREIFUSS

Dreifuss: I would like to preface the remarks pointing out that in 1964 a group of potential epilepsy study collaborators met at the National Institutes of Health to work out the methodology for collaborative studies. The absence seizures were chosen as a model because 'everybody knows all about absence and can basically agree'. Ten years later, we were still struggling with the definition of absence seizures. I hope that we will have more unanimity here than has previously been achieved. The following reviews will be discussed:

P. Loiseau — Reviewer — Petit Mal Absence
C.A. Tassinari — Reviewer — Myoclonic Absences
P. Jeavons — Reviewer — Photosensitive Epilepsies

Dreifuss: On looking at the prognostic criteria which allow one to predict a good prognosis group and seizures which are likely to persist, there are certain factors which may be helpful. One of these is not so much the regularity of the spike and wave discharge but the normality or slowing of the EEG background, as of course, are the other factors which distinguish the truly primary epilepsies from the lesional and which include normal intelligence, absence of abnormal neurological findings, the absence of other seizure types, etc.

Gastaut: I agree with Tassinari and have nothing to add to his presentation. Concerning the review presented by Loiseau, I wish to remark on the symptomatology. In 1951 and in 1956 (in a book prefaced by Penfield), I noted that it was necessary to distinguish between simple and complex absences, the latter with automatisms, hypertonia, atonia, myoclonia and autonomic symptoms. I was surprised when Penry, Porter and Dreifuss found few simple absences and a predominance of complex absences and now this point of view is confirmed by Loiseau. If there are 60 per cent of absences with automatisms in petit mal, then there are also 60 per cent of absences with automatisms in temporal lobe epilepsy and that makes for a very difficult differential diagnosis, yet I make this diagnosis entirely by questioning the patients, in 100 per cent of the cases. I find automatisms in petit mal absences to be different from those of temporal seizures. While I once saw a child who climbed on a piano during an absence attack which lasted three minutes, the usual petit mal absences last 15 seconds, hardly enough time to put your hand in your pocket. Perhaps someone is able to walk during a petit mal absence but during a temporal lobe seizure he runs (procursive absence). In many patients, 60 per cent have simple absences which can include small automatisms. Another point is terminology: Should one speak of petit mal epilepsy, petit mal absences or primary generalized epilepsy with absence? The latter allows us to have a place for the myoclonic primary generalized epilepsies or myoclonic petit mal and for the grand mal primary generalized epilepsy. Regarding evolution, I have seen about 10 patients between 40 and 49 whom I have followed for 35 years and who continue to have pyknolepsy while working, driving their car, and so on.

I have a question to Jeavons: one cannot define a single photosensitive epilepsy; they are rather epilepsies which are photosensitive. On one simple point I do not agree. Ames stated that in self-induced absence, the hand movement was a part of the attack. The hand movement precedes the absence and not vice versa. Microabsences upon closure of the eyes do exist and I have about 20 cases of that. They may be benign or severe. They consist of attacks lasting 2-3 seconds with a palpebral flutter and occur only when the eyes are closed and only in children.

Henriksen: If I understood correctly, you asked why not use the word 'petit mal'? In Scandinavia and many other countries the term petit mal is grossly misused by many physicians. That is why I prefer to use 'absence'.

Dreifuss: Fortunately, there is going to be an animal model for the primary generalized epilepsies, whether these be absence or phctically-stimulated seizures, and this will allow one to study these at a more basic level; in the absence seizures, perhaps, the penicillin model in the cat and in the case of the photic sensitive seizures by manipulating the biochemical environment with glutamic acid dehydrogenase and with the administration of dopamine receptor agonists which affect this particular type of epilepsy.

Binnie: For photosensitivity we use the same criteria, the same equipment, the same method of photic stimulation and we obtain virtually the same results as Jeavons. Much disagreement in the literature is not on the basis of true disagreement but because of lack of precise definitions. For example, Doose, using a broader definition, describes an iceberg of which Jeavons and I describe only the clinically evident top.

If one looks for subgroups which might form interesting syndromes, one conceivable candidate might be pattern-sensitive epilepsies, variety of which might be artifactual because of the commonly used checkerboard stimulus which is virtually ineffectual in pattern-sensitive epilepsy. In grid patterns, 40 per cent are sensitive to static patterns and over 60 per cent to oscillating patterns among the photosensitive group. The true incidence is hard to define because the correct questions are rarely asked. For example, if a child has seizures when going to bed, one may not get the answer unless one asks whether his bedroom wallpaper is striped.

Jeavons suggested eyelid myoclonus as a possible separate category. A lot of patients complain of ocular discomfort when exposed to potentially epileptogenic stimuli and many of these may have eyelid myoclonus. There may also be some confusion between what Jeavons calls eyelid myoclonus and what we have found to be self-induction by slow eyelid closure. On telemetry, some 25 per cent of photosensitive patients show this phenomenon of slow-eye-closure followed by epileptic discharges provided they are exposed to bright light. When questioned, some 60 per cent admit to deriving a pleasant sensation form doing this. Some patients begin with slow eye closure and then use the hand movements to make this phenomenon persist. Ames's cinephotos show just this.

If pattern stimulation is carried out in one or other field, we were quite excited some years ago to find focal discharges in the contralateral occipital region and this response was frequently quite asymmetrical and this is just as common in patients with primary generalized epilepsy as in those with partial or secondary generalized epilepsies.

Photic sensitivity is common in both primary generalized epilepsies where there may be heavy genetic weighting as well as in secondary generalized epilepsies with focal cerebral lesions who have nothing in common with the first group other than a favorable response to valproate and I can see no basis for using the presence of photic sensitivity as a basis for classification into primary or secondary epilepsies.

Oller-Daurella: I would like to show a film with unilaterally predominant absences. We have recorded 210 patients with absences and we have found unilaterally predominant absences in 36 per cent. We have divided them into four groups, absences with versive movements, absences with unilateral myoclonus, absences with unilateral atonia, and absences with unilateral hypertonia. In the first example, there are right-sided myoclonic jerks with right-sided turning movements a little slower than 3 c/s, accompanied by bilateral synchronous spike and wave, interictal EEGs with discharges clearly predominant on the controlateral side. These versive absences account for about 17 per cent. Secondly, absences with predominantly unilateral myoclonus make up about 11 per cent. The third group make up approximately 4 per cent with unilateral loss of tone. It is necessary to record patients with their arms raised in the air. Unilateral hypertonia is the rarest example and we only have two examples with thigh extension.

The prognosis is less good than in typical petit mal. For all these absences, 75 per cent are controlled in the first year, in the versive absences 61 per cent, in the myoclonic absences 38 per cent and tonic and atonic absences have the worst prognosis.

Munari: Concerning classical petit mal absence, everybody can agree, but regarding complex absences one must remember that some manifestations akin to petit mal 2-3 per second spike-waves can be provoked by stimulation of the mesial frontal lobe. Moreover, in partial seizures automatisms may not have the same significance in all cases and their localizational value may differ according to their clinical appearance and their time of occurrence during the seizure. The cases of Oller are interesting but raise a lot of questions regarding the difference between spike-waves in the scalp EEG and what might be seen with depth recordings. Is one really justified to include versive seizures.

Dreifuss: To enlarge a little on the relationship between absence and automatisms, this relationship is not only described by Porter, Penry and myself but is frequently observed, particularly when seizures are studied with video tape which can be reviewed repeatedly. In this way one can study what happens when one manipulates the patients internal and external environment in the hope of better identifying and classifying the automatisms that result from interfering with the patient's milieu during the seizure. One sees two types of automatisms in absence seizures. In one, continuation of activity which is ongoing at the onset of the absence seizures. These are perseverative automatisms, and they may be quite elaborate in their manifestations. The patient may wander around in response to his seizure which overtook him while walking or he may pick things up and put them down such as cans on a supermarket shelf which he would not do were he not in such a milieu during the seizure and the nature of the automatisms is determined by the nature of his environment. We have actually caused a patient to chew vigorously in response to having put chewing gum in her mouth during a seizure. We induced automatisms in almost 100 per cent of patients whose seizures lasted in excess of 10 seconds. Of course we know that patients in absence status live in an automatism. The other interesting thing about automatisms is that if the patient engages in a continuous task, he may continue the task accurately for the first few seconds of the spike wave bursts, his performance then drops off and may recover before the electrographic seizure is at an end. In other words, the 3 per second spike and wave bursts is an epiphenomenon and the response during seizures is in the shape of a trough without a sudden onset or termination.

Wolf: I would agree with Gastaut that there are several kinds of epilepsy with a different load of photic sensitivity. There is rather good correlation with pyknoleptic absences and there is no correlation with the nonpyknoleptic, there is great correlation with impulsive petit mal and there is some correlation with grand mal on awakening. We have been interested in the spatial distribution of spike wave discharges that is whether there was frontal predominance, occipital predominance or no predominance and found the only correlation to exist with occipital predominance. I have here a video of a patient who had a history of falling and who showed a myoclonic response to light without any EEG correlation. This is a clinical, visible response but not an epileptic one.

Binnie: As regards the topography, one can manipulate the epileptogenicity of the stimulus by, for example, pattern stimulation. One may see an occipital discharge and if the intensity is increased one may see a generalized discharge with frontal predominance. Conversely one can modify the topography by medicating the patient converting what was a generalized discharge with frontal predominance to a more localized posterior discharge.

Jeavons: With regard to myoclonic absences, in our experience the only effective treatment is the combination of valproate and ethosuximide which may work better than either drug given alone.

Wolf: On the topic of absences, Tassinari and Loiseau paid much attention to different kinds of myoclonic phenomena with absence. I would like to know how valid the distinction between mild clonic components and myoclonic absence really is. For example, are there more tonic-clonic seizures in this group of patients than in the remainder of the absence category which would imply a worse prognosis in this group of patients.

Tassinari: There should be no confusion between absences with mild clonic components and myoclonic absence. In the latter, eyelid twitching may be absent and there is something completely different about the myoclonus. It is not a continuum. They do have pyknoleptic characteristics in that they occur several times every day. This group is not particularly distinguished by the presence of tonic-clonic seizures.

Doose: In general, I do not believe myoclonic absence has such a poor prognosis. In our experience, the early onset myoclonic absence and especially those who also have grand mal, or would start with grand mal, do badly. For 20 years, we have distinguished three types of absence epilepsies. First, typical pyknolepsy starting between 5 and 8 years of age, predominantly in girls. Secondly, juvenile absence epilepsy affecting both

240

sexes equally and more often combined with grand mal and which has a poorer prognosis. The third type is early childhood absence epilepsy affecting boys predominantly, beginning often as grand mal and has a poor long-term prognosis. The three types have a different hereditary predisposition.

Seino: Two hundred and five patients with photic convulsive responses were divided into three groups according to the Bickford Classification. 16 had environmentally produced photic seizures (Group A), 31 had seizures induced by photic stimulation only in the laboratory (Group B) and 158 had photic-induced paroxysmal discharges without clinical seizures (Group C). In Group A, 81 per cent had onset of epilepsy below 3 years of age, in Group B 29 per cent and in Group C 28 per cent. 100 per cent of Group A patients were mentally retarded, 61 per cent of Group B and 39 per cent of Group C. Of the 205 patients, 84 had secondary generalized epilepsy; 33 Lennox-Gastaut syndrome, 13 myoclonus epilepsy and 38 secondary generalized epilepsy with failed to fulfil the Lennox-Gastaut syndrome criteria. Of these 38 patients, 27 had combined myoclonic absences, myoclonic jerks and generalized tonic-clonic convulsions.

These were tentatively classified as photosensitive myoclonic epilepsy. The common features of photosensitive myoclonic epilepsy included mental retardation in 100 per cent, a positive past medical history with no family history in 44 per cent, onset of seizures before 3 years of age in 82 per cent and a uniform resistance to pharmacotherapy. The EEGs were characterized by slow background and short bursts of irregular spike and wave at faster than 3 c/s. We regard photosensitive myoclonic epilepsy as a syndrome related to the severe myoclonic epilepsy proposed by Dravet *et al.* (1981).

Epileptic syndromes in infancy, child-
hood and adolescence. J. Roger,
C. Dravet, M. Bureau, F.E.
Dreifuss and P. Wolf. John Libbey
Eurotext Ltd ©1985.

Chapter 27
Juvenile Absence Epilepsy

Peter WOLF

*Abteilung Neurologie, Klinikum Charlottenburg der FU Berlin, Spandauer Damm 130, D-1000 Berlin
19, Federal Republic of Germany*

Summary

Juvenile absence epilepsy is a syndrome of idiopathic generalized epilepsy with age-related
onset. The absences do not differ from those of childhood but absences with retropulsive movements are, perhaps, less common. Age of onset is around puberty. The seizure frequency is low,
the absences not occurring every day and usually sporadic. The sex distribution is equal. If there
are generalized tonic-clonic seizures (GTCS), they mostly occur on awakening. Not
infrequently, the patient may also have myoclonic seizures. The EEG mostly shows rapid (> 3
c/s) spikes and waves. Therapy response is good.

Synonyms: Epilepsy with non-pyknoleptic absences
Epilepsy with spanioleptic absences (greek $\sigma\pi\alpha\nu\iota o\zeta$ = rare)

History

Absences were among the first types of epileptic seizures other than generalized tonic-
clonic that were clearly recognized and described (Tissot, 1770). Since the introduction
of the EEG, the use of the term became restricted to the absences of generalized epilepsy that were now clearly defined by the bilateral spike-and-wave discharge.
Previously, the brief lapses of consciousness that may occur in temporal lobe epilepsies
would also have been called absences. On the other hand, it had long been argued
whether all absences were epileptic. This discussion had concentrated upon the disorder named 'pyknolepsy' (for an account of this discussion see Janz, 1969). Not long
before the introduction of the EEG, this had led to the conclusion that pyknolepsy was
indeed an epileptic syndrome defined by absences that occurred several to many times
every day. In its course, grand mal seizures could develop. A relevant form of seizure
status, the 'status pyknolepticus' (Ratner, 1927) had also been described. The EEG
added the last and decisive feature to that syndrome when Jung (1939) reported that
the EEG of pyknoleptic children showed exactly the same type of spike-wave-discharge
'as in petit mal seizures of true epilepsy'.

It was only after the definite establishment of pyknolepsy as an epileptic syndrome
that more attention was paid to patients who had absences of the same clinical appear-

ance as pyknolepsy, with identical EEG but recurring much less frequently. Probably the first paper that is aware of this is Janz and Christian (1957).

Doose *et al.* (1965) conducted a study with the purpose of determining whether all cases of 'spike-wave-absences' belonged to one syndrome or not. They found that apart from pyknolepsy with a peak age of onset from 4 to 8 years and a female preponderance there were cases with earlier or later onset, and these were in some respects clinically different. Particularly, these authors found a second manifestation peak for absences from ages 10 to 12. For these patients, there was no sex difference, and the recurrence of absences was infrequent especially when the patient also had grand mal seizures. The recurrence could be 'cycloleptic' (in clusters of seizures) or 'spanioleptic' (from $\sigma\pi\alpha\nu\iota o\zeta$ = rare), for randomly-recurring seizures.

Description

Prevalence: In the study of Janz (1969) of 1169 patients suffering from 'epilepsies with age-related minor seizures' there were 197 or 17 per cent that did not belong to the 'petit mal quartet', the latter comprising West syndrome (114 patients or 10 per cent), myoclonic-astatic petit mal (idiopathic and symptomatic forms, 73 patients or 6 per cent), pyknoleptic petit mal (505 patients or 43 per cent) and impulsive petit mal (or juvenile myoclonic epilepsy, see next chapter, 280 patients or 23 per cent).

Of these, 116 (ie, 10 per cent of all age-related epilepsies with minor seizures, or 59 per cent of those not belonging to the 'petit mal quartet') had their first seizures — all absences — between the 10th and 17th year of age, and were thus regarded as cases of juvenile absence epilepsy.

In Wolf and Inoue's study (1984) on the therapeutic response of 229 absence patients from a seizure clinic for adolescents and adults, 122 had pyknoleptic, and 107 had non-pyknoleptic absences recurrence. Obviously, in this age group, many patients with pyknoleptic absences are already cured, and the relative frequency of both syndromes is, thus, much dependent on the age of the investigated patient group. It can thus be assumed, that the syndrome of childhood absences is considerably more frequent than that of juvenile absences.

Sex distribution: Whereas in childhood absence epilepsy there is a female preponderance, this has not been found in juvenile absence epilepsy. In the material of Janz, there are 62 females (53 per cent) and 54 males (47 per cent). In the investigation of Wolf and Inoue, there are 48 females (45 per cent) and 59 males (55 per cent). The respective figure for childhood or pyknoleptic absences in both investigations was 56 per cent females and 44 per cent males (Table 1). In both investigations, however, the difference in the sex distribution of the two absence syndromes is not statistically significant.

Genetics: In the cohort investigated by Janz (1969) there was a report of epilepsy in the families of 11.2 per cent of patients (the percentage for childhood absence epilepsy of the same investigation is 13.9 per cent, for 'impulsive petit mal' 25 per cent). It appears that the syndrome has not otherwise been studied genetically.

Age of onset: In the group studied by Janz, the absences had, by definition, manifested after the 10th birthday. He found that the age of onset ranged from 10-17 with only occasional later onset. Doose *et al.* (1965) found in their pediatric material, which in general does not include cases over the age of 15 years, a peak age of onset of 7-12.

Table 1. Pyknoleptic and non-pyknoleptic absence epilepsy (Wolf and Inoue, 1984).

Mode of recurrence	Age of onset	Rate of females	Retroversive movements	Association with myoclonic seizures
Pyknoleptic (n = 122)	8.3 ± 4.5	68 (56%)	28 (23%)	10 (8.2%)
Non-pyknoleptic (n = 107)	14.8 ± 8.3	48 (45%)	2 (2%)	17(15.9%)
Significance:	< 0.001	n.s.	< 0.001	> 0.05 <.1

Wolf and Inoue (1984) who defined their patient group only by the criterion of non-pyknoleptic seizure recurrence (Table 1) found a mean age of onset of absences at 14.8 ± 8.3 years (range 2-47), and mean manifestation age for these patients' epilepsy of 13.4 ± 7.0 years (range 1-47). Pyknoleptic absences in this study became manifest at 8.3 ± 4.5 years (range 2-27) the epilepsies of the patients at 8.1 ± 4.5 years (range 1-27).

Clinical features: As in childhood absences, abnormal physical and mental signs and symptoms occur only exceptionally, and do not form part of the syndrome. The same is true for exogenous etiological signs. The neuropathology of generalized idiopathic epilepsies will be discussed in the chapter on epilepsy with grand mal on awakening.

Thus far, no preponderance of one or the other subtype of absences of the International Classification of Epileptic Seizures (1981) has been demonstrated in this syndrome. Janz (1969) pointed out that absences with retropulsive movements, a type which in the International Classification has no special niche, are, here, much less common than in pyknolepsy (3 versus 54 per cent). In the study of Wolf and Inoue (1984), retropulsive movements in absence were known in 28 out of 122 patients with childhood absences but only 2 of 107 patients with juvenile absences (Table 1). In order to obtain more exact data about subgroups of absence, more studies including video- registration of absences are still necessary.

The majority of patients also have generalized tonic-clonic seizures (83 as compared to 66.5 per cent of patients with pyknolepsy, Janz, 1969). Some reservation, however, is appropriate as there is reason to believe that many patients with pure juvenile absences do not see a doctor as the condition does not disturb them, and may even pass unnoticed by themselves and their relatives. This is deduced from patients who, after a period with absences only, seek treatment as a consequence of GTCS manifestation.

Chronobiological analysis of the GTCS of the syndrome revealed that 75 per cent belonged to the awakening grand mal group, 14 per cent had GTCS during sleep, and 11 per cent in random distribution (Janz, 1969). In the investigation of Wolf and Inoue (1984), the figures are 82 per cent awakening grand mal and 9 per cent each sleep and random grand mal. The figures for childhood absences were almost identical (83, 9 and 8 per cent).

Association with myoclonic seizures of the type of juvenile myoclonic epilepsy was found in 15.9 per cent of the juvenile absence patients of Wolf and Inoue but only in 8.2 per cent of their childhood absence patients. This difference is not statistically significant (Table 1). It must be kept in mind, however, that the childhood absence patients of this study are a selection of patients with absences persisting after puberty, and with a bias towards cases with more than one seizure type. Janz (1969) found only

13 patients out of 461 with pyknolepsy (2.8 per cent) developed myoclonic seizures, but not all his pyknoleptic patients had already passed puberty. Combinations with other seizure types have not been reported.

EEG: The background activity is usually normal. The characteristic epileptic feature of the ictal and interictal EEG is generalized symmetric spike-and-wave discharge with frontal accentuation. The spike-wave frequency is usually a little faster than 3 c/s (3.5-4 c/s), the first complex of a group sometimes being even faster. Often, the slow wave is preceded by two or, less commonly, three spikes. The spike-wave discharge is easily precipitated by sleep withdrawal and by hyperventilation.

Remarkably, photosensitivity is much less common than in other idiopathic generalized epilepsies (Table 2). When patients who had additional myoclonic seizures were not considered, Goosses (1984) found photosensitivity only in six of 80 patients with juvenile absences (7.5 per cent) as compared with the 18 per cent in childhood absences and 30.6 per cent of juvenile myoclonic epilepsy. This finding could not be explained by differences in sex ratio or investigation age.

Evolutionary aspects: The manifestation sequence in patients with additional GTCS is much less uniform than in childhood absence epilepsy: Of the 96 combined cases of Janz (1969), only 46 began with absences, and 38 with GTCS; in 12 patients, the mode of onset could not be determined.

Response to therapy: Therapy response in the majority of cases is good in spite of the frequent combination with GTCS which is usually a negative prognostic factor. In the investigation of Wolf and Inoue (1984), non-pyknoleptic absences responded better to therapy than pyknoleptic absences ($P < 0.02$) and only 16 of 107 patients with juvenile absence epilepsy (15.8 per cent) did not become seizure free, although 102 had also GTCS. The respective rate for childhood absences in this study was 20.5 per cent, but here again, combination with GTCS was frequent (106 of 122 patients) which accounts for the relatively high rate of non-responders. In both groups, all patients that had no GTCS ($N = 21$) became seizure-free.

Combination with myoclonic seizures did not affect the prognosis. If there was complete control of absences, the same was true for GTCS in 93 per cent whereas GTCS

Table 2. Photosensitivity in age-related generalized idiopathic epilepsies (after Goosses, 1984)

Syndrome diagnosis	n	Non-photosensitive patients			Photosensitive patients		
		Females	Males	Total	Females	Males	Total
Childhood absences	94	44	33	77 (82 %)	9	8	17 (18%)
Juvenile absences	80	35	39	74 (92.5%)	4	2	6 (7.5%)
Juvenile myoclonic epilepsy	121	35	49	84 (69.5%)	25	12	37 (30.5%)
GTCS on awakening	270	121	114	235 (87%)	22	13	35 (13%)

These patients belong to a total of 1044 epileptics, 103 of whom (9.9 per cent) were photosensitive. Photosensitivity was statistically correlated with childhood absences ($P < 0.01$), juvenile myoclonic epilepsy ($P < 0.001$) and generalized tonic-clonic seizures on awakening ($P < 0.01$) but not with juvenile absences.

control was only reached in 60 per cent of patients with incomplete absence control (P < 0.0005).

Nosological place of the syndrome

Considered from a developmental or biological standpoint, the various syndromes of generalized idiopathic epilepsy have a number of traits in common: exogenous pathogenetic factors are infrequent; there is a relatively high hereditary predisposition, a background of undisturbed physical and mental development, a high propensity to seizure precipitation by sleep withdrawal; peak occurrence of seizures in the period after awakening; in the EEG, bilateral symmetric discharge of epileptic activity against a background that is fundamentally normal.

The course of such disorders is usually benign, and the therapeutic response good. The differences between the various syndromes mostly concern seizure type, type of epileptic discharge, and age of onset. The possibility cannot be excluded that there is one disease, idiopathic generalized epilepsy, that takes various appearances according to the age of onset, the hypothesis being that it is the same pathological process that is active but interacts with the healthy brain differently at the different steps of the maturation of the central nervous system.

Whether this be true or not, juvenile absence epilepsy appears as an intermediate syndrome between childhood absence epilepsy and juvenile myoclonic epilepsy. With the first, it shares the seizure type (perhaps with a difference regarding retropulsive movements in the absence) differing from it mainly in age of onset and seizure frequency. With the latter it shares the approximate age-relation and seizure frequency, however, the seizure type is very different. The EEG findings of this syndrome also have an intermediate position between the 3 c/s single spike-and-wave most typical for childhood absences, and the more rapid polyspike-and-wave most characteristic for the juvenile myoclonic epilepsy. Between the syndromes of juvenile absences and of juvenile myoclonic seizures there is considerable overlap as a significant proportion of patients has both seizure types. The presence or absence of photosensitivity seems to have an important influence on the composition of the syndrome when a generalized idiopathic epilepsy manifests early in the second decade.

There is also an overlap with awakening grand mal epilepsy (see that chapter). In many instances, it will be an arbitrary decision to class an individual patient either according to the absence or to the grand mal syndrome. No rules can be given for this as for different purposes either of the two may be a more suitable category.

References

Doose, H., Völzke, E., Scheffner, D. (1965): Verlaufsformen kindlicher Epilepsien mit Spike-Wave-Absencen. *Arch. Psychiat. Nervenkrh.* **207**, 394-415.
Goosses, R. (1984): *Die Beziehung der Fotosensibilität zu den verschiedenen epileptischen Syndromen.* Thesis, West Berlin.
Janz, D. (1969): *Die Epilepsien.* Thieme: Stuttgart.
Janz, D., Christian, W. (1957): Impulsiv-Petit mal. *J. Neurol.* **176**, 346-386.
Jung, R. (1939): Elektroencephalographische Befunde bei der Epilepsie und ihren Grenzgebieten. *Zbl. ges. Neurol. Psychiat.* **91**, 199-200.
Ratner, J. (1927): Beitrag zur Klinik und Pathogenese der Pyknolepsie. *Mschr. Psychiat. Neurol.* **64**, 283-298.
Wolf, P., Inoue, Y. (1984): Therapeutic response of absence seizures in patients of an epilepsy clinic for adolescents and adults. *J. Neurol.* **231**, 225-229.

Epileptic syndromes in infancy, childhood and adolescence. J. Roger, C. Dravet, M. Bureau, F.E. Dreifuss and P. Wolf. John Libbey Eurotext Ltd ©1985.

Chapter 28
Juvenile Myoclonic Epilepsy

Peter WOLF

Abteilung Neurologie, Klinikum Charlottenburg der FU Berlin, Spandauer Damm 130, D-1000 Berlin 19, Federal Republic of Germany

Summary

Juvenile myoclonic epilepsy (JME) is a syndrome of idiopathic generalized epilepsy with age-related onset (pre- to postpuberty). It is characterized by seizures with bilateral, single or repetitive, arrhythmic, irregular myoclonic jerks, predominantly in the arms. A minority of patients may suddenly fall from a jerk. No disturbance of consciousness can be noticed. The etiology is not known. In some cases, the disorder is inherited.

The sex distribution is equal. Often, there are additional generalized tonic-clonic seizures — less often absences of usually infrequent repetition. The seizures of all types occur predominantly shortly after awakening and are often precipitated by sleep withdrawal.

The ictal EEG shows rapid (> 3 c/s) generalized, often irregular spike waves and polyspike waves that are also found interictally. There is no close phase correlation|between'EEG spikes and the jerks.

Frequently, the patients are photosensitive. The response to appropriate antiepileptic drugs is good.

Synonyms: Impulsive petit mal
                        Herpin-Janz Syndrome
                        Jerk epilepsy
                        Intermittent sporadic myoclonic epilepsy
                        Myoclonic petit mal

History

The first extensive report of a patient with the syndrome was by Herpin (1867; complete quotation in Janz 1969), although many other authors of the 19th century (Delasiauve, Reynolds, Féré, Binswanger, Gowers) also mention myoclonic jerks as heralding symptom of generalized tonic-clonic seizures or as isolated events. Lundborg (1903) differentiated this 'intermittent sporadic myoclonic epilepsy' from the 'progressive familial myoclonic epilepsies'. Terms like 'myoclonic epilepsy' (Lennox 1945) and 'myoclonic petit mal' came into use around the middle of this century but seemed not to be specific as there are other minor epileptic seizures with myoclonic symptoms (Gastaut, 1973). Lennox's (1960) expression 'jerk epilepsy', however, more precisely covers this syndrome.

Janz and Christian (1957) gave the first detailed description that was based on the study of a substantial group of patients, and suggested the term 'impulsive-petit mal' as a homage to Herpin who had talked of 'impulsions'.

Description

Prevalence: In Janz (1969) the 280 patients with impulsive petit mal represent 4.3 per cent of all epileptic patients (6500) or 24 per cent of the 1169 patients with 'age-related epilepsies with minor seizures'.

Tsuboi (1977) found 399 such patients (5.4 per cent) amongst the 7400 epileptics that were in — and out — patients of the Heidelberg University Department of Neurology on 1.8. 1970. The 37 patients of Simonsen *et al.* (1976) represent only 3.4 per cent — after statistical correction at least 2.8 per cent — of 1100 patients with epilepsy. This, however, is not a figure of ambulant but hospitalized patients.

In the study of Goosses (1984) on 1069 patients from a seizure clinic for adolescents and adults that had video-EEG investigations, there were 126 patients with impulsive petit mal (11.9 per cent of the total, or 20.6 per cent of patients with generalized epilepsies and 36 per cent of patients with various forms of generalized minor seizures). Asconapé and Penry (1984) found the syndrome in 4 per cent of 275 epileptic patients referred in a three-year period.

Sex ratio: In the three largest of the studies just mentioned, the sex distribution was about equal (Table 1).

Table 1. Distribution, by sex, of juvenile myoclonic epilepsy

Author	Male	Female	Total
Janz	149 (53%)	131 (47%)	280
Tsuboi	195 (49%)	204 (51%)	399
Goosses	61 (50%)	60 (50%)	121

Genetics: Of the 280 patients of Janz (1969), 70 (25 per cent) had a family history of epilepsy which was the highest rate of all epileptic syndromes he had investigated. Tsuboi (1977), in his comprehensive study of the syndrome, discussed its genetics in more detail. He found a positive family history in 27.3 per cent of the 319, out of a total of 399 patients, who provided a reliable family history. These 319 patients had 1618 relatives of first degree, 66 of which (4.1 per cent) had seizures; age correction gave a morbid risk of 5 per cent. As only 390 of the 1618 relatives could be personally investigated (including EEG) these results must still be considered as preliminary. The EEG investigation of these 390 relatives revealed epileptic discharge in 59, or 15 per cent. Female relatives were more often affected, and the same was true for the relatives of female patients.

Furthermore, the seizure types of affected relatives were generalized tonic-clonic in 85.3 per cent (68.1 per cent occasional seizures plus 17.2 per cent repetitive all on awakening), 'myoclonic petit mal' in 14.7 per cent, non-pyknoleptic absences in 11.2 per cent, and pyknolepsy in 3.4 per cent. There was only one relative with Lennox syndrome, and one with 'psychomotor epilepsy'.

Tsuboi concluded that the mode of inheritance is most probably polygenic with a lower manifestation threshold for females.

Age of onset: Janz found that the age of onset varied between 8 and 26, but in 79 per cent ranged from 12 to 18. In the Tsuboi investigation, 72.7 per cent of myoclonic seizures started between 12 and 19 years, and the mean age of onset was 16.7 years. In the study of Goosses (1984) the mean age of onset of 37 such patients who were photosensitive was 12.6, of the 84 non-photosensitive patients, 16.0 (total mean: 15.0 years). This difference is not statistically significant. The mean age of onset of myoclonic jerks in the small study of Asconapé and Penry (1984) was 14.7 ± 1.95 years (range 11-18 years).

Clinical features: The characterizing feature of the syndrome are the myoclonic jerks that are bilateral, mostly but not always symmetric, single or repetitive, rapid and of variable amplitude. They are always most pronounced in and often restricted to the arms where they seem to mostly affect the extensor muscles. If they are multiple, they are usually arrhythmic. The facial muscles are usually not involved but some patients report that the jerks may extend to the legs, and sometimes cause a sudden fall. The actual fall is remembered, and consciousness is retained during the seizures. Occasionally, however, patients are in doubt regarding the state of consciousness or believe it momentarily disturbed.

The seizures are precipitated by sleep withdrawal and mostly occur shortly after awakening, a feature that has been noticed by many observers, and most systematically discussed by Janz and Christian (1957). Touchon (1982) in his study on the circadian distribution of these seizures in 33 patients found 51 manifestation peaks (1.55 per patient) half of which (26) were after morning awakening and 10 at nocturnal awakenings. Six peaks each were in the evening relaxation period and during sleep, the last three at sleep onset.

Some patients report seizure precipitation by intermittent light stimuli.

Physical investigations fail to reveal any grossly pathological findings. If slight abnormalities are considered, minor dysplasias of the body build and signs of lability of vegetative functions are increased in comparison with other epileptic patients as well as a control group (Helmchen, 1958). X-rays reveal a significant increase of the diameter of the skull bone as well as frequent calvarial hyperostoses (Kammerer, 1961).

Similarly, major mental defects or aberrations are uncommon but many of these patients are noticeable for an attractive but unstable, suggestible and unreliable, rather immature personality that often results in inadequate social adjustment. Unsatisfactory sleep habits also may contribute to seizure precipitation, and dissimulation may prove an important obstacle to compliance and successful therapy (Janz, 1969).

While this description is merely based on clinical observation, a small controlled study of 33 patients confirmed these characterological traits and showed a non-significant trend towards social maladjustment (Reintoft *et al.,* 1976).

Most of the patients who come for treatment, also have generalized tonic-clonic seizures (GTCS): 253 or 90 per cent of 280, of the patients studied by Janz (1969), 381 of 399 (95 per cent) in the Tsuboi (1977) investigation. Chronobiologically, the GTCS are almost exclusively of the awakening type: 94 per cent of all patients with GTCS in both investigations. GTCS of these patients are often preceded by a series of jerks, and there are a few patients who have the jerks only before a GTCS.

The other seizure type that may be associated with juvenile myoclonic epilepsy is absence. In the Janz material, 10 per cent of the patients had absences of the juvenile type with infrequent recurrence (see previous chapter); Tsuboi found these in 56 or 14 per cent of his patients. Janz mentions 13 patients (4.6 per cent) where the syndrome evolved out of pyknolepsy (childhood absences with daily seizures) after several years of illness when the patients reached the manifestation age of myoclonic seizures. (These 13 patients represent 2.8 per cent of his patients with pyknolepsy. Not all his patients with pyknolepsy, however, had reached puberty at the time of this investigation). Tsuboi gives a proportion of 30 (7.5 per cent) patients with pyknoleptic petit mal without, however, going into evolutional details. He found, further, an association with Lennox syndrome in eight patients (2 per cent). Whereas Janz never observed a combination with any kind of focal seizures, amongst the patients of Tsuboi there were 15 (3.7 per cent) with 'psychomotor epilepsy'.

EEG: When Janz and Christian (1957) published their first series of 47 patients, 38 of them had had a total of 63 EEG investigations. Methods of provocation included hyperventilation and sleep withdrawal, but only occasionally intermittent light stimulation. In 15 patients (39 per cent) ictal EEGs were obtained, and in most others positive interictal findings. The EEG was unrevealing only in two patients who were on high antiepileptic drug doses.

It was noted that background activity was normal in all but four patients. The typical and pathognomonic type of epileptic discharge was the polyspike-wave (PSW) complex of which several varieties were mentioned and demonstrated (Figs. 1-3). The number of spikes varied between 5 and 20, and it seemed to be correlated not with the duration but the intensity of the clinical seizures. It was not said how many of the patients showed this type of discharge but the authors did not observe a clinical seizure that was not accompanied by PSW (Fig. 1). The EEG discharges often lasted longer than the clinical seizures, and these seemed mostly to coincide with the onset of the multiple spikes (see, however, Fig. 2).

PSW were also found interictally but, here, the slow wave was often preceded by not more than 2 or 3 spikes (Fig. 3). The complexes were more rapid than the 3 c/s SW of absence patients but, in patients who also had pyknoleptic absences, the latter could be found in addition to PSW (Janz, 1969).

More extensive data were collected by Tsuboi (1977) who reported EEG data of 381 of his 399 patients with 1 to 27 investigations with an average of 4.1 per patient. His analysis of this material that was compared with findings of 466 controls with other epileptic syndromes is extensive, and covers too many aspects to be reviewed in detail here. In comparison with the findings of Janz and Christian (1957), Tsuboi found epileptic discharge in 93 per cent of his patients, but only in 70 per cent it was of one of the various SW types. PSW (including double-SW) was still the most characteristic finding but was only present in 37 per cent of the patients. Rapid SW were found in 21.5 per cent, 3 c/s SW in 11 per cent and irregular SW in 12 per cent. It must be kept in mind, however, that almost all these patients were on medication. As regards the EEG background activity, Tsuboi noted increase of high voltage alpha activity, beta activity and slow waves, the beta presumably being explained by barbiturate therapy. The response to hyperventilation was usually intense.

All these findings were of the same type as those in awakening grand mal epilepsy and pyknolepsy but usually more pronounced in myoclonic epilepsy.

No mention was made of photosensitivity, but photic stimulation was not performed routinely in these patients.

Sensitivity to intermittent light stimulation and eye closure (Fig. 4): Asconapé and Penry (1984) found a 'photoconvulsive response' in four of their 12 patients (1/3). The rela-

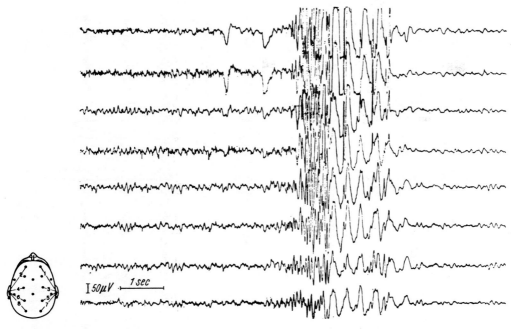

Fig. 1. Ictal EEG of JME: A myoclonic jerk is accompanied by a P-SW burst. It follows closure of the eyes that had been opened for a second.

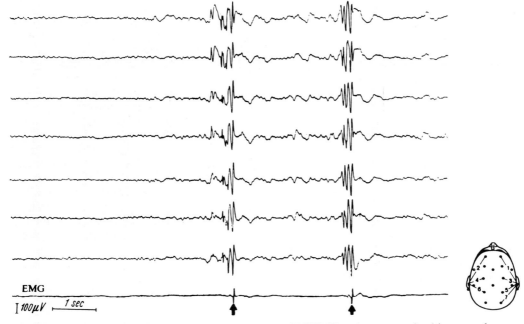

Fig. 2. A myoclonic status in JME with short bursts of PSW. The slow waves in this example are of unusually low voltage (note small gain). The EMG shows no close relation between EEG spikes and myoclonus.

251

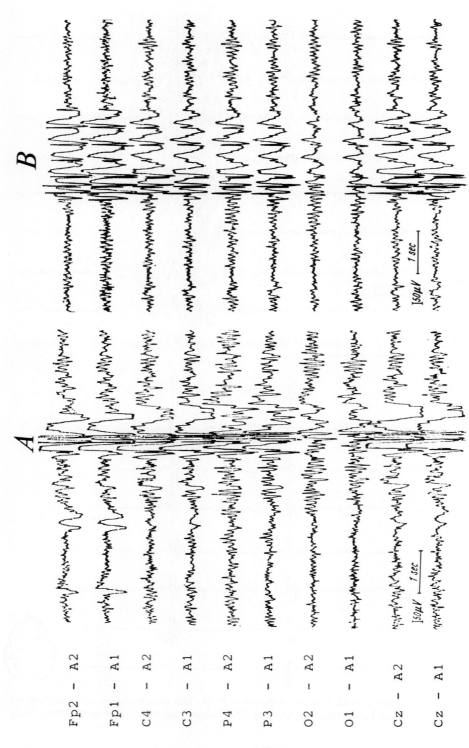

Fig. 3. A-C. Variants of interictal PSW discharge in JME. (Fig. 3C is on the following page).

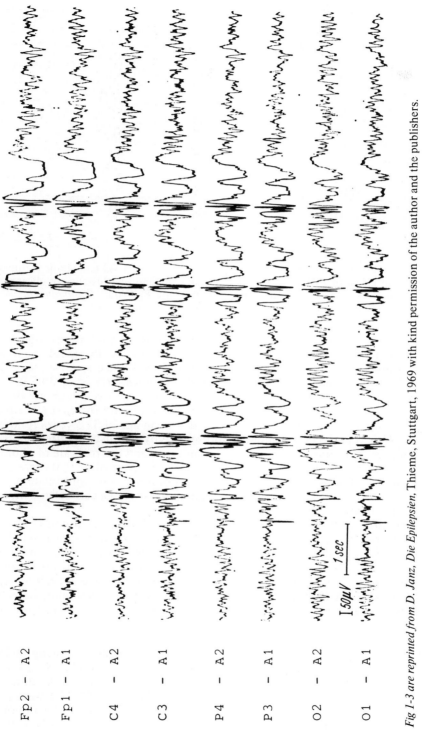

Fig 1-3 are reprinted from D. Janz, Die Epilepsien, Thieme, Stuttgart, 1969 with kind permission of the author and the publishers.

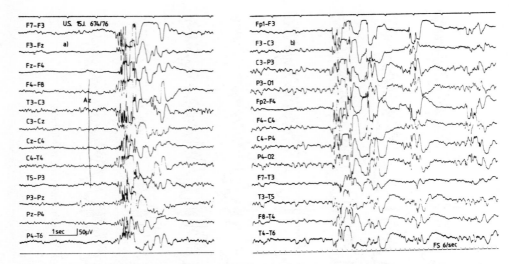

Fig. 4 A and B. Precipitation of PSW discharge by eye closure (Az) and photic stimulation (F) in a 16-year-old girl with JME, two GTCS on awakening and one instance of absence status (no isolated absences ever observed). (Reprinted from: P. Wolf, *Einführung in die praktische Epileptologie,* 1984, by courtesy of Beltz Verlag, Weinheim and Basel.)

tion of photosensitivity to various epileptic syndromes was investigated by Goosses (1984) who found that no other epileptic syndrome was as closely related to photosensitivity as juvenile myoclonic epilepsy (see: Juvenile absence epilepsy, table 2). Of 115 patients with this syndrome that were included in his study, 35 or 30.5 per cent were photosensitive; in female patients, the percentage was even higher (40 per cent). Almost all these patients were already on medication, and the first available EEG of the non-photosensitive patients was taken at a mean age of 32.5 years (photosensitive patients: 23.6 years), an age when photosensitivity has usually already disappeared. These figures therefore represent only a minimum, and the real rate of photosensitivity in this syndrome is presumably still higher. It seems possible that there exists a still unexplained pathogenetic relation between photosensitivity and bilateral myoclonic jerks as photosensitivity is also very common in dyssynergia cerebellaris myoclonica as well as some forms of progressive myoclonus epilepsy.

Precipitation of PSW discharge and jerks by eye closure was found in one patient of Asconapé and Penry (1984), and had not been reported before in studies of this syndrome. Two of the EEG examples of Janz (1969), however, show this feature (Figs. 1 and 3A). It is, as far as the EEG discharge goes, by no means uncommon but was found in 26 (20.6 per cent) of the patients with juvenile myoclonic epilepsy of Goosses (1984). In 20, it coexisted with photosensitivity. As in photosensitivity, this feature was most frequent in juvenile myoclonic epilepsy, of all epileptic syndromes (Table 2).

Polygraphic studies: Touchon *et al.* (1982) investigated nocturnal sleep of 18 patients (12 females) with this syndrome (11 with and seven without GTCS). In all patients, seizures were 'satisfactorily controlled' by medication of VPA alone (isolated myoclonic seizures) or in combination with phenobarbital (if GTCS were present). It appears, however, that all these patients still had PSW discharge. The aim of the study was to find relationships between states of alertness and epileptic EEG activity. These

Table 2. Sensitivity to intermittent light stimuli and to eye closure in the various syndromes of age-related generalized idiopathic epilepsy (after Goosses, 1984)

Syndrome diagnosis	n	Photo-sensitive only	Light and eye closure sensitive	Eye closure sensitive only	Total photo-sensitive	Total eye closure-sensitive
Childhood absence epilepsy	94	2 (2%)	15 (16%)	2 (2%)	17 (18%)	17 (18%)
Juvenile absence epilepsy	80	0	6 (7.5%)	6 (7.5%)	6 (7.5%)	12 (15%)
Juvenile myoclonic epilepsy	121	17 (14%)	20 (16.5%)	6 (5.5%)	37 (30.5%)	26 (21%)
GTCS on awakening	270	12 (4.5%)	23 (8.5%)	5 (2%)	35 (13%)	28 (10.5%)

In all other epileptic syndromes, sensitivity to eye closure was extremely rare. Of the two juvenile syndromes (juvenile absence epilepsy and juvenile myoclonic epilepsy) only JME is related both to photosensitivity and to eye closure sensitivity ($P < 0.01$). There is an overlap between the first three syndromes and GTCS on awakening but not between the first three as cases of absences plus myoclonic jerks are all included in JME.

were indeed found, the rate of PSW discharge being highest during nocturnal awakening followed by morning awakenings, relaxed waking state before sleep onset, and sleep stage I. There was some discharge in stage REM, and very little in stage II. It seems that no PSW were observed in deep NREM sleep stages.

It was further found that provoked awakenings were followed by a higher discharge rate than spontaneous awakenings. This provocative effect of artificial awakenings was more intense when the interrupted sleep phases were unstable ones (such as REM sleep of early night and stage II of end of night) as compared with more stable phases such as REM sleep of end of night and stage II of early night.

Finally, it was noted that the discharge rate following morning awakening (spontaneous) was significantly higher after a night's sleep that had been disturbed by repeated provoked awakening than after an undisturbed night. In another paper, Touchon (1982) was able to add a group of 15 patients with this syndrome whose seizure control was 'unsatisfactory'. Qualitatively, the relation of their PSW frequency to the different states of alertness was the same as in the 'well-controlled' group. However, the 'non-satisfactory' group had less epileptic discharge than the well-controlled patients. It is further reported that the circadian peak seizure occurrence differed in both groups. The exact nature of this difference, however, is not clear.

Neuropathology: The neuropathology of generalized idiopathic epilepsies is discussed, in the next chapter. So far, only three cases of juvenile myoclonic epilepsy have been autopsied (Janz and Neimanis, 1961; Meencke and Janz, 1984).

Pathogenesis and evolution

In the study of Tsuboi (1977), possible exogenous factors were found in 78 of 399 patients (19.5 per cent). These included such dubious factors as 'head trauma with loss of consciousness' without further specification (34 patients) and poliomyelitis (four patients). Forty-seven patients (11.8 per cent), had had birth complications and 8 (2 per cent) cerebral diseases or damage. Thirteen of 78 patients also had a positive family history. Exogenous factors appear to be of minor importance, presumably only as manifestation factors on a genetic predisposition. In 15 patients (3.8 per cent) of the Tsuboi investigation the disease started with 'childhood convulsions' that were not further differentiated. If there was an association with absences (no differentiation of subtypes was attempted), these manifested later than the absences of a control group, the peak age of onset being 12 - 14 years. The manifestation sequence was not noted. Of the 381 patients with associated GTCS, these preceded the myoclonic seizures in 17 per cent and followed them in 18 per cent; in 65 per cent both seizure types are said to have appeared 'simultaneously'.

GTCS were increased in the age group 12 - 19, which was, again, later than in a control group of GTCS on awakening without associated myoclonic seizures (8 - 15 years).

Different figures are given by Janz (1969) who found that myoclonic seizures preceded GTCS in 50 per cent, and followed them in 37 per cent, whereas in 13 per cent only, both seizure types began roughly at the same time. As regards the associated absences, these preceded the myoclonic seizures in all 13 patients with associated pyknolepsy, whereas non-pyknoleptic absences appeared at the same time or before the myoclonic seizures. Of the 10 combinations of myoclonic epilepsy and GTCS of Asconapé and Penry (1984) the GTCS of one patient preceded, and of 9 followed myoclonic seizures, the GTCS age of onset being 16.4 ± 3 (range 8 - 24 years).

Therapy

As seizure precipitation by sleep withdrawal is particularly common in the syndrome, therapy must be based on regulation of the sleep-waking habits. Photosensitive patients must be counselled to avoid the appropriate stimuli. For patients with infrequent seizures, this may be sufficient. Early studies on drug action (before the introduction of valproic acid, and without control of drug levels) showed that primidone and phenobarbital were the most efficient drugs both for the myoclonic and the concomitant GTCS (Janz, 1969).

It would now appear that sodium valproate is the drug of first choice, but no report on a larger series of patients thus treated has yet been given. Of the 11 patients followed by Asconapé and Penry (1984), six (54.5 per cent) had complete seizure control by valproate monotherapy. Jeavons et al. (1980) achieved 100 per cent seizure-control by valproate alone in 13 of 17 patients (76 per cent) with juvenile myoclonic seizures but did not indicate how long the patients were followed. Of 27 patients with myoclonic seizures in association with absences, grand mal, or both, 18 (67 per cent) became seizure free with valproate alone in a study of Feuerstein et al. (1983). Here, the follow-up period was 43 ± 16 months.

Seventy five per cent of 49 patients with juvenile myoclonic and GTCS became seizure free for at least 2 years in the study of Janz et al. (1983). This investigation which. does not report drug regimens indicated that good therapeutic response of these patients does not signify definite cure as 91 per cent of them had a relapse when medication was later partially or completely withdrawn. This was the highest rate of relapse of all common epileptic syndromes.

Differential diagnosis

Historically, the main differential diagnosis was the progressive myoclonic epilepsy of Unverricht and Lundborg. This would clinically be based on the clear mode of inheritance (usually autosomal recessive) of the latter and the mental deterioration accompanying it. In the EEG, the progressive diseases have a pathological background activity, pathological discharge of a type different from PSW, and no close correlation of myoclonic phenomena to the EEG discharge.

The harmless jerks that may occur at the onset of sleep, especially in young persons, are strictly bound to this moment of the day whereas epileptic myoclonus will also occur at other times even in the rare cases (Touchon, 1982) who have only one peak occurrence at sleep onset. In the former, the EEG is normal, and there are no other seizures. Juvenile myoclonic epilepsies are typically distinguished from myoclonic-astatic seizures by the ages of onset. There is, occasionally, an unusually early onset of the one, and an unusually late onset of the other syndrome that may pose problems of differential diagnosis. The decisive features will be exemption of facial muscles, arrhythmic repetition of jerks, and undisturbed consciousness in juvenile myoclonic epilepsy, and also its SW discharges that are, at least, rapid even if they are not of the PSW type.

Some patients with myoclonic absences are aware of part of their jerks, and the ages of onset overlap. In these patients, however, the jerks involve the face, are rhythmic and strictly phase-locked to the spike-waves that are, again, rhythmic, regular, and of 3 c/s frequency. If consciousness during the seizures is tested it is detected that there is an actual lapse. These seizures occur more frequently, and often have a poorer therapy response.

There are some very rare patients, however, who seem to present true transitional forms of myoclonic absence and juvenile myoclonic epilepsy presenting some features of the one, and some of the other syndrome. Such cases should not be forced into one of the categories — which could only be done arbitrarily — but recognized as the intermediate forms whose existence is to be expected if the concept of phenotypical determination of generalized idiopathic seizure syndromes by the state of brain maturation at their first manifestation is valid.

Nosological place

In the chapter on juvenile absence epilepsy, the nosological relationship of the various syndromes of generalized idiopathic epilepsy has already been discussed. In this group of syndromes, juvenile myoclonic epilepsy is one of the three syndromes manifesting around puberty with considerable overlap. It differs from juvenile absence epilepsy by seizure type, somewhat later age of onset, and the frequent finding of photosensitivity. From epilepsy with generalized tonic-clonic seizures on awakening, no strict separation is either possible or necessary as most patients also belong to the latter syndrome, and so few patients with isolated myoclonic seizures are known to doctors that possible differences between these and those with additional GTCS could not yet be studied.

References

Asconapé, J., Penry, J.K. (1984): Some clinical and EEG aspects of benign juvenile myoclonic epilepsy. *Epilepsia* **25**, 108-114.

Feuerstein, J., Revol, M., Roger, J., Sallou, C., Truelle, J.L., Vercelletto, P., Weber, M. (1983): La monothérapie par le valproate de sodium dans les épilepsies généralisées primaires. *Sem. Hôp. Paris* **59**, 1263-1274.

Gastaut, H. (1973): *Dictionary of epilepsy*. WHO: Geneva.

Goosses, R. (1984): Die Beziehung der Fotosensibilität zu den verschiedenen epileptischen Syndromen. Thesis, West Berlin.

Helmchen, H. (1958): Beitrag zur konstitutionellen Differenzierung im Bereich genuiner Epilepsien. *J. Neurol.* **178**, 541-582.

Janz, D. (1969): *Die Epilepsien*. Thieme: Stuttgart.

Janz, D., Christian, W. (1957): Impulsiv-Petit mal. *J. Neurol.* **176**, 346-386.

Janz, D., Neimanis, G. (1961): Clinico-anatomical study of a case of idiopathic epilepsy with impulsive petit mal and grand mal on awakening. *Epilepsia* **2**, 251-269.

Janz, D., Kern, A., Mössinger, H.-J., Puhlmann, H.-U. (1983): Rückfallprognose während und nach Reduktion der Medikamente bei Epilepsie behandlung. In *Epilepsie 1981*, pp 17-24, ed H. Remschmidt, R. Rentz and J. Jungmann. Thieme: Stuttgart.

Jeavons, P.M., Covanis, A., Gupta, A.K., Clark, J.E. (1980): Monotherapy with sodium valproate in childhood epilepsy. In *The place of sodium valproate in the treatment of epilepsy*, pp 53-58, ed M.J. Parsonage and A.D.S. Caldwell. Academic Press: London, and Grune and Stratton: New York.

Kammerer, Th. (1961): Untersuchungen am Schädelröntgenbild bei genuiner Epilepsie. *J. Neurol.* **182**, 13-33.

Lennox, W.G. (1945): The petit mal epilepsies. Their treatment with tridione. *J. Am. Med. Ass.* **129**, 1069-1073.

Lennox, W.G. (1960): *Epilepsy and related disorders*. Little and Brown: Boston

Meencke, H.J., Janz, D. (1984): Neuropathological findings in primary generalized epilepsy: a study of eight cases. *Epilepsia* **25**, 8-21.

Reintoft, H., Simonsen, N., Lund, M. (1976): A controlled sociological study of juvenile myoclonic epilepsy. In *Epileptology*, pp. 48-50, ed D. Janz, Thieme: Stuttgart.

Simonsen, N., Møllgaard, V., Lund, M. (1976): A controlled clinical and electroencephalographic study of myoclonic epilepsy (impulsiv-Petit mal). In *Epileptology*, pp 41-48, ed D. Janz. Thieme: Stuttgart.

Touchon, J. (1982): Effect of awakening on epileptic activity in primary generalized myoclonic epilepsy. In *Sleep and epilepsy*, pp 239-248. ed M.B. Sterman, M.N. Shouse, P. Passouant. Academic Press: New York.

Touchon, J., Besset, A., Billiard, M., Baldy-Moulinier, M. (1982): Effects of spontaneous and provoked awakening on the frequency of polyspike and wave discharges in 'Bilateral Massive Epileptic Myoclonus'. In *Advances in epileptology*, pp 269-272. XIIIth Epilepsy International Symposium, ed H. Akimoto, H. Kazamatsuri, M. Seino, A.A. Ward. Raven Press: New York.

Tsuboi, T. (1977): *Primary generalized epilepsy with sporadic myoclonias of myoclonic Petit Mal type*. Thieme: Stuttgart.

*　　　　*　　　　*

Discussion pages 271-273

Epileptic syndromes in infancy, childhood and adolescence. J. Roger, C. Dravet, M. Bureau, F.E. Dreifuss and P. Wolf. John Libbey Eurotext Ltd ©1985.

Chapter 29
Epilepsy with Grand Mal
on Awakening

Peter WOLF

Abteilung Neurologie, Klinikum Charlottenburg der FU Berlin, Spandauer Damm 130, D-1000 Berlin 19, Federal Republic of Germany

Summary

Epilepsy with grand mal on awakening is a syndrome of generalized idiopathic epilepsy with GM seizures, presumably mostly generalized tonic-clonic, manifesting exclusively or predominantly (over 90 per cent) shortly after awakening (regardless of the time of day) or in a second seizure peak in the evening period of relaxation. The onset is mostly in the second decade. The etiology is usually unknown. Genetic predisposition is relatively frequent. If there are other seizures these are mostly absences or myoclonic seizures as in juvenile myoclonic epilepsy. Seizures may be precipitated by sleep withdrawal and other external factors. The EEG shows one of the patterns of generalized idiopathic epilepsies. There is a significant correlation with photosensitivity.

History

A relationship of grand mal[1] seizures to the circadian rhythm was already noticed by the classical authors. Originally, the interest focused mainly on GM seizures during sleep but Gowers (1881) first mentioned patients whose attacks occurred only in the early morning and who accounted for 5 per cent of his material. Langdon-Down and Brain (1929) divided their patients into three groups: diurnal, nocturnal and diffused. They noted peak occurrences of seizures in the first two groups. For the diurnal group, the most important peak was shortly after awakening. The patients presenting this peak accounted for 24.2 per cent of their material of 66 patients, all but five suffering from idiopathic epilepsy. The authors, however, did not separate them from the rest of the diurnal group that was the largest of the three, representing 42.5 per cent of their patients.

Patry (1931) in a group of 31 patients, 27 of whom had idiopathic epilepsy, duplicated most of the findings of Langdon-Down and Brain, and noticed that the seizure peaks were not influenced by drugs.

---

[1] The term 'grand mal' is used, here, to cover all seizures with generalized convulsions (tonic, clonic, tonic-clonic etc) both without and with focal onset.

Hopkins (1933) reported on 302 out-patients of various ages, etiologies and durations of epilepsy. She confirmed the above observations of seizure peaks, and found that they were characteristic enough to separate two groups: patients with seizures during sleep (about one-half of all patients) and in the period of awakening (defined as the first hour after arousal from sleep; about 1/3 of all patients). The remaining 1/6 ('diurnal') had their seizures 'from the end of the awakening period to the resumption of sleep'. Relations to afternoon naps were not considered by this author.

Griffiths and Fox (1938) followed the suggestion of Hopkins and differentiated, in a group of 104 institutionalized patients, 'night fitters' (38.5 per cent), 'day fitters' (37.5 per cent), 'rising fitters' (10.5 per cent), and 'diffused' (13.5 per cent). They made the point that, if patients were prone to series of seizures, no peaks became apparent as long as each individual seizure was indiscriminately charted. 'If, however, we take only the first fit of a series, and fits that occur singly the fits are really not diffuse at all but have a clear and definite peak time, and it would be sound to regard all the fits of a series subsequent to the first as part of the epileptic manifestation that started with the first fit'. Further, 'rising fitters' impressed these authors as a particularly intelligent group.

Janz (1953) wrote the first paper that was dedicated to what he now called 'awakening epilepsy'. Going into the details of circadian seizure distribution he found that many of these patients had a second seizure peak in the later afternoon or evening hours of leisure and relaxation, and there was a small group for whom this evening peak was the main or even exclusive seizure peak. Patients with long-lasting epilepsy can be categorized less easily — although belonging to the awakening epilepsy group, some had a tendency to start having seizures during sleep. To define the biorhythmicity, it was therefore advisable to evaluate the circadian distribution of seizures in the first years of the disease.

Patients who belonged to the 'awakening epilepsy' group thus defined, rarely had any indication of a symptomatic etiology and seemed to form a syndrome of idiopathic epilepsy. The following syndromatic traits could be added. For most of these patients waking up was a prolonged process rather than an event; they were late and difficult raisers; seizure precipitation by sleep withdrawal (but also by other external factors) was much more common in these patients than in others with grand mal seizures; precipitating factors seemed especially important for the first seizure manifestation. Unlike sleep epilepsy, awakening epilepsy had a characteristic manifestation age; there was little tendency to dementia, but many patients were remarkable for their unsteady life style, unreliability and instability.

The patients studied by Janz had not yet been investigated with EEGs, and other significant traits of the syndrome such as the relative frequency of different types of minor seizures were only added in later publications by this author (Janz, 1962).

French investigations were reviewed by Loiseau (1964). He mentioned a case report by Delasiauve (1854), and referred to the writings of Barré (1946) Marchand and Ajuriaguerra (1948) and Roger et al. (1950). Two theses of the early 1950s had defended the opposite views: that seizures at awakening did not represent a separate syndrome (Le Camus, 1951), and that awakening epilepsy constituted a homogeneous syndrome (David, 1955). Loiseau (1964) concluded that seizures of different kinds could be related to the awakening situation but there was still one syndrome of awakening epilepsy grouped around grand mal seizures of this biorhythmic peculiarity, sometimes associated with myoclonic seizures or absences, and with generalized epileptic EEG discharges.

It is in the French tradition that the most elaborate sleep investigations were made on this syndrome (Billiard, 1982). Thus, the French and German literature evidences more familiarity with the syndrome whereas it has received little attention in Anglo-

Saxon writings after the papers of Langdon-Down and Brain, Patry and Hopkins.

Description

Prevalence: Janz (1969) reviewed five papers on the chronobiology of GM seizures using the triple distinction of grand mal on awakening (GMA), grand mal during sleep (GMS) and grand mal of random distribution or diffuse GM. The percentage of GMA varied from 22 to 37 per cent. Of the total 2825 patients of these papers, 924 or 33 per cent had GM seizures on awakening, 1246 or 44 per cent during sleep, and 655 or 23 per cent at random. Billiard (1982) divided 77 patients with GM epilepsy into four groups: epilepsy on awakening (16.8 per cent), day-time epilepsies (36.3 per cent), sleep epilepsies (28.5 per cent) and day and sleep epilepsies (18.1 per cent). The opposite extreme of this low figure of GMA is the study of Goosses (1984), in which there were 512 patients with GM epilepsy. Of these, 137 (27 per cent) had GM during sleep, 270 (53 per cent) on awakening, 40 (8 per cent) in the evening leisure period and 65 (13 per cent) in random distribution.

Tsuboi and Christian (1976) found among 318 GM epilepsies 147 on awakening (46 per cent), 89 during sleep (28 per cent), and 82 at random (26 per cent). The reasons for these considerable differences are not clear. They may be related to differences in the diagnosis but also to differently selected patient groups.

Sex distribution: As for most epileptic syndromes, a slight male preponderance was found in the three studies giving information about this (see Table 1).

Table 1. Epilepsy with GMA, sex distribution

Authors	Males	Females	Total
Tsuboi & Christian	84(57%)	63(43%)	147
Goosses:			
on awakening	143(53%)	127(47%)	270*
evening leisure	26(65%)	14(35%)	40*
Beyer & Jovanovic	65(54%)	55(46%)	120

*Difference not significant (Chi-square test).

Genetics: Of the 719 patients with GMA studied by Janz (1969), a family history of epilepsy was reported in 90 cases (12.5 per cent) which was considerably more than in the groups of GMS (73 out of 946 = 7.7 per cent) or GM at random (17 of 445 = 3.8 per cent). GMA differs from the rest with $P < 0.0005$.

Sixteen of the 147 patients with GMA (10.9 per cent) studied by Tsuboi and Christian (1976) had a familial predisposition in contrast to 6.7 per cent in GMS, and 7.3 per cent in random GM. In this much smaller cohort, although the percentages are similar, the differences are not statistically significant.

Age of onset: Compared with the rather narrow manifestation peaks of age-related epilepsies with minor seizures (see preceeding chapters), the range is broader, here. Sixty-six per cent of GMA cases became manifest between ages 9 and 24 (Janz, 1969). Tsuboi and Christian (1976) report 78 per cent onset in ages 6-22. Of the 120 patients of Beyer and Jovanovic (1966), 50 (41.7 per cent) manifested between the ages of 11 and 15 and 86 (71.7 per cent) between the ages of 6 and 20. Of 100 patients of David (1955), 88 had started between 10 and 25.

In all studies, there is a clear peak age of onset around puberty — significantly different from epilepsies with GM of different chronobiology that have, on the whole, no typical age of onset (in GMS, subgroups might still be discovered that have).

Seizure syndrome: GM seizures without aura are the constituent seizure type of the syndrome. From the case histories it appears that the usual kind of generalized convulsive seizure in this syndrome is generalized tonic-clonic. However, there has never been a video investigation to confirm this. Many patients have, in addition, minor generalized seizures, either absence or myoclonic or both (Table 2). In such cases, it is

Table 2. GM on awakening, association with other seizure syndromes

	Janz (1969)	Beyer & Jovanovic	Tsuboi & Christian
Ratio pure GM: GM + other seizures	? (1962: 320:399)	53:67	90:49
GMA + pyknoleptic absences	272 (33.5%)	42 (63%)	22 (45%)
GMA + non-pyknoleptic absences	106 (13%)		
GMA + JME	238 (29%)	4 (6%)	13 (27%)
GMA + other generalized seizures	20 (2.5%)	6 (9%)	4 (8%)
GMA + complex focal seizures	127 (15.5%)	15 (22%)	8 (16%)
GMA + other focal seizures	49 (6%)	0	2 (4%)

In all these papers, the possibility of several kinds of minor seizures associated with GMA is not discussed.

not uncommon that the individual GM seizure is preceded by a series of absences or a volley of bilateral jerks in clear consciousness. In some such patients, the GM is always preceded by minor seizures, and in some of these, as well as in some others, minor seizures are never isolated but are always followed by a convulsive seizure. If the preceding minor seizures are absences, the preparoxysmal condition may be one of a twilight state due to absence status. If the period of repetitive minor seizures preceding the convulsive seizure in such composite seizure events is long, the biorhythmicity may be veiled as the convulsive seizure seems no longer related to the awakening condition. The event, however, should be regarded as a whole, and the biorhythmicity evaluated according to the onset of the initial signs and symptoms. The same applies to GM in series and GM status. These are rare and mainly caused by drug withdrawal.

It has not been investigated whether there are differences in the relation of GMA to childhood or juvenile absences or to absence subtypes.

According to Loiseau (1964), cases of GM with associated myoclonic seizures are the most characteristic manifestation of epilepsy on awakening. Association with other seizure types is rare; its significance will be discussed below.

Clinical examinations: As in other syndromes of generalized idiopathic epilepsy, the presence of gross physical or mental abnormalities is rare. Helmchen (1958) compared the bodily constitution of 50 patients with GMA and 33 patients with GMS of unknown aetiology. The body build of the GMA patients was more often of the leptosome-asthenic, that of GMS patients more often of the dysplastic type. Within the GMA group, the subgroup with seizures strictly bound to the awakening period differed from those wtih seizures also or predominantly in the evening period of leisure in that they were taller (Table 3). The GMA group was further remarkable for frequent signs of vasomotor and other vegetative lability (respiratory arrhythmia, acrocyanosis, intense dermographism, increased transpiration) and relatively early onset of puberty. Many of these signs were even more noticeable in patients with GMA plus myoclonic seizures.

Table 3. Epilepsy with GMA, patients with different seizure peaks (modified from Helmchen)

	n	Age of onset*		Body height**	
		$\leqslant 19\,years$	$> 19\,years$	$< 165\,cm$	$> 165\,cm$
Only seizure peak on awakening	28	21	7	5	23
Various peaks or evening leisure peak	22	5	17	10	12

Chi-square tests: *P < 0.0005 **P < 0.05

Psychologically, Janz (1953) had noted that the patients with this epileptic syndrome were, as a rule, very different from what had long been considered the typical personality of 'genuine epileptics' (slow, circumstantial and irritable, utterly pedantic and obstinate, having difficulty changing the subject of conversation, prone to hypochondria). In the colourful description by Janz, however, patients with GMA belong to an almost opposite type, unstable, unreliable, inconsiderately neglectful of their duties but equally their own interests, always ready to follow the slightest temptation even against their better judgement.

The clinical observation of Janz was followed by a psychological investigation of Leder (1967), who studied a group of 34 patients with GMA and 55 with GMS. From these, two groups of 10 persons each were extracted for statistical evaluation. These selected groups were matched for sex, age, seizure frequency, association with minor seizures, intelligence, lack of etiological clues, and social status. They were investigated with two personality tests, the Rorschach and Szondi tests, and several significant differences between the groups could be found. Their interpretation describes patients with GMA as extroverted with difficulty delineating themselves from the external world. Often they have little ability to suppress, to contradict and to renounce; conflicts, tensions and disinclinations are usually momentarily disposed of by denial. These patients will follow simultaneously the most divergent and irreconcilable aims without being aware of any difficulties.

The Leder investigation has often been criticized for its methodology, Rorschach and Szondi tests are regarded with reserve by many psychologists. The unprejudiced reader, however, will be reminded, by this description, of many of his patients with generalized idiopathic epilepsy whose lack of discipline is often an obstacle to successful therapy. Their unstable sleep behaviour may precipitate seizures, and sleep withdrawal is often the cause of the first seizure. It therefore seems possible that unstable personalitites of this kind are so frequent in GMA because such a personality is a manifestation factor for a seizure predisposition which may often remain latent in people of a more regular life-style. Comparative psychological investigations of patients and predisposed but unaffected relatives could elucidate this question.

Seizure precipitation: The high liability to seizure precipitation by influences such as sleep withdrawal had already been identified as a constituent of the syndrome by Janz (1953). Helmchen (1958) confirmed that precipitating factors were much more frequent in patients with GMA, and JME with GMA than in those with GMS and 'oral petit mal' (= complex focal seizures with oro-alimentary automatisms). The most important factors were sleep deficit, excessive alcohol intake, and sudden external arousal; female patients often reported increased seizure frequency just before and during menstruation. This, unlike the previous factors, could not be confirmed by Loiseau (1964). Often, combinations of several of these factors were responsible for seizure precipitation. Beyer and Jovanovic (1966) found precipitating factors in 99 (88.5 per cent) of 120 patients with GMA. From these, however, 15 per cent should perhaps be subtracted who thought that the weather was the provocative factor (curiously, no patient of this study seems to have had more than one precipitating factor). Many patients feel that seizures can be precipitated by annoying events but when their reported examples are analysed in detail, it is most often found that sleep disturbance was the mediating factor. David (1955) considers this as the central factor involved in all other modes of precipitation.

For photosensitivity, see below.

Chronobiology: The definition of GMA requires that, for this diagnosis, at least 90 per cent of seizures must occur in the first two hours after awakening (regardless of the time of day), or in the second seizure peak, during the evening relaxation phase. In a total of 40 (13 per cent) of 310 patients with this syndrome studied by Goosses (1984) this other seizure peak was the main one. Until now, nothing has been found to indicate that this is more than a subvariety. In the Goosses study, patients with the evening mode of distribution had somewhat higher manifestation age, were more often males, and less often photosensitive (Table 4). None of these differences, however, was statistically significant, and they could be interrelated. It is interesting, however, that Helmchen (1958) already noted that after age 19 the syndrome manifested more often with an important or predominant evening peak, and a Chi-square test done with his figures reveals that they are statistically significant (Table 3).

Table 4. Epilepsy with GMA, patients with different seizure peaks (modified from Goosses)

Main seizure peak	% males	Mean age of onset	% photosensitive
On awakening (n = 270)	53	15.1 years	13
Evening leisure (n = 40)	62	20.1 years	10

All differences are not significant (Chi-square and U-tests)

EEG and polygraphy

Christian (1960) was the first author who studied the EEG of GMA (in comparison with GMS). He compared four groups of 150 patients each: GMA alone, GMA with minor seizures, GMS alone, and GMS with minor seizures. The two GMA groups contrasted clearly with GMS groups. Whereas of the latter, 57 per cent of the pure and 23 per cent of the combined patients had a completely normal EEG, this was only true for 18 per cent of those with pure, and 3 per cent of those with combined GMA. The most frequent findings in GMA were increased slow waves (76 per cent), disorganized background activity with steep transients (63 per cent) and generalized spike-wave activity (41.3 per cent). In patients with additional minor seizures, spike-waves were found in 70 per cent. Another 12.6 per cent, and respectively, 10 per cent developed spike waves during hyperventilation. Focal abnormalities were extremely rare (two respectively 2.6 per cent). In contrast, the abnormalities found in GMS included temporal sharp waves in 3 per cent, and other focal abnormalities in 12.6 per cent, whereas 3 per cent only had spike-wave activity. Several subtypes of spike-wave discharge were observed in this study but not further analysed; they included spike-wave frequencies from 2.5 — 4 c/s, and polyspike-wave. It seems that their predominant type depends mainly on the associated minor seizures. Loiseau (1964) reported bilateral SW in 76 per cent of his patients but noted the rarity of perfectly regular 3 c/s SW; polySW, irregular shapes of complexes and shifting asymmetries were common findings. No study has yet compared the epileptic discharge of pure GMA with that of cases with associated absences or myoclonic seizures. In contrast to other grand mal syndromes, GMA is one of the epileptic syndromes that are related to photosensitivity (Table 5).

Table 5. Different grand mal syndromes and photosensitivity (modified from Goosses)

Syndrome	n	% photos.	Males (n)	% photos.	Females (n)	% photos.
GM during sleep	137	4.4	80	2.5	57	7.0
GM on awakening	270	13.0	143	9.1	127	17.3
GM in evening	40	10.0	26	3.8	14	21.4
GM at random	65	4.6	37	5.4	28	3.6

GMA is positively (P < 0.01) correlated, and GMS negatively (P < 0.05) correlated with photosensitivity

Billiard (1982) reviewed the findings of the Montpellier group on sleep polygraphy in 77 patients with GM only, 13 of which were of the awakening type; further patients with GMA seem to be included in his 32 patients with absences, and 32 patients with JME. The exact figures, however, cannot be derived from this report. The 13 patients with only GMA were noted for frequently presenting epileptic discharge at sleep onset and during night or morning awakenings. Only to a lesser extent was it found in daytime routine EEG and NREM sleep.

Some other papers that report polygraphic findings in GMA are difficult to evaluate because of methodological problems. They have been discussed by Wolf and Röder (1982). Some of them are also concerned with the sleep structure, an issue that seemed interesting in view of the peculiarities of sleep behaviour of these patients (see historical introduction).

The matter has been studied in untreated epileptic patients by our own group. Wolf and Röder (1982) published some preliminary results, and Danninger (1982) reported on spontaneous sleep after two adaptation nights in a group of 43 patients wih various kinds of epilepsy. The patients in this program were reinvestigated with antiepileptic drugs at various stages, and Wolf *et al.* (1984) compared the influences of phenobarbital and phenytoin monotherapy shortly after adjustment to therapeutic steady states.

Of Danninger's patients, 19 were diagnosed as having generalized idiopathic epilepsy, 12 of them had GMA associated or not with minor seizures, and 15 could be grouped as 'awakening epilepsy' because they had absence, JME or GMA or combinations of these. Various comparisons were made with other patient groups (but not with healthy controls), and it appeared that patients with GMA, awakening epilepsy or generalized idiopathic epilepsy were conspicuous, above all, by an increase of deep sleep. This could not convincingly be explained by age differences, but Danninger was able to demonstrate that the difference was entirely caused by the subgroup of photosensitive patients. Non-photosensitive subjects with generalized and awakening epilepsies did not differ at all from other patients.

Wolf *et al.* (1984), however, reported that the response of patients with awakening epilepsy to antiepileptic drugs differed from other patients. It appeared that, in them, the early sleep cycles of the night were particularly affected by either drug: much above average increase of deep NREM sleep in first cycle with phenobarbital and, unlike patients with focal epilepsy, decrease of stage 2 and of cycle duration in the first and second cycle with phenytoin. These studies indicate that the hypothesis (Christian, 1960; Janz, 1962) of a specific sleep disorganization in GMA must probably be replaced by the hypothesis that the sleep of these patients is particularly unstable and modifiable by external influences. This is an interesting parallel to their propensity to seizure precipitation by external stimuli as reported above.

Neuropathological findings

Gross anatomical lesions are a strong argument against classifying an epileptic disorder as idiopathic, although chance coexistence of a genetically determined epilepsy and an exogenous brain lesion is not a priori impossible. The widespread assumption that there is no neuropathology of idiopathic epilepsy extrapolates from absence of gross lesions demonstrable in vivo, and is merely based on theoretical considerations that view idiopathic generalized epilepsy as a primarily functional disturbance of a neurophysiological order. Morphological evidence to support this assumption is, however, lacking because, until very recently, autopsy reports on patients with some form of idiopathic generalized epilepsy were restricted to two cases, one with 'frequent' absences and one GM seizure (Cohn, 1968), and one with JME and seven convulsions of GMA (Janz and Neimanis, 1961). Recently, Meencke and Janz (1984) have reported eight cases of GMA with absences, two of which had myoclonic seizures in addition. Still, the total of neuropathological reports on this group of epileptic syndromes is restricted to 10 cases. This seems to be due to two reasons:

First, that autopsies are rarely performed in disorders that are usually benign; second, neuropathologists in general seem not to be aware that there are open problems about idiopathic epilepsies.

The causes of death in the 10 reported cases were suicide (three), anti-epileptic drug toxicity, heart failure, and carcinoma (one each). In four cases, death occurred unexpectedly, and the cause could not be established with certainty. The ages of death ranged from 13 to 71 years (mean: 30.1 years). All these patients had had some kind of generalized minor seizures, and the nine patients with repeated grand mal, GMA. Patients with small (< 20) as well as very large numbers of GM seizures (including one GM status) are represented.

Remarkably, even in the three patients who suffered between 400 and 900 GM seizures in their life time, as well as the one with about 160 GM seizures and one status epilepticus with a subsequent psychotic state, Meencke and Janz were unable to demonstrate lesions of the type generally considered to be caused by seizures ('Krampfschäden', elective parenchymal necrosis) which casts doubt on the pathogenetic interpretation of such findings in subjects with other kinds of epilepsies.

Janz and Neimanis (1961) in a patient with only seven convulsive seizures were struck by the importance of findings that seemed to be attributable to injuries caused by seizures. They took great pains to find explanations for possible excessive ictogenic hypoxia in this individual patient, and pointed to the unusual distribution of the supposed ictogenic lesions (mainly cerebellar cortex, dentate nucleus, and nucleus ruber). This, however, was not duplicated in the Meencke and Janz series.

Meencke and Janz (1984) drew attention to the findings of microdysgenesias in seven of their eight cases. These comprise:
- immediately subpial rows of uni- and bipolar nerve cells
- increased nerve cell density in the stratum moleculare
- in addition to this, indistinct boundary between lamina 2 and stratum moleculare
- protrusion of nervous tissue containing well-differentiated neurons, into the pia
- displaced modes of columnar cortical neuronal architecture
- increased nerve cells in the white matter
- increase of large nerve cells marked by satellitosis in the stratum radiatum of hippocampus together with indistinct transitions from stratum pyramidale to stratum oriens.
- Purkinje cell dystopias (also reported by Janz and Neimanis, 1961)

As far as these dysgenesias that reflect disturbances of brain maturation can be related to certain stages of fetal development, they seem all to belong to the period between the 7th month of pregnancy and the neonatal period. Their etiology is not determined, and both hereditary and exogenous factors (viral embryopathies, respiratory disturbances) can be discussed.

Discussions of such findings mostly concentrate on the question of their significance as they can also be found in subjects who have clinically been healthy. Meencke and Janz (1984) review the literature on the relative frequency of microdysgenesias in different groups of persons. For one of the dysgenesias, the dystopic neurons in the white matter, Meencke (1983) has performed a controlled morphometric study in the inferior frontal gyrus. Six cases of generalized idiopathic epilepsy (GMA + absences) were compared with eight traumatic epilepsies and 22 non-epileptic controls. The age factor was corrected. The density of dystopic neurons in idiopathic generalized epilepsy was 3.5 times that of non-epileptic controls, and 2.5 times of traumatic epilepsy, and these differences were statistically highly significant. Interestingly, the density in traumatic epilepsy was still 1.4 times that of controls ($P < 0.01$). An innate seizure disposition of some degree may well be one pathogenetic factor of traumatic epilepsy. Thus, the findings of Meencke could indeed be connected with a primary seizure disposition.

Nothing is known about the discharging properties and connections of such dystopic neurons nor their inhibition. But one is puzzled if there might even be a very close relation of these dystopias to the functional disorder of generalized epilepsy. This hypothesis is the more attractive as the findings refer to a phylogenetically very young area, and generalized idiopathic epilepsies of the kind discussed here are exclusively human diseases. However, the Meencke investigation marks mainly the onset of a new mode of neuropathological approach to the problem of idiopathic generalized epilepsy, and studies of other areas are necessary before a more complete morphological pattern allows for more detailed hypotheses.

Pathogenesis and evolution

Tsuboi and Christian (1976) found possible exogenous factors in 7.5 per cent of 147 patients with GMA which meant a significant decrease in comparison with all other epileptic syndromes. No specification of these factors was given.

Janz (1962) reported 2110 patients with GM seizures, 719 (34 per cent) of which had GMA. Of 106 patients with perinatal damage, however, only 14 per cent had GMA, among 227 traumatic epilepsies 14 per cent, among 77 epilepsies due to a tumor only 8 per cent, and among 117 other symptomatic epilepsies, 14 per cent. In other words, 10 per cent of all GMA patients were diagnosed as having symptomatic epilepsy in contrast to 23 per cent of patients with GMS, and 53 per cent of those with GM at random. The same figure of 10 per cent with pathogenetic clues was found by Loiseau (1964). Thus, although GMA, as a syndrome, clearly belongs to the idiopathic epilepsies with frequent genetic predisposition, in the individual case exogenous pathogenic factors are not excluded automatically. The border between idiopathic and symptomatic epilepsies is by no means sharp. Even in JME (see previous chapter), the syndrome of idiopathic epilepsy with the highest genetic predisposition, the penetrance is far from complete, and exogenous influences can be detected. Influences of manifestation factors (that may be endogenous or exogenous) are presumably the rule rather than the exception in idiopathic epilepsies. It would probably be better to talk about 'predominantly idiopathic' and 'predominantly symptomatic' epilepsies suggesting multifactorial pathogenesis in a substantial proportion of cases. The association of GMA with focal seizures which will be discussed below, is pertinent to this question.

Association with other generalized seizure types has been discussed. The manifestation sequences in such cases have not been investigated. For the manifestation sequence in juvenile absences and JME with GM seizures (which are predominantly of the awakening type), see the relevant chapters. Among the patients with pyknolepsy plus GM seizures (GMA in 88 per cent) of Janz (1969), absences had not been noticed before the first GM seizure in only 12.5 per cent. As is pointed out by the author, even this does not necessarily mean that absences were not present before as they may have passed unnoticed. No information is given about the ages of onset of seizures in this small group of doubtful manifestation sequence.

The tendency, within the group of GMA, to evening seizure-peaks in patients of later age of onset has been mentioned above. If seizure control is not achieved, changes of the circadian distribution may occur in the course of the disease as was pointed out by Janz (1962), and Loiseau (1964). Thus, the epilepsy of patients with GMA who had only one seizure peak, had lasted 10.0 years on average but that of those with two peaks 12.2 years (Janz, 1962; significance levels not given). It was further pointed out that of the cases that began as GMA, 17 per cent turned later into GMS, and 6 per cent into a random seizure distribution. On the other hand, no cases of initial random distribution or relation to sleep evolved to GMA which is a rather strong argument in favour of the syndromatic significance of the chronobiology of GMA. The reasons for such secondary changes of circadian seizure distribution are not known. The hypothesis of Janz (1962) that they were due to traumatic or ictogenic lesions has never since adequately been investigated.

Therapy and prognosis

Avoidance of precipitating factors (see above) is as important a base for therapy as in JME. Thus, patients may have to avoid a job or profession that requires shift work.

Vocational rehabilitation must then be included in the therapeutic plan.

Retrospective investigations on the relative efficacy of various antiepileptic drugs suggested that barbiturates were perhaps more efficient in these patients than hydantoins and carbamazepine (Janz, 1969; Beyer and Jovanovic, 1966; Schmidt, 1982). There are, however, no controlled studies or studies involving determinations of serum drug levels in GMA. According to the data given by Janz (1969), complete seizure control could be expected in at least 65 per cent of patients with only GMA. Loiseau (1964) reported complete seizure control in 52 of 83 patients with GMA (62.7 per cent). Of his 47 patients with GM only, however, 37 or 79 per cent were completely controlled.

The investigation of Janz *et al.* (1983) about relapse following dose-reduction or withdrawal in seizure-free patients found this to be particularly high in GMA (63 patients, 83 per cent relapses), significantly higher than in other GM epilepsies.

Nosological place

The close syndromatic relations of both absence syndromes, JME and GMA have been discussed in the previous chapters. They are confirmed by the rate of associated seizures in Table 2. The papers reviewed in that table also indicate association with psychomotor or complex partial seizures in as many as 15-22 per cent of patients with GMA. It should be pointed out, however, that in all these studies, the diagnosis of seizure types was based on reports of patients and witnesses, interictal EEG, occasional direct observations but never split screen recordings. It is possible that some of the supposed complex partial seizures in reality were absences with automatisms. Presumably, this would not account for all cases. Another possibility is the co-existence of hereditary and symptomatic factors that was discussed above. Lange and Rabe (1978) reported some such patients who had both focal and generalized clinical and EEG signs. Some patients with GMA and partial seizures may belong to the same category, but at the moment detailed reports of such cases do not seem to exist. Theoretically, there would be no problem in accepting that, in individuals with an innate predisposition to seizures, additional exogenous pathogenetic factors may sometimes not only contribute to the actual manifestation of an epileptic disorder but also exact a determining influence on its symptomatology. In such instances that will often appear as epilepsies with generalized and focal features, the present author would regard a link of GM seizures to the awakening situation as an indicator of an idiopathic generalized predisposition.

References

Barre, J.A. (1946): De l'utilité du dénombrement de l'épilepsie banale et classique. *Rev. Neurol.* **78**, 376-378.

Beyer, L., Jovanovic, U.J. (1966): Elektrencephalographische und klinische Korrelate bei Aufwachepileptikern mit besonderer Berücksichtigung der therapeutischen Probleme. *Nervenazzt* **37**, 333-336.

Billiard, M. (1983): Epilepsies and the Sleep-Wake Cycle. In *Sleep and epilepsy,* pp 269-286. ed M.B. Sterman, M.N. Shouse, P. Passouant. Academic Press: New York.

Christian, W. (1960): Bioelektrische Charakteristik tagesperiodisch gebundener Verlaufsformen epileptischer Erkrankungen. *J. Neurol.* **181**, 413-444.

Cohn, R. (1968): A neuropathological study of a case of petit mal epilepsy. *Electroenceph. Clin. Neurophysiol.* **24**, 282.

Danninger, Th. (1982): Polygraphische Untersuchung des Schlafes unbehandelter Epilepsiepatienten. Thesis, West Berlin.

David, J. (1955): L'épilepsie du réveil. Thèse, Lyon.

Goosses, R. (1984): Die Beziehung der Fotosensibilität zu den verschiedenen epileptischen Syndromen. Thesis, West Berlin.

Gowers, W.R. (1881): *Epilepsy and other chronic convulsive diseases: their causes, symptoms and treatment.* Reprint 1966. Dover: New York.

Griffiths, G.N., Fox, J.T. (1938): Rhythm in Epilepsy. *Lancet* **234**, 409-416.

Helmchen, H. (1958): Beitrag zur konstitutionellen Differenzierung im Bereich genuiner Epilepsien. *J. Neurol.* **178**, 541-582.

Hopkins, H. (1933): The time of appearance of epileptic seizures in relation to age, duration and type of the syndrome. *J. Nerv. Ment. Dis.* **77**, 153-162.

Janz, D. (1953): 'Aufwach'-Epilepsien. (Als Ausdruck einer den 'Nacht'-oder 'Schlaf' Epilepsien gegenüberzustellenden Verlaufsform epileptischer Erkrankungen). *Arch. Psychiat. Nervenkrh.* **191**, 73-98.

Janz, D. (1962): The Grand Mal Epilepsies and the sleeping-waking cycle. *Epilepsia* **3**, 69-109.

Janz, D. (1969): *Die Epilepsien. Spezielle Pathologie und Therapie.* Thieme: Stuttgart.

Janz, D., Kern, A. Mössinger, H.J., Puhlmann, H.U. (1983): Rückfallprognose während und nach Reduktion der Medikamente bei Epilepsiebehandlung. In *Epilepsie 1981. Verlauf und Prognose, neuropsychologische und psychologische Aspekte,* pp 17-24. ed H. Remschmidt, R. Rentz, J. Jungmann. Thieme: Stuttgart.

Janz, D., Neimanis, G. (1961): Clinico-anatomical Study of a Case of Idiopathic Epilepsy with Impulsive Petit Mal ('Impulsiv-Petit mal') and Grand Mal on Awakening ('Aufwach-Grand mal'). *Epilepsia* **2**, 251-269.

Langdon-Down, M., Brain, W.R. (1929): Time of day in relation to convulsions in Epilepsy. *Lancet* **1**, 1029-1032.

Lange, H.U., Rabe, F. (1978): Zur Frage 'symptomatischer' Pyknolepsien und Impulsiv-Petit-mal. *Nervenarzt* **49**, 41-46.

Le Camus. (1951): L'épilepsie du réveil. Thèse, Paris.

Leder, A. (1967): Zur Psychopathologie der Schlaf-und Aufwachepilepsie (Eine psychodiagnostische Untersuchung). *Nervenarzt* **38**, 434-442.

Loiseau, P. (1964): Crises épileptiques survenant au réveil et épilepsie du réveil. *Sud Médical et Chirurgical* **99**, 11492-11502.

Marchand, L., Ajuriaguerra, J. (1948): *Epilepsies.* Desclée de Brouwer: Paris.

Meencke, H.J. (1983): The density of dystopic neurons in the white matter of the gyrus frontalis inferior in epilepsies. *J. Neurol.* **230**, 171-181.

Meencke, H.J., Janz, D. (1984): Neuropathological findings in primary generalized epilepsy: a study of eight cases. *Epilepsia* **25**, 8-21.

Patry, F.L. (1931): The relation of time of day, sleep and other factors to the incidence of epileptic seizures. *Am. J. Psychiat.* **10**, 789-813.

Roger, H., Cornil, L., Paillas, J. (1950): *Les épilepsies.* Flammarion: Paris.

Schmidt, D. (1981): *Behandlung der Epilepsien.* Thieme: Stuttgart.

Tsuboi, T., Christian, W. (1976): *Epilepsy. A clinical, electroencephalographic and statistical study of 466 patients. Springer: Berlin, Heidelberg, New York.*

Wolf, P., Röder, U.U. (1982): Sleep patterns in untreated epileptic patients with seizures during sleep or after awakening. In *Sleep and epilepsy,* pp 411-419. ed M.B. Sterman, M.N. Shouse, P. Passouant. Academic Press: New York.

Wolf, P., Röder-Wanner, U.U., Brede, M. (1984): Influence of therapeutic phenobarbital and phenytoin medication on the polygraphic sleep of patients with epilepsy. *Epilepsia* **25**, 467-475.

*　　　　*　　　　*

Discussion pages 271-273

Epileptic syndromes in infancy, child-hood and adolescence. J. Roger, C. Dravet, M. Bureau, F.E. Dreifuss and P. Wolf. John Libbey Eurotext Ltd ©1985.

Discussion of
Epilepsies with Generalized
Convulsive Seizures
(Chapters 14, 28 & 29)

Summarized by Peter WOLF

In the discussion following the review of juvenile myoclonic epilepsy (JME), epilepsy with grand mal on awakening (GMA), and epilepsy with generalized convulsive sei-zures in childhood, a variety of points were touched upon.

The syndrome of JME was discussed by *Dreifuss, Jeavons, Lerman, O'Donohoe, Roger* and *Sorel.* There was unanimous agreement with the description of the syn-drome and its inclusion in the idiopathic generalized epilepsies. JME was considered the most appropriate terminology.

Jeavons pointed out that, in female patients, the seizures had a tendency to occur before and at menstruation, and stop during pregnancies. *Dreifuss* drew attention to the role of alcohol as a triggering factor in this, as in other syndromes of adolescence. He mentioned two instances of fatal car accidents caused by alcohol-induced seizures in otherwise well-controlled patients.

Wolf thought that, in such cases, the sleep withdrawal that usually accompanies alcohol excess was perhaps the more important factor.

Lerman also found this factor important especially for grand mal manifestation in this syndrome.

Sorel raised the question of the manifestation sequence of different seizure types in this syndrome. The printed manuscript includes information thereon. Sorel felt that myoclonic seizures usually preceded grand mal seizures, and that an inverse sequence may indicate a less favourable prognosis.

Jeavons underlined the diagnostic importance of directly asking patients if they had jerks as many will not report them spontaneously. He reminded that there are two types of benign myoclonic epilepsy, one of small children, and one of puberty, mani-festing at the same age as photosensitivity. Sensitivty to eye closure and its possible re-lation to photosensitivity was briefly discussed by *Roger* and *Wolf.*

Oller Daurella commented on epilepsy with grand mal seizures in adolescence, without special reference to GMA. He reported from his material that GM seizures (not includ-

271

ing single seizures) most frequently began in the age-group 12-18, and that in idiopathic generalized epilepsies of earlier manifestation, adolescence was often an age when GM seizures manifested as an additional seizure type. This was true in 38 of 86 patients (out of a total of 168 primary generalized epilepsies with onset before age 12) who had not had GM seizures before that age. If GM was the only seizure type, the prognosis was good in 83 per cent, and mental development was unaffected in all cases. Of the patients who also had absences, only 55.8 per cent had a good prognosis and, mental deterioration was sometimes observed.

Seino asked which proportion of seizures occurring during sleep or after awakening was required for a diagnosis of sleep grand mal (SGM) or GMA, and *Wolf* gave the figure of at least 90 per cent.

Seino asked further if any interictal EEG findings were typical for SGM, and if SGM should be considered as belonging to the idiopathic generalized epilepsies.

Wolf replied that he did not think that SGM was a homogeneous group, and that the EEG findings of various subgroups differ.

Tassinari and *Wolf* exchanged words to the effect that the term 'grand mal' did not necessarily mean seizures that were generalized from the beginning but also included partial seizures evolving to generalized tonic-clonic, or GM of focal onset.

Jeavons remarked that the terms grand mal and petit mal should be avoided altogether.

Roger warned against too rapidly assuming a diagnosis of idiopathic generalized epilepsy. According to him, there was no doubt about that diagnosis in cases of pyknoleptic absences manifesting at early school age, with sudden onset and termination of seizures, and 3 c/s spike-wave, nor was there a doubt in cases with GMA, accompanied or not by myoclonic seizures, manifesting in adolescence and with poly-spikes in the EEG. He thought that cases different from these, such as early combinations of absences and GM plus, eventually, myoclonic seizures, or GM followed by absences, having a less good prognosis and a higher tendency to develop psychiatric complications, did not necessarily belong to idiopathic generalized epilepsy. They could belong to heterogeneous subgroups. Some could represent mild forms of symptomatic generalized epilepsy with late manifestation. In others, seizures of focal origin in both frontal lobes could be detected. The first group often had EEG signs reminiscent of Lennox-Gastaut syndrome (slow spike-wave, rapid rhythmic discharge during sleep). Also for the second group, the sleep EEG was considered important for the detection of focal abnormalities. *Roger* recommended that care be taken in rating such patients and all of them should be investigated with modern equipment (video, sleep EEG, longterm monitoring).

Cavazzuti said he had the impression that in cases of the kind indicated by Roger there was often some unilateral ventricular enlargement. *Roger* was of the same opinion and even thought that, sometimes, longtitudinal studies revealed an atrophic process. This was supported by *Dulac* who thought this warning applied especially to children younger than 5 years of age.

Aicardi, however, thought that rare generalized seizures of early childhood following febrile convulsions definitely did not belong here and had an excellent prognosis.

Beaumanoir said that a good response to therapy also indicated to which category a patient belonged. *Roger* thought this argument was limited to a good response to minimal therapy.

A final point was raised by *O'Donohoe*. Did focal abnormalities in patients with rare grand mal seizures always exclude a diagnosis of idiopathic generalized epilepsy and indicate an unfavourable prognosis? *Oller Daurella* held that interictal focal abnormalities indicate a focal onset of GM seizures. Neither he nor *Roger*, however, were positive that this excluded that the epilepsy syndrome was primarily one of idiopathic generalized epilepsy. *Dulac* mentioned patients with both rolandic spikes and generalized discharge and, most often, photosensitivity, who have a good prognosis even if focal or unilateral seizures occur. *O'Donohoe* found that Gloor's concept of cortico-reticular epilepsy could explain such cases: in them, cortex and reticular system could be equally involved, and the focal finding at the surface could be a functional disturbance in the cortex that might trigger the system to produce generalized seizures. His conclusion was, again, that focal interictal discharge did not exclude idiopathic generalized epilepsy.

Epileptic syndromes in infancy, childhood and adolescence. J. Roger, C. Dravet, M. Bureau, F.E. Dreifuss and P. Wolf. John Libbey Eurotext Ltd ©1985.

Chapter 30
Benign Partial Seizures of Adolescence

Pierre LOISEAU and Pierre LOUISET

Hôpital Pellegrin/ Tripode, Place Amélie-Raba-Léon, 33076 Bordeaux, France

Summary

A syndrome of benign partial epileptic seizures in the adolescent is characterized as follows: an onset between 10 and 20 years of age, with a peak at 13 to 14 years of age; a predominance in boys; no family history of epilepsy; neither neurological nor psychic impairment; either simple or complex partial seizures mainly with motor and/or sensory symptoms, and frequently with secondary generalization; a single seizure, or a cluster of 2 to 5 seizures in less than 24 hours; a normal electroencephalogram or with mild abnormalities.

Introduction

Epileptic seizures are far from being infrequent in adolescents. The average annual incidence rate of epilepsy has been calculated as 24.7/100,000 between the ages of 10 and 14 years and 18.6/100,000 between the ages of 15 and 19 years (Kurland, 1959). Epilepsies with an onset between the ages of 10 and 14 years have been reported to represent 15 per cent and those with an onset between the ages of 15 and 19 years 11 per cent of all epilepsies (Lennox and Lennox, 1960; Gudmundsson, 1966; Beaussart *et al.,* 1980).

Forty-five per cent of adolescents' seizures have a focal onset (Loiseau and Dartigues, 1981). A brain tumor is suspected every time partial seizures occur in patients without previously known brain damage. However 77 per cent of epilepsies with an onset during adolescence remain without aetiology (Watanabe & Fukushima, 1978) and brain tumors at this age are very rare :2.6 per cent of patients (Loiseau & Dartigues, 1981). The prognosis of partial seizures is a controversial matter (Rodin, 1968). However when occurring during adolescence these attacks may have an excellent prognosis (Loiseau *et al.,* 1983). A syndrome of benign focal epileptic seizures in teenagers was thus described (Loiseau & Orgogozo, 1978). We up-dated the material on which this report was based. The records of 108 patients followed up for five years or more were reviewed.

Description

1. *Prevalence.* Benign partial seizures would represent 24 per cent of all partial seizures with an onset between the ages of 12 and 18 years.

2. *Sex ratio.* A higher incidence among males is striking: 71.2 per cent of patients.

3. *Genetics.* A family history of epilepsy was very rare (3 per cent) as was a personal history predisposing to epilepsy. Possible acquired factors existed in 4 per cent of cases. No special event appears to provoke a seizure.

4. *Age of occurrence.* Seizures were unequally distributed during adolescence: age 10-11: 12 per cent; 11-12: 10.2 per cent; 12-13: 13.9 per cent; 13-14: 18.5 per cent; 14-15: 15.8 per cent; 15-16: 11.1 per cent; 16-17: 6.4 per cent; 17-18: 10.2 per cent; 18-19: 1.90 per cent. The syndrome peaks at 13-14 years of age, appears to be exceptional after the age of 20, but can probably exist before the age of 10.

5. *Clinical symptomatology.* Seizures are characterized by a succession of symptoms and/or signs associated with a stepwise involvement of primary or secondary cortical areas and very seldom of temporal structures. Combined signs or symptoms were noted in 57 per cent of seizures. They were mainly motor signs (110 seizures) or sensory symptoms (79 seizures). Motor signs were mainly without march (49 seizures), less often versive (28 seizures). Only 10 Jacksonian seizures were reported. Phonatory signs were noted in 27 seizures. Somato-sensory symptoms were frequent (44 seizures). Visual symptoms were present in 24 seizures and vertigo in 11 seizures. Auditory, olfactory and gustatory symptoms were never reported. Autonomic symptoms were reported in 20 seizures. Psychic symptoms were reported in only 6 seizures. These attacks were diurnal in 87 per cent of cases.

According to the revised clinical and electroencephalographic classification of epileptic seizures (1981) there were:
- simple partial seizures: 14.5 per cent
- complex partial seizures:
    simple partial onset followed by impairment of consciousness: 22.5 per cent
    with impairment of consciousness at onset: 6 per cent
- partial seizures evolving to secondarily generalized seizures:
    after a simple partial onset: 34.2 per cent
    after a complex onset: 6.8 per cent
    after a simple onset evolving to complex partial: 16.2 per cent

The interictal neurological and mental status was normal in almost all cases (97 per cent of patients).

6. *Electroencephalogram.* A normal interictal EEG or an EEG showing only non-specific and non-focal abnormalities is mandatory for the diagnosis of benign partial epileptic seizure in adolescents. The record is usually normal at rest or showing some slight diffuse abnormalities. Bilateral posterior or diffuse slow waves may be found when the EEG is recorded within the first days after the seizure. A mild slow dysrhythmia is not infrequent on hyperventilation. However no typical spike-wave complex is seen in any case, nor any focal abnormality.

7. *Evolution.* There was an isolated seizure in 79.6 per cent of patients. In the others, a cluster of 2 to 5 attacks occurred in less than thirty-six hours. During a follow-up period ranging from 5 to 20 years (mean: 9.5 years) no recurrence was noted.

Discussion

Epilepsy is defined as a state of chronically recurrent seizures. In the above syndrome a single seizure occurs in most cases and, when several seizures occur, they are never in a chronic repetition. Therefore the term benign partial epileptic seizures of adolescence must be preferred to the term benign partial epilepsy.

When doctors are confronted with a first seizure they have to decide what examinations are to be done, and whether or not treatment is necessary. They have to answer the patient's or his family's questions. They cannot wait for several months to determine if this seizure is an isolated event or the first manifestation of an epilepsy. It is valuable to have some immediate predictors of outcome. A cluster of symptoms and signs allows a diagnosis of benign epileptic seizures of adolescence to be made. Unfortunately no specific clinical or electroencephalographic signs characterize this syndrome. Errors are not infrequent. Just after the seizure a benign epilepsy may only be suspected. A one or two years outcome is necessary for diagnosis. However when a strong suspicion exists, unnecessary investigation and anticonvulsant drug therapy are to be avoided.

Rèfèrences

Beaussart, M., Faou, R., Defayes J. (1980): Epidémiologie de l'épilepsie dans la région du Nord-Pas-de-Calais (à propos de 12 290 cas). *Lille Médical* **25**, 183-191.

Commission on Classification and Terminology of the International League Against Epilepsy (1981): Proposal for revised clinical and electroencephalographic classification of epileptic seizures. *Epilepsia* **22**, 489-501.

Gudmundsson, G. (1966): Epilepsy in Iceland. A clinical and epidemiological investigation. *Acta Neurol. Scand.* **43**, suppl. 25, 124 pp.

Kurland, L.T. (1959): The incidence and prevalence of convulsive disorders in a small urban community. *Epilepsia* **1**, 143-161.

Lennox, W.G., Lennox, M.A. (1960): *Epilepsy and related disorders.* (Vol. I). Little, Brown and Co: Boston.

Loiseau, P., Dartigues J.F. (1981): Formes électro-cliniques et évolutions des épilepsies de l'adolescence. *Rev. EEG Neurophysiol.* **11**, 493-501.

Loiseau, P., Dartigues, J.F., Pestre M. (1983): Prognosis of partial epileptic seizures in the adolescent. *Epilepsia* **24**, 472-481.

Loiseau, P., Orgogozo, J.M. (1978): An unrecognized syndrome of benign focal epileptic seizures in teenagers. *Lancet* **2**, 1070-1071.

Rodin, E.A. (1968): *The prognosis of patients with epilepsy.* Charles C. Thomas: Springfield, Ill.

Watanabe, S., Fukushima, Y. (1978): A study on adolescence epilepsy. *Brain Nerve* **30**, 63-68.

Discussion
Summarized by Pierre LOISEAU

Beaumanoir: The question is to decide if we are dealing with an epileptic syndrome, in order to recognize it.

Munari: Is a single such event sufficient for us to speak of epilepsy?

Wolf: I think we should keep to calling epilepsy something for which there have been several seizures, and not merely one.

Jeavons: It is definitely important to know that such an entity exists in order to better manage such cases. In the United Kingdom, it is of great practical importance that one does not say a single seizure is epilepsy. Because if you say somebody has epilepsy, you have to wait two years to get a driving licence. But if you have a single seizure you only have to wait one year. Epilepsy is a tendency to recurrent seizures. One seizure is, therefore, not epilepsy but a fit is a fit.

Dalla Bernardina: If we do not classify these facts, we shall lose them and we shall continue to lack sound diagnosis and prognosis criteria.

Soulayrol: This discussion is very important from a practical point of view. You may classify this syndrome as an epileptic syndrome in your silent laboratories. However to tell a patient he has epilepsy is very serious. I do not think it is possible to assign an epileptic label after a single seizure. If this is an epileptic seizure, is this an epileptic patient?

Tassinari: Do you have EEG sleep records?

Bureau: We did three sleep records. Two patients had some generalized spike-waves immediately after a seizure. The other patient, 45 days later, had a strictly normal EEG.

Epileptic syndromes in infancy, childhood and adolescence. J. Roger, C. Dravet, M. Bureau, F.E. Dreifuss and P. Wolf. John Libbey Eurotext Ltd ©1985.

Chapter 31
Lesional Epilepsies with Partial Seizures

Michel REVOL

Service d'Explorations Fonctionnelles du Système Nerveux, Centre Hospitalier Lyon Sud, 69310 Pierre-Bénite, France

Summary

In contrast to idiopathic benign partial epilepsy (particularly BECT), partial epilepsies in childhood secondary to cerebral lesions do not appear to constitute an epileptic syndrome because of the variability in their age of onset, etiology, semiology and prognosis. The nosological outline is itself unclear, the lesional feature of the epilepsy does not necessarily imply a particular prognosis and the existence of a cerebral lesion does not exclude the possibility that the patient has a benign idiopathic epilepsy. In addition, some cerebral lesions may not be evident and others not detectable. However, one can make a certain number of observations relating to the elements of a diagnosis of a partial lesional epilepsy. Certain types of seizures and EEG patterns seem to be related to them and on the other hand some prognostic factors can be specified.

Among childhood epilepsies, partial epilepsies (PE) are undoubtedly those which, in everyday practice, give rise to the majority of problems because of their frequency (over 40 per cent of epilepsies in children under 15 years of age, Gastaut *et al.*, 1975; Cavazzuti, 1980), of the diversity of the etiological and semiological aspects and the place which seizures may play in the life of the child.

It is certainly a debatable point whether it is possible to tackle partial lesional epilepsies (PLE) as a whole within the scope of this workshop devoted to 'epileptic syndromes'. It is indeed difficult to differentiate syndromes, as has been done for 'benign' (or 'mainly' functional, Gastaut, 1981) partial epilepsies on semiological, evolutive, but also etiological bases. Several remarks are, however, worth making.

Nosological aspects

What is meant by 'lesional epilepsy'? Electroclinical and neuroradiological data are frequently insufficient to allow the lesional nature of an epilepsy to be revealed.

Even though the introduction of computerized tomography (CT) has enabled the number of epilepsies without any known lesional cause to be reduced by making the neuroradiological examination easier, this technique suffers from certain drawbacks which should not be overlooked: high percentage of normal examinations (30-90 per cent normal examinations depending on the authors — Angeleri *et al.,* 1980; Yang, 1979; Gandon *et al.,* 1983) in PE in the child; existence of modifications which should be interpreted with caution — in particular discrete diffuse modifications, transitory focal signs.

Epilepsy surgery, after SEEG location, allows the lesional nature of any epilepsy to be affirmed when it reveals the existence of an anatomical lesion connected with an epileptogenic zone, even though the lesion may not be visible on CT examination. We may recall the data reported by Talairach *et al.* (1974), the value of which has not been much modified by the introduction of CT: out of 146 patients operated on for epilepsy, a probable etiology could be suspected from the electroclinical and neuroradiological findings in only 56.2 per cent of cases, but in 85 per cent of the patients, the operative record disclosed an 'anatomical change' and therefore a lesion. Anatomopathological examination can, in addition, reveal lesions which are not visible macroscopically.

Given these considerations, a few questions may be raised:

— should we retain the existence of non-benign but also non-lesional partial epilepsies? If so, can we differentiate them from PLE?

— in discussing on the one hand partial lesional epilepsy, and, on the other, benign partial epilepsy there is a risk of confusing anatomical lesions with their functional expression, which may or may not be transitory. This ambiguity is clearly noticeable, particularly in epilepsies with characteristics of benign partial epilepsy — epilepsy with centro-temporal spikes (BECT), or other types (BPE) — which may be seen in children with cerebral lesions, particularly with cerebral palsy.

Furthermore, the benign character of benign partial epilepsy cannot always be established as was pointed out recently by Newton and Aicardi (1983) with regard to certain occipital spike-wave epilepsies (Gastaut, 1982).

Etiological aspects

Without repeating what has been covered of the various etiologies in general reviews (O'Donohoe, 1979) the major points are as follows.

The problem of etiology is generally dominated by the existence of static cerebral lesions occurring before the appearance of seizures (e.g. scars, gliosis, sclerosis...). However, more frequently than admitted up to now, an expansive lesional etiology can be considered. In the case of ante-natal or neonatal pathology, the etiology varies, the electroclinical features of partial epilepsies do not have specific characteristics for a given etiology. Some are a little better individualised than others, for example, Sturge-Weber's disease, because in the majority of cases seizures have an early occurrence and they are hemicorporal in nature. Another distinguishable epilepsy is that of complex partial seizures due to atrophic parieto-occipital lesions related to vascular damage in the peri or post-natal period (Remillard *et al.* 1974; Roger *et al.* 1977).

Regarding acquired pathology, there have been attempts to particularize individual syndromes based on certain elements of etiology; the value in being able to identify a tumoral epilepsy is obvious from a diagnostic point of view. Unfortunately, epilepsy due to tumours does not have any specific characteristics, particularly when considering the semiology of seizures, as shown by Aicardi *et al.,* 1970 and Blume *et al.,* 1982.

One of the best described entities is post-unilateral status epilepticus syndrome with or without permanent deficit i.e. HHE (hemiconvulsion hemiplegia and epilepsy) syndrome (Gastaut *et al.* 1960). The characteristics of consecutive epilepsy, that is partial seizures of delayed onset after status epilepticus, are features which we found in a study on post status epilepticus (SE) infantile cerebral hemiplegias (Roger *et al.* 1972).

Semiological aspects

What does an analysis of seizures in terms of their semiology, mode of recurrence and triggering mechanisms, contribute towards the diagnosis of PLE?

Any type of partial seizure may be symptomatic of a PLE. However, some features more than others lead to a search for a lesional process, e.g. complex partial seizures, irrespective of the type (Aicardi, 1983); certain simple partial seizures, particularly crural; mixed seizures; combined seizures, e.g. those in which simple and complex partial symptoms are successive or associated (which may be compared with complex partial motor seizures described by Roger *et al.* 1981). The association of several types of seizures and a change of ictal semiology should all give rise to a suspicion of a lesional process.

A lesional process cannot formally be excluded if we consider only descriptions of seizures which are normally part of the BPE semiology (hemifacial seizures, fits of terror).

The trigger factors can be the same irrespective of the type of epilepsy: for example changes in arousal; vigilance and psychological factors. The special case of startle epilepsies, found in children with cerebral palsy, can however be distinguished. The problem of the value of ictal symptoms when considering prognosis will be discussed later.

EEG aspects

The position of the 'conventional' EEG has in general become clearer in the interpretation of the epilepsies when considering ictal or interictal features, by the introduction of the comparison between surface EEG and SEEG (Bancaud *et al.*, 1973).

The value of an ictal EEG recording is beyond question (Fig. 1). However, its value in the diagnosis of a lesional epilepsy presents the same problems as the analysis of the seizure in terms of clinical signs (Ambrosetto and Gobbi, 1975). Certain features have been generally considered as indicative of PLE; for example, ictal activity consisting of rhythmical slow waves and electrically silent seizures (Bancaud *et al.*, 1973). The occurrence of signs of post-ictal sufferance are rare in non-lesional epilepsies. (Dalla Bernardina *et al.*, 1980; Dulac and Arthuis, 1980).

Concerning interictal EEG, a few more observations can be made:

- The absence of abnormalities does not eliminate a lesional epilepsy. Besides, some abnormalities sometimes transiently disappear during treatment with anticonvulsants or other drugs, even in cases of tumour.

- Certain non-paroxysmal changes have great value, because they are related to the etiology rather than the epileptic phenomenon. They include abnormal basic rhythm, focalized polymorphic or even monorhythmic slow waves, localized or extensive depression of rhythms in one hemisphere, asymmetry of rhythms during hyperventilation and sleep, changes induced by the injection of medication.

- Paroxysmal abnormalities, depending on their features, have a variable value in

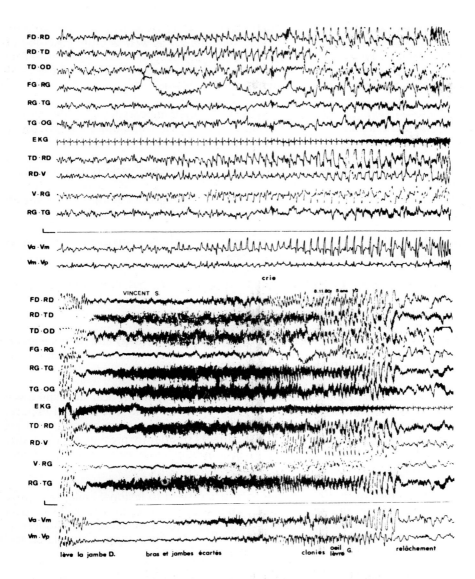

Fig. 1 Child 51/2 years-old at the time of recording, who had suffered multiple seizures daily for several weeks starting with a violent sensation of fear, without any hallucinatory phenomenon; after about 30s tonic type motor signs appeared, rapidly becoming bilateral, which also lasted 30s, accompanied by loss of contact. The two parts of the figure (top and above) are continuous. Two types of ictal EEG abnormalities are to be noted, which differ by their nature and by their localization, during the two successive phases of the seizure. In the first phase there are rhythmical slow spikes in the right fronto-central area and in the vertex; in the second phase there are fast rhythms with low amplitude in the vertex, becoming progressively slower. The clinical and neuroradiological report did not show evidence of any cerebral lesion in this epilepsy, which appeared to originate in the right frontal region. After three years, the seizures persisted despite different antiepileptic medication and were accompanied by increasing difficulties at school.

identifying lesional features of a partial epilepsy. Their analysis must take into account recording conditions (e.g. sleep, age etc. . .) as well as other EEG features, background activity, non-paroxysmal abnormalities, ictal activity. Furthermore, the relationship between the paroxysmal focalized abnormalities of the lesional type and the epileptogenic zone can present problems.

Unifocal spike-waves have a diagnostic value when their appearance differentiates them clearly from spike-waves of the BPE and, particularly, from those of epilepsy with centro-temporal spikes, according to their:

- Morphology and grouping: non-repetitive spike-waves of various morphology;

- Localization: fixed localization mainly frontal, or anterior temporal, localizations which are not normally found in BPE;

- Evolution, related to activation: no increase, or only a slight one, in frequency during sleep, but with a possibility of spreading.

- Relation with slow focalized abnormalities, particularly polymorphous

Multifocal spike-waves raise the same problems:

- They may represent multifocal epilepsy: by their morphology and their steady-state localization. This problem mainly concerns temporal foci and is difficult to solve by conventional EEG (Bancaud *et al.*, 1973).

- A further complex problem is the significance of the multifocal slow spike-waves reported by Noriega Sanchez and Markand (1976) in severe lesional epilepsies. These changes observed chiefly in the waking state are asynchronous and blend into a slow background activity. These patients frequently present with a picture of encephalopathy with bilateral cerebral lesions which may have previously been accompanied by hypsarrhythmia, or by diffuse slow spike-waves.

- These two types of multifocal abnormalities related to lesional epilepsies must be differentiated from multifocal spike-waves with the morphology and significance of typical centro-temporal spikes, which may also be observed in children with cerebral palsy. Their localization is not stable and they cannot be related to the cerebral lesions (Loiseau and Cohadon, 1981).

Paroxysmal bilateral synchronous abnormalities are sometimes seen in PLE under various circumstances:

- Paroxysms of bilateral synchronous spike-waves either are associated with focal paroxysmal or non-paroxysmal abnormalities or exist without localized abnormality. They are sometimes related to a familial predisposition. Photic stimulation and/or drowsiness can increase their frequency. They are of no diagnostic value and are misleading if interpreted as suggesting functional epilepsy.

- On the other hand, the significance of bilateral spike-waves predominating in both frontal regions — symmetrical or not, and related to frontal lesional epilepsy — is quite different. These abnormalities sometimes display features of rhythmic spike-wave discharges. The pattern of bilateral abnormalities is due to the ability of bilateral diffusion from a frontal unilateral focus or to the presence of bilateral frontal foci.

- Among bilateral abnormalities should be mentioned diffuse polyspikes, polyspike-waves and bursts of fast rhythms, analogous to those observed in Lennox-Gastaut syndrome, which can be seen in sleep recordings in children with severe PLE but never in BPE.

Evolution and prognosis

The influence of epilepsy on the life of a child depends on many factors, not only his seizures and their treatment but also their somatic and psychic context and the reactions of those around him. These influences are more important in cases of PLE than in primary generalized epilepsy or BPE. Several types of seizure evolution may occur, but their respective frequency is hard to define as studies generally include all partial epilepsies. According to Latinville and Loiseau (1975), and Gastaut (1981), one can say that about half the cases have a favourable evolution, more in simple partial seizures and less in cases of complex partial seizures.

The non-recurrence of seizures after cessation of treatment is seen above all in simple partial seizures, single or rare hemicorporal seizures, seizures grouped together in a single episode, epilepsies which are difficult to classify with regard to BPE. (see Oller-Daurella, chapter 14 and Loiseau and Louiset, chapter 30).

The need to maintain treatment because of recurrences upon withdrawal but also the persistence of seizures during treatment is seen particularly with complex partial seizures. Worthy of note is the spontaneous recurrence of seizures, sometimes after a long period of remission.

The persistence of seizures in spite of treatment may be accompanied by a disturbing evolution, very rarely associated with a progressive process (eg partial status epilepticus or development of a Lennox-Gastaut syndrome) but more often because of an interference with school performance and the development of psychopathological problems.

Based on these evolutional schemes, several authors have been able to evaluate the prognostic value of different parameters as described by Rodin (1968), Holowach et al. (1972), Lindsay et al. (1979), Roger et al. (1981), Pazzaglia et al. (1982), and Scarpa and Carassini (1982).

The following factors are most often held to represent an unfavourable prognosis:

- a known etiology
- seizures with early onset
- complex partial seizures
- seizures of several types
- a change in the type of seizures during evolution
- associated generalized seizures (rather than a secondary generalization)
- frequent seizures
- interictal EEG abnormalities, both frequent and various and not ressembling those found in epilepsy with centro-temporal spikes
- the presence of ictal discharges on routine recordings
- associated neurological and psychopathological signs.

Some of the data reported by Roger et al. (1981) are mentioned in Table 1 and are particularly illustrative of the prognostic value of the semiological features of seizures.

Table 1 Partial epilepsies in children. 119 cases according to Roger (1981)

Type of seizures	Type of evolution			
	I (n = 20)	II (n = 33)	III (n = 21)	IV (n = 45)
BECT	10			
SPS	5	22	18	21
CPS	3	8	10	17
CMPS		3	6	19
Unclassifiable	2			
Several types	1	17	11	38
Gen. assoc. seizures	0	8	2	14
Sudden fall	0	2	4	18
Reflex triggering	0	0	0	5
Onset of fits before 3 years	0	8	8	23
Existence of symptoms of encephalopathy	4	12	10	25

Frequency of different parameters in four groups depending on the severity of epilepsy.

I   Complete recovery and withdrawal of treatment (mean follow-up 4 years after the withdrawal).
II   No seizures with treatment (mean follow-up 5 years 10 months).
III Persistent occasional seizures with treatment.
IV   Frequent seizures and more pronounced seizures.

References

Aicardi, J., Praud, E., Bancaud, J., Mises, J., Chevrie, J.J. (1970): Epilepsies cliniquement primitives et tumeurs cérébrales chez l'enfant. *Archs Franç. Péd.* **27**, 1041-1055.

Aicardi, J. (1983): Complex partial seizures in childhood. In *Advances in epileptology,* the XIVth Epilepsy International Symposium, ed M. Parsonage, A.G. Craig, R.H.E. Grant, A.A. Ward, pp 237-242. Raven Press: New York.

Ambrosetto, G., Gobbi, G. (1975): Benign epilepsy of childhood with rolandic spikes or a lesion? EEG during a seizure. *Epilepsia* **16**, 793-796.

Angeleri, F., Provinciali, L., Salvolini, V. (1980): Computerized tomography in partial epilepsy. In *Advances in epileptology,* the XIth Epilepsy International Symposium, ed R. Canger, F. Angeleri, J.K. Penry, pp 53-64. Raven Press: New York.

Bancaud, J., Talairach, J., Geier, S., Scarabin, J.M. (1973): *EEG et SEEG dans les tumeurs cérébrales et l'épilepsie.* Edifor: Paris.

Blume, W.T., Girvin, J.P., Kaufmann, J.C.E. (1982): Childhood brain tumours presenting as chronic uncontrolled focal seizure disorders. *Ann. Neurol.* **12**, 538-541.

Cavazzuti, G.B. (1980): Epidemiology of different types of epilepsy in school age children of Modena, Italy. *Epilepsia* **21**, 57-62.

Dalla Bernardina, B., Bureau, M., Dravet, C., Dulac, O., Tassinari, C.A. (1980): Epilepsie bénigne de l'enfant avec crises à sémiologie affective. *Rev. E.E.G. Neurophysiol.* **10**, 8-18.

Dulac, O., Arthuis, M. (1980): Epilepsie psychomotrice bénigne de l'enfant. *Journées Parisiennes de Pédiatrie,* pp 211-219, Flammarion, Paris.

Gandon, Y., Baraton, J., Aicardi, J., Goutières, F. (1983): Efficacité de la scanographie dans les convulsions et épilepsies de l'enfant. *Ann. Pédiat.* **30**, 195-200.

Gastaut, H. (1981): Individualisation des épilepsies dites bénignes ou fonctionnelles aux différents âges de la vie. *Rev. E.E.G. Neurophysiol.* **11**, 346-366.

Gastaut, H. (1982): L'épilepsie bénigne de l'enfant à pointe-ondes occipitales *Rev. E.E.G. Neurophysiol.* **12**, 179-201.

Gastaut, H., Poirier, F., Payan, H., Salamon, G., Toga, M., Vigouroux, M. (1960): H.H.E. syndrome: hémiconvulsions, hémiplegia, epilepsy. *Epilepsia* **1**, 418-447.

Gastaut, H., Gastaut, J.L., Gonçalves e Silva, G.E., Fernandez Sanchez, G.R. (1975): Relative frequency of different types of epilepsy: a study employing the classification of the international league against epilepsy. *Epilepsia* **16**, 457-461.

Holowach, J., Thurston, D.L., O'Leary, J. (1972): Prognosis of childhood epilepsy. *New Engl. J. Med.* **286**, 169-174.

Holowach, J., Thurston, D.L., Hixon, B.B., Keller, A.J. (1982): Prognosis in childhood epilepsy. Additional follow-up. *New Engl. J. Med.* **306**, 831-836.

Latinville D., Loiseau, P. (1975): Evolution et pronostic de l'épilepsie chez l'enfant. *Bordeaux Médical* **8**, 2237-2257.

Lindsay, J., Ounsted, C., Richards, P. (1979): Long-term outcome in children with temporal lobe seizures; social outcome and childhood factors. *Develop. Med. Child. Neurol.* **21**, 285-298.

Loiseau, P., Cohadon, S. (1981): Les épilepsies à foyers E.E.G. intercritiques multiples. *Rev. E.E.G. Neurophysiol.* **11**, 259-266.

Newton, R., Aicardi, J. (1983): Clinical findings in children with occipital spike-wave complexes suppressed by eye-opening. *Neurology* **33**, 1526-1529.

Noriega-Sanchez, A., Markand, O.N. (1976): Clinical and electroencephalographic correlation of independent multifocal spike discharges. *Neurology* **26**, 667-672.

O'Donohoe, N.V. (1979): *Epilepsies of childhood.* Postgraduate Paediatrics Series. Butterworths: London.

Pazzaglia, P., D'Alessandro, R.,Lozito, A., Lugaresi, E. (1982): Classification of partial epilepsies according to the symptomatology of seizures: practical value and prognostic implications. *Epilepsia* **23**, 343-350.

Remillard, G., Ethier, R., Andermann, F. (1974): Temporal lobe epilepsy and perinatal occlusion of the posterior cerebral artery. *Neurology* **24**, 1001-1009.

Rodin, E.A. (1968): *The prognosis of patients with epilepsy.* Thomas: Springfield.

Roger, J., Bureau, M., Dravet, C., Dalla Bernardina, B., Tassinari, C.A., Revol, M., Challamel, M.J., Taillandier, P. (1972): Les données E.E.G. et les manifestations épileptiques en relation avec l'hémiplégie cérébrale infantile. *Rev. E.E.G. Neurophysiol.* **2**, 5-28.

Roger, J., Gastaut, J.L., Dravet, C., Tassinari, C.A., Gastaut, H. (1972): Epilepsie partielle à sémiologie complexe et lésions atrophiques occipito-pariétales. Intérêt de l'examen tacoencéphalographique. *Rev. Neurol.* **133**, 41-53.

Roger, J., Dravet, C., Menendez, P., Bureau, M. (1981): Les épilepsies partielles de l'enfant. Evolution et facteurs de pronostic. *Rev. E.E.G. Neurophysiol.* **11**, 431-437.

Scarpa, P., Carassini, B. (1982): Partial epilepsy in childhood: clinical and EEG study of 261 cases. *Epilepsia* **23**, 333-341.

Talairach, J., Bancaud, J., Szikla, G., Bonis, A., Geier, S., Vedrenne, C. (1974): Approche nouvelle de la neurochirurgie de l'épilepsie. *Neurochirurgie* **20**, (Suppl. 1) 240 pp.

Yang, P.J., Berger, P.E., Cohen, M.E., Duffner, P.K. (1979): Computed tomography and childhood seizure disorders. *Neurology* **29**, 1084-1088.

*   *   *

Discussion pages 299-301

Epileptic syndromes in infancy, childhood and adolescence. J. Roger, C. Dravet, M. Bureau, F.E. Dreifuss and P. Wolf. John Libbey Eurotext Ltd ©1985.

Chapter 32
Kojewnikow's Syndrome (Epilepsia Partialis Continua) in Children

Jean BANCAUD

INSERM U-97, 2 ter Rue d'Alésia — 75014 Paris, France

Summary

Kojewnikow's syndrome (KS), or Epilepsia Partialis Continua, has been studied in children on the bases of 22 personal cases and from the cases reported in the literature. Two electroclinical groups can be distinguished. The first group corresponds to classical KS: in children with a previous rolandic fixed lesion, for which the aetiology is usually known, and with a stable neurologic deficit, partial motor seizures occur, followed after a variable interval by well localized myoclonic jerks. In these patients the EEG shows only focal abnormalities, more often in the central area. This epilepsy is not progressive and neurosurgical treatment can be effective. The second type occurs in previously normal children. It is characterized by partial motor seizures, which become rapidly associated with myoclonic jerks, and are variable in topography. The EEG shows abnormalities in the background activity and focal and diffuse paroxysmal abnormalities. Evolution is progressive: appearance of a neurological deficit, other types of seizures, mental impairment and inflammatory pathological finding on brain biopsy are some of the elements which suggest that this second type is due to a 'chronic encephalitis'.

Introduction

The original definition of 'epilepsia partialis continua' (EPC) given by Kojewnikow (1895) includes an association of localized 'epileptic jerks' with more or less continuous Jacksonian seizures.

The majority of authors admit that Kojewnikow's syndrome (KS) is relatively rare. The etiological factors are very diverse (Dereux 1955): infection, vascular causes and tumours. However a process described as 'encephalitis' seems to be the most frequent aetiological factor, more than 50 per cent of 102 cases collected by Dereux (1955), thus confirming the initial hypothesis proposed by Kojewnikow.

Souques (1922) considered that dysfunction of the motor cortex was the cause of focal motor seizures, but that the localized myoclonias must be of sub-cortical origin.

Juul-Jensen and Denny-Brown (1966) suggested that subcortical lesions are frequent in KS and could be an important feature of the clinical picture.

The unequivocal cortical origin of these two elements of KS appear substantiated in man on the basis of clinical (Bancaud, 1967), electrophysiological (Bancaud *et al.,* 1967; Buser *et al.,* 1971) and neurosurgical evidence (Bancaud *et al.,* 1970; Bancaud, 1980). In addition an epileptogenic lesion of the central cortex can provoke in monkeys the appearance of a typical KS (Amand *et al.,* 1973; Chauvel and Lamarche, 1975).

It is well known that KS is particularly resistant to treatment. This is why a number of patients have been admitted to our department for surgical treatment.

Patients and methods

The inclusion criteria for patients in this study is that they show the association of two types of clinical features characteristic of KS: (a) localized muscle jerks, semicontinuous or permanent, and most often limited to a small group of muscles; and (b) unilateral somatomotor seizures, associated or not with other types of seizures.

The second criterion is that KS began before the age of 10 years.

We have studied 22 patients admitted into the Neurosurgery Service B of the Hôpital St-Anne (Prof. J. Talairach and Prof. J.P. Chodkiewicz) eventually for surgical treatment.

The methodology allows definition of the precise indications for stereo-EEG exploration and eventually surgical intervention, as described previously (Bancaud *et al.,* 1965; Talairach *et al.,* 1974; Bonis *et al.,* 1981). We would like to emphasize however the fundamental importance that we attach to the clinical study of our patients.

The preliminary investigation always includes:

(a) questions on the exact age at the start of seizures, the first clinical symptoms, the evolution of the ictal symptomatology;

(b) a neurological and neuropsychological examination of patients in the interictal, ictal and postictal periods;

(c) an average of 10 EEG recordings, ictal and interictal, with observation and description of the seizures by the neurologist and with video recording.

Eight patients have had pneumoencephalography, eight a CT scan. Fifteen subjects have had stereotactic identification of cerebral structures (Talairach *et al.,* 1974; Szikla *et al.,* 1977).

Nine patients have been operated on the basis of SEEG data. In five of them a cortical biopsy was carried out.

Results

In our previous study (Bancaud *et al.,* 1982) we have studied 23 cases of KS of all ages. It was apparent that one could also class nearly all of the patients (22/23) into two groups.

Group I (11 out of 23 cases) including patients of all ages (average age of appearance of KS: 20 years), in which the ictal symptomatology is of a KS generally with a known aetiology and for which the neurological state is not affected in the course of its evolution. The EEG of these patients shows only focal abnormalities, most often central, EEG paroxysms were not frequent. In cases where neurosurgical intervention has been possible, it has led to a cure of the KS.

Group II (11 out of 23 cases) have the following features: KS always appeared before 10 years old. It was often associated with other types of seizures. The syndrome appeared early, the myoclonias were often diffuse. The aetiology was unknown. The neurological and mental state of the patient deteriorated, often progressively, during its evolution. In the EEG, there were abnormalities in the background rhythm, paroxysmal abnormalities were extensive, infraclinical ictal discharges were frequent. No patient in this group had any long-lasting benefit from surgery.

Using the same criteria we have divided our present population of 22 patients into two groups (as defined in our previous study).

Five subjects belong to the first group, 17 to the second.

(1) Clinical symptomatology (Table 1)

The average age is much lower in group II and the onset could be very early in life (8 months).

Table 1. Clinical symptomatology

	Group I	Group II
Age at onset:	30 months — 10 years (m : 6.4 years)	8 months — 10 years (m : 5 years)
Aetiology:		
unknown	2	17
neonatal anoxia	2	-
trauma	1	-
Frequency of seizures:		
≤ 1/day	5	-
> 1/day	-	2
> 20/day	-	15
Ictal discharge:		
well localized (central area)	5	1
central secondarily spreading	-	10
multifocal (or bilateral)	-	6
Delay seizures/myoclonic jerks:		
< 1 year	3	14 (< 4months: 11)
> 5 years	2	3
Neurological deficit:		
absent	1	-
discrete (localized)	2	-
hemiplegia	2	17
Other than motor	-	4
Mental impairment:		
absent	5	2
mild	-	2
severe	-	13

The aetiology is unknown in all patients in group II.

The frequency of seizures is around one a day in the patients in group I. In group II, almost all the patients have, at least in certain periods, more than 20 seizures per day.

The myoclonic jerks appear early in the evolution of the syndrome in patients of group II (in the first year in 14 and in the first four months in 11).

All the subjects of group II have severe motor deficit, which is associated with other neurological problems in four.

A significant mental retardation exists in 13 patients of group II, which is not found in any subjects in group I.

(2) EEG symptomatology

(a) interictal symptomatology (Table II): The background activity is very abnormal in all the patients of group II and only in one case in group I.

Fourteen patients of group II have a practically continuous high voltage delta activity, in a very extensive area of the scalp and often bilateral. 'Irritative' interictal abnormalities are well localized in 4/5 cases in group I and in no cases of group II.

One can observe these isolated interictal spikes, more or less rhythmically (Fig. 1). The myoclonic jerks do not often have an evident chronological relationship with the interictal spikes, and they are generally asynchronous among the various muscles examined (Fig. 2).

Table 2. Interictal Symptomatology

	Group I	Group II
Background activity:		
normal	4	-
asymmetrical	1	7
absent (or very slow)	-	10
Delta waves:		
absent	1	-
localized	3	3
widespread	1	6
diffuse (or bilateral)	-	8
Spikes and/or spikes and waves:		
localized	4	-
widespread	1	3
diffuse (or bilateral)	-	14
Subclinical paroxysmal discharges:	-	17
(> 10'')		(bilat: 13)

(b) Ictal symptomatology: The ictal discharges remained limited to the central region in all patients in group I. In the patients of group II, the discharge is localized in the central region in only one case. In the other cases, the discharge was widespread (10 cases) and multifocal and/or bilateral in six cases.

The ictal discharge could be seen on the EEG recording at the start of seizure (Fig. 3). During the seizure, the muscle artifacts often made an interpretation of the discharge difficult in the scalp EEG (Fig. 4). The clonic jerks involve different muscles according to a type of march which is not a classical Jacksonian march. In several cases the topography is difficult to recognize, and it seems to be of a much higher voltage in the secondarily-involved hemisphere (Fig. 5). In spite of the duration of the seizure, the patients could remain perfectly conscious, capable of talking during the seizure (Fig. 6) and carrying out orders (Fig. 7). The end of the jerks could coincide with the end of the discharge (Fig. 8a). Bilateral synchronous jerks could appear some seconds after the end of the seizure (Fig. 8b).

An examination by stereo-EEG (Fig. 9) permits an exact identification of the origin of the discharge (Fig. 10) and a study of the chronological relationship between the evolution of the discharge and the ictal muscle symptoms. The end of a significant

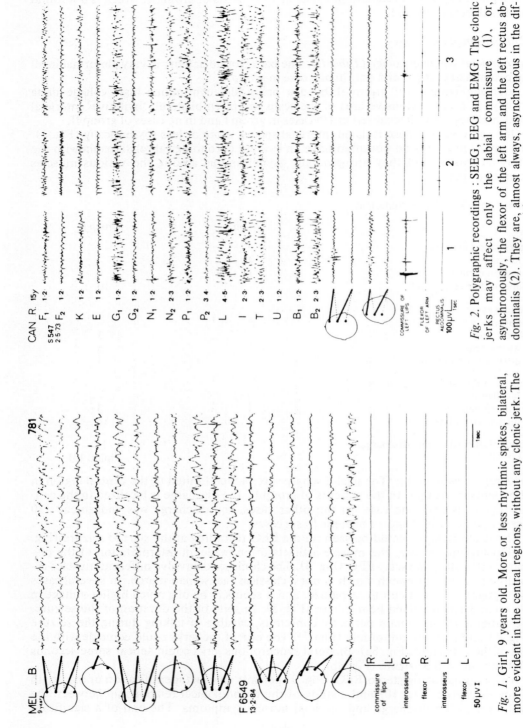

Fig. 1. Girl, 9 years old. More or less rhythmic spikes, bilateral, more evident in the central regions, without any clonic jerk. The background activity is of very low voltage.

Fig. 2. Polygraphic recordings : SEEG, EEG and EMG. The clonic jerks may affect only the labial commissure (1), or, asynchronously, the flexor of the left arm and the left rectus abdominalis (2). They are, almost always, asynchronous in the different explored muscles (3).

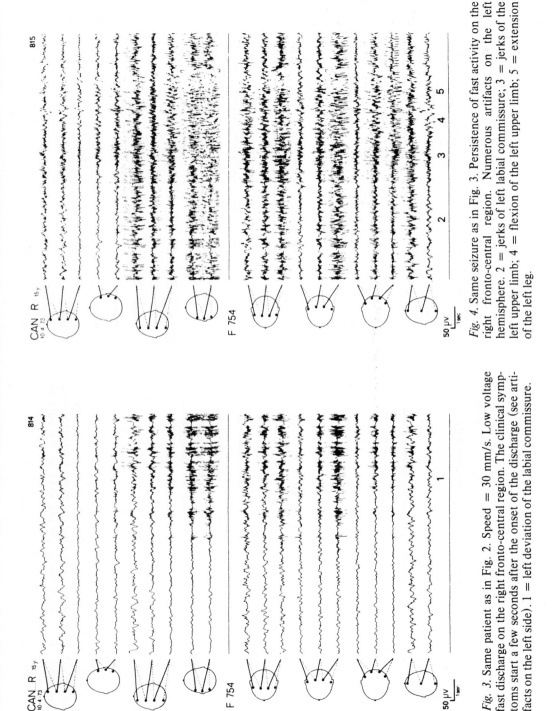

Fig. 3. Same patient as in Fig. 2. Speed = 30 mm/s. Low voltage fast discharge on the right fronto-central region. The clinical symptoms start a few seconds after the onset of the discharge (see artifacts on the left side). 1 = left deviation of the labial commissure.

Fig. 4. Same seizure as in Fig. 3. Persistence of fast activity on the right fronto-central region. Numerous artifacts on the left hemisphere. 2 = jerks of left labial commissure; 3 = jerks of the left upper limb; 4 = flexion of the left upper limb; 5 = extension of the left leg.

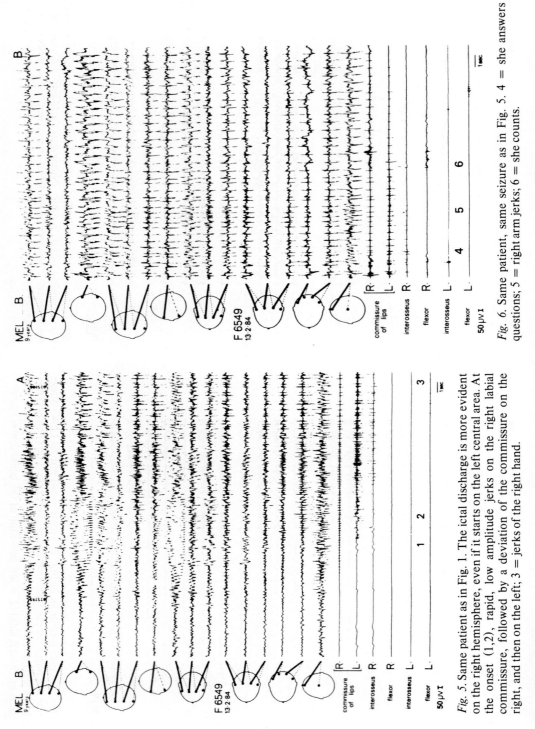

Fig. 5. Same patient as in Fig. 1. The ictal discharge is more evident on the right hemisphere, even if it starts on the left central area. At the onset (1,2), rapid, low amplitude jerks on the right labial commissure, followed by a deviation of the commissure on the right, and then on the left; 3 = jerks of the right hand.

Fig. 6. Same patient, same seizure as in Fig. 5. 4 = she answers questions; 5 = right arm jerks; 6 = she counts.

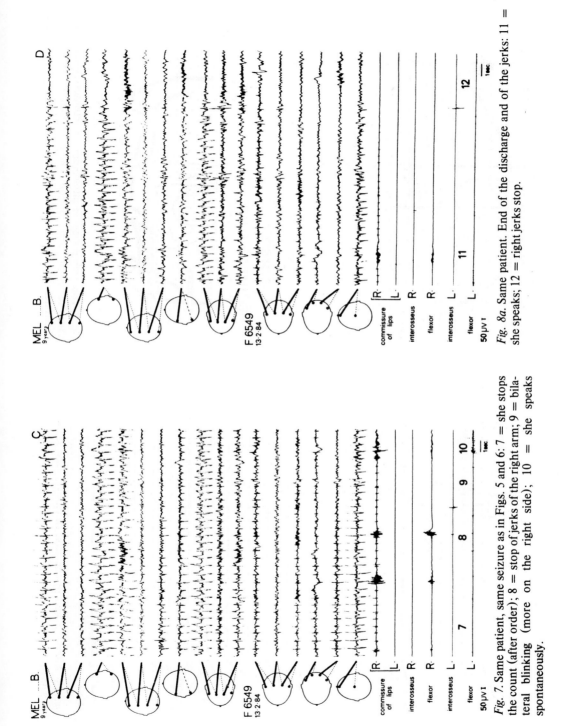

Fig. 8a. Same patient. End of the discharge and of the jerks: 11 = she speaks; 12 = right jerks stop.

Fig. 7. Same patient, same seizure as in Figs. 5 and 6: 7 = she stops the count (after order); 8 = stop of jerks of the right arm; 9 = bilateral blinking (more on the right side); 10 = she speaks spontaneously.

293

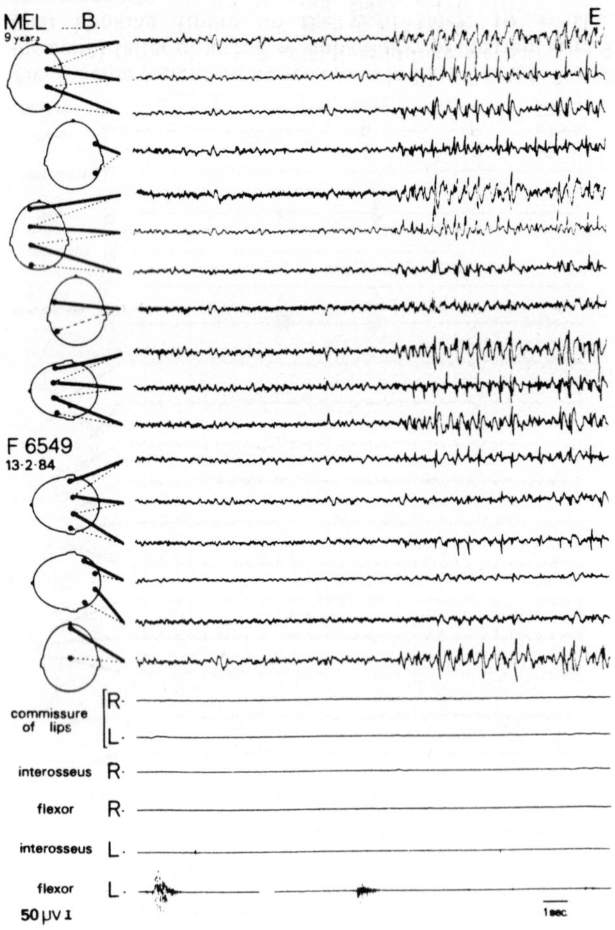

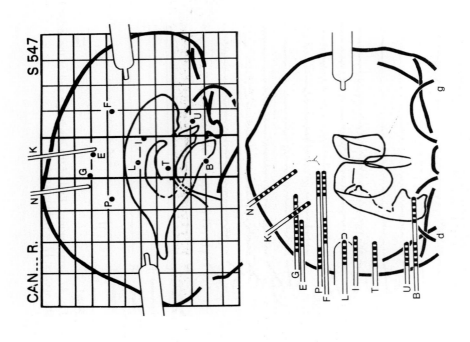

Fig. 9. Top: lateral view of intracerebral electrodes exploring large centro-temporal area. Bottom: antero-posterior view of the electrodes. The right frontal horn is dilated.

Fig. 8b. After the end of the ictal discharge, rare asynchronous jerks, predominantly on the left side.

294

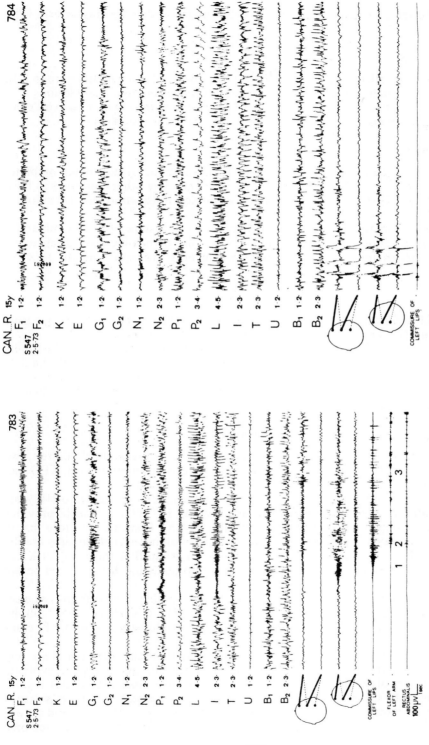

Fig. 10. Same patient of Fig. 9. Fast, low voltage discharge on a large cerebral area (F1, P1, I but also E and P2). On the scalp it is very difficult to appreciate the onset of the discharge. The contraction of the left labial commissure occurs very early, and it is followed by jerks of the left arm and of the left rectus abdominalis.

Fig. 11. Same patient, same seizure. Progressive end of clonic jerks, and of the discharge.

intra-cerebral discharge may or may not coincide with the end of the muscle jerks (Fig. 11).

(3) Neuroradiology

The existence of a cortico-subcortical scar has been observed in a patient in group I. In the four others, neuradiological examination has not shown any significant lesions.

In group II, a relatively localized lesion has been found in only two cases. An extensive lesion existed in eight cases, and some bilateral or diffuse lesions in seven.

(4) Surgical results

Two patients of group I have been operated on. In one of them seizures have completely disappeared (with a remission of more than 10 years). The other continues to have only rare nocturnal clonic jerks of the right hand (surgical intervention has been voluntarily incomplete).

Among the 17 patients of the group II, five have had a stereo EEG examination, four have had operations. In all of them, seizures and myoclonic jerks disappeared during a 1-8 month follow-up period after which both types of epileptic seizures reoccurred.

(5) Evolution

A follow up of more than 12 years has not resulted in the detection of a progressive deterioration in the 5 patients of group I. They seem well stabilized.

Four patients from group II have been followed up for less than a year. The others have been followed for less than 12 years, generally less than 7 years. In all, the data from the neurological, neuropsychological and EEG examinations show evidence of a progression of the lesional process. Three of four who were operated on have died (1, 2 and 9 years after the operation).

Discussion

This study confirms the results of our work of 1982. There exist among children, two distinct groups of patients suffering from KS which have different clinical, EEG, aetiological and evolutive signs.

Our observations, limited to the cases of KS appearing before the age of 10 years old, showed an increased proportion of cases in group II (17/23), than in previous statistics which grouped together cases of all ages (11/23). It seems therefore that in cases of KS of early onset, those which begin with an evolving encephalopathy are the most frequent. It further seems that one can maintain group II as the group of KS of early onset: in all the cases of group II of our previous statistics, KS appeared before the age of 10.

While in the majority of cases of group I, an exact aetiology can be found, as elsewhere in the majority of cases in the literature, e.g. 92/102 of Dereux (1955), all the cases of Thomas et al. (1977), no discernable aetiology could be found in the 17 cases of group II.

This confirms in this paediatric group, our previous proposals: there exists a group of patients suffering from KS (our group II) which clearly appears to have an evolving disorder, which involves progressively other cortical areas than the central region. This is evidenced by the association (or the ultimate appearance) of types of seizures other than partial motor seizures, the widespread abnormalities in the EEG and the existence of subclinical EEG paroxysms which could be seen in various cortical regions.

This was described many years ago by Rasmussen *et al.,* (1958) who described similar EEG patterns in one of their three patients (a child).

Our findings were recently confirmed by Dulac *et al.,* (1983). These authors report 26 cases of KS, observed before the age of 15 years (a certain number of these cases described by Dulac *et al.* overlap our group of observations). Dulac *et al.* also divided their patients into two groups : 11 belong to our group I, 11 to our group II, four have not been classified precisely. They provide the following complementary data.

(i) The cases in group I, (average age 1 year 11 months) most often begin with generalized or unilateral convulsions. Status epilepticus is frequent before the start of KS (7/11 cases) which then appears over a variable period (up to 5 years later). The motor deficit, often preexistent to KS, is stable. Neuroradiological examination is positive in 8/11 cases: one intracerebral haematoma, cerebral atrophy in seven, diffuse (four) or unilateral (three). The repetition of these examinations has not shown any evolution of these lesions.

(ii) In the case of group II, the onset, more delayed than in our group II (average age 6 years) occurs in normal children with partial motor seizures, the frequency of which increases rapidly and involves more and more extensive muscle regions. The delay to the onset of KS is much shorter (on average 10 months). Other types of seizures are associated with partial motor seizures. In all cases except one, the evolution appears as a progressive deterioration of the neurological and psychological state (appearance of a hemiplegia, language difficulties and mental deterioration). One child died 4 months after the onset. Neuroradiological investigation showed extensive lesions. In three out of four cases where investigations were repeated, they showed the appearance of cerebral atrophy and its deterioration. Finally in three out of six cases where the CSF had been examined, the protein electrophoresis showed oligoclonal features with a raised IgG index in two cases.

It therefore emerges that the majority of cases of KS appearing in childhood can be classified into two groups.

Group I does not pose any special problems. It is a classical picture of KS, most often related to a stable cerebral lesion, of a central location of prenatal, perinatal or postnatal origin.

Group II remains much more 'mysterious'. It seems that in these cases, the KS is evidence of a cerebral disorder of a progressive evolution. The hypothesis has been proposed that this is an encephalitis of slow evolution (Rasmussen *et al.* 1958) on biopsy data (perivascular inflammatory infiltrates). The findings of Dulac *et al.* (1983) of a type of inflammatory abnormalities of the CSF are in agreement. This hypothesis has always been maintained, since Kojewnikow (1895), by Russian authors, who have described a large number of cases of KS following encephalitis transmitted by ticks. Moreover, they have observed various motor problems (localized convulsions, abnormal movements) after intracerebral inoculation of a virus of tick-borne encephalitis. These results have been confirmed by Asher (1978).

Acknowledgements
This work was achieved with the collaboration of C. Munari, O. Dulac, J. Talairach, A. Bonis and S. Trottier.

References

Amand, G., Demoulin, A., Lamarche, M., (1973): Réponses évoquées multisensorielles chez le singe porteur d'un foyer épileptogène rolandique. *Rev. E.E.G. Neurophysiol.* **3**, 321-326.

Asher, D.M. (1975): Movements disorders in Rhesus Monkeys after infection with Tick-Borne encephalitis Virus. In *Advances in Neurology,* vol. 10, pp. 277-289, ed B. Meldrum, C.D. Marsden. Raven Press: New York.

Bancaud, J., Talairach, J., Bonis, A., Szikla, G., Schaub, C., Morel, P., Bordas-Ferrer, M. (1965): *La stéréoencéphalographie dans l'épilepsie.* Masson: Paris.

Bancaud, J. (1967): Origine focale multiple de certaines épilepsies corticales. *Rev. Neurol.* **117**, 222-243.

Bancaud, J., Talairach, J., Bonis, A. (1967): Physiopathogénie du syndrome de Kojewnikow (interprétation des données électrographiques). *Rev. Neurol.* **117**, 507.

Bancaud, J., Bonis, A., Talairach, J., Bordas-Ferrer, M., Buser, P. (1970): Syndrome de Kojewnikow et accès somatomoteurs (étude clinique, E.E.G., E.M.G. et S.E.E.G.). *L'Encéphale* **5**, 391-438.

Bancaud, J. (1980): Surgery of epilepsy based on sterotaxic investigations. The plan of the S.E.E.G. investigations. *Acta Neurochir.* suppl. **30**, 25-34.

Bancaud, J., Bonis, A., Trottier, S., Talairach, J., Dulac, O. (1982): L'épilepsie partielle continue: syndrome et maladie. *Rev. Neurol.* **138**, 802-814.

Bonis, A., Chodkiewicz, J.P., Munari, C., Szikla, G., Bancaud, J., Talairach, J. (1981): La chirurgie de l'épilepsie. Méthodologie stéréotaxique, résultats et indications. *Gaz. Méd. France* **88**, 4125-4130.

Buser, P., Bancaud, J., Bonis, A., Talairach, J. (1971): Etude électrophysiologique d'un syndrome de Kojewnikow. *Rev. EEG Neurophysiol.* **1**, 369-378.

Chauvel, P., Lamarche, M. (1975): Analyse d'une "épilepsie du mouvement" chez un singe porteur d'un foyer rolandique. *Neurochirurgie* **21**, 121-127.

Dereux, J. (1955): Le syndrome de Kojewnikow (épilepsie partielle continue). Thèse, Paris.

Dulac, O., Dravet, C., Plouin, P., Bureau, M., Ponsot, G., Gerbaut, L., Roger, J., Arthuis, H. (1983): Aspects nosologiques des épilepsies partielles continues chez l'enfant. *Archs Fr. Pédiatr.* **40**, 689-695.

Juul-Jensen, P., Denny-Brown, D. (1966): Epilepsia partialis continua. *Archs Neurol.* **15**, 563-578.

Kojewnikow, L. (1895): Eine besondere Form von corticaler Epilepsie. *Neurologisches Centralblatt.* **14**, 47-48.

Rasmussen, T., Olszewski, J., Lloyd-Smith, D. (1958): Focal seizures due to chronic localized encephalities. *Neurology* **8**, 435-445.

Souques, M.A. (1922): Dissociation des paroxysmes convulsifs et des secousses interparoxystiques dans l'E.P.C. et interprétation de cette dissociation. *Rev. Neurol.* **1**, 61-63.

Szikla, G., Bouvier, G., Hori, T., Petrov, V. (1977): *Angiography of the human brain cortex. Atlas of Vascular patterns and stereotactic cortical localization.* Springer: Berlin-Heidelberg-New York.

Talairach, J., Szikla, G., Tounoux, P., Prosalentis, A., Bordas-Ferrer, M., Covello, L., Jacob, M., Mempel, E. (1967): *Atlas d'anatomie stéréotaxique du télencéphale.* Masson: Paris.

Talairach, J., Szikla, G. (1980): Application of stereotactic concepts to the surgery of epilepsy. *Acta. Neurochir.* suppl. **30**, 35-54.

Thomas, J., Reggan, J., Klass, D. (1977): Epilepsia partialis continua. A review of 32 cases. *Archs Neurol.* **34**, 266-275.

* * *

Discussion pages 299-301

Epileptic syndromes in infancy, childhood and adolescence. J. Roger, C. Dravet, M. Bureau, F.E. Dreifuss and P. Wolf. John Libbey Eurotext Ltd ©1985.

Discussion of Lesional Partial Epilepsies

(Chapters 31 and 32)

Summarized by Claudio MUNARI

Dulac: Fully agrees with the paper of Bancaud on Kojewnikow's syndrome (KS). He stresses the following three points:
(a) the most important difference from the North American papers is the exclusion, in the French papers, of acute, symptomatic, epileptic status;
(b) in his personal experience, more than half of patients of the group I (good prognosis) had an epileptic status before the appearance of the EPC;
(c) the existence, in many children with KS with poor prognosis, of oligo-clonal features of IgG in the CSF.

Later on, *Dulac* presented a film of KS showing the stability of clonic jerks in a patient in Bancaud's group I.

Another example shows that the clonic jerks are erratic, persist during sleep and are increased by voluntary movements in a patient of group II.

In one case (from group I) it is possible to see strict correlations between the spikes recorded on the scalp and the myoclonias.

Roger: Raises the problem of the prognosis of partial seizures of 'lesional' origin in children. A group of 119 patients was classified in the following subgroups according to the evolution of the seizures:
(1) suppression of seizures even after the cessation of anti-epileptic drugs (AED);
(2) control of seizures with AED:
(3) some rare seizures with AED:
(4) numerous seizures in spite of AED.

Among the factors probably related to a poor prognosis, Roger considers:
(a) the very early onset of the seizures (before 3 years);
(b) the high frequency of seizures;
(c) the occurrence of multiple types of seizures;
(d) the existence of an encephalopathy.

The seizure pattern, apparently characterizing the worse evolution, would be the association, during the same seizure, of a loss of consciousness and of somatomotor, almost always bilateral, manifestations. When such 'complex partial motor' seizures (a term certainly inadequate) exist the prognosis is always poor whereas this type of seizure seems to be very rare in the course of the epilepsies with a favourable course. The other clinical ictal symptoms worsening the prognosis are the initial violent falls and the so-called 'reflex' seizures, as in the 'startle' epilepsies. In the EEG, an ictal pattern showing a bilateral flattening of rhythm is also an indication of a poor prognosis.

Roger thinks it is important to define the prognosis as soon as possible, so that one does not have to wait too long before surgical treatment. He considers that surgical intervention in a 25-year-old patient suffering from epilepsy since he was 3 years old could cure the epilepsy, but not the other psychosocial and social problems that have been created by this epilepsy.

Loiseau: Does not agree with the terminology used by *Revol:* there is no reason any longer to use the terms 'functional' and 'lesional', considering that all seizures are a 'functional' disorder. His proposal is to return to the older terms 'symptomatic' and 'idiopathic'.

Beaumanoir: Emphasized that the spikes, as well as the seizures, are also 'functional'.

Munari: Said that *Bancaud* and he have the same objection to use terms such as 'lesional' and 'functional'. During this meeting, there has not been any discussion concerning a 'syndromic' classification of different patterns of seizures. It may be difficult to establish clear electro-clinical relationships during the seizures of the newborn, but it is feasible in children and in adolescents.

For him, it is evident that an ictal discharge involving the frontal lobe will be accompanied by clinical symptoms different from those linked to a discharge starting in the occipital or in the temporal lobe. Moreover, considering that 'the discharges do not know the limits separating the different lobes', a careful analysis of clinical symptoms may help in understanding the spatial evolution of the electrical discharge.

Dulac: Observed the same seizure patterns described by *Roger* and asks *Munari* if he has some experience on the surgery of this type of seizures.

Munari: Is not sure that he understood what kind of seizures *Roger* calls 'complex partial motor seizures'. He stresses the importance of the direct observation of the chronology of the clinical symptoms. In fact, if the somatomotor manifestations only occur at the end of the seizure, this fact itself does not exclude a possible surgical procedure.

On the contrary, if the motor symptoms occur very early in the seizure, in a patient without any motor deficit, such a patient cannot be considered as a candidate for surgery.

And finally, the impairment of consciousness, not having a precise localizing value, does not by itself permit the selection or rejection of patients for surgery.

Dravet: Shows and comments on a brief film of a 3-year-old child whose motor manifestations may affect, independently and in different sequences, all his limbs. She points out that the consciousness is not impaired many seconds after the onset of the motor signs, even if he has a forced laugh.

Cavazzuti: Asks *Roger* if all his patients with violent falls have a 'temporal focus' like those observed by himself. The second question — is the fall followed, or not, by motor phenomena?

Roger: Says that the recorded seizures and the interictal abnormalities seem to indicate that the epilepsies he described are above all extra-temporal, and probably frontal. After the fall, there may be either tonic manifestations or purposeless movements of the limbs.

Munari: Replying to a previous question from *Dulac* said that in the experience of the St Anne group, the seizures which started and remained in the temporal lobe are not associated with somatomotor lateralized seizures: Bossi *et al.* (1982) showed that somatomotor symptoms only occur in less than 20 per cent of true temporal seizures, when the discharges spread outside of the temporal lobe.

He emphasizes the need to distinguish 'temporal lobe seizures', 'psychomotor seizures' and 'complex partial seizures' and not to regard these as synonymous.

Dreifuss: Agrees with the importance of this distinction.

Dulac: Points out that gelastic seizures with clonias of the upper eyelids should be recognized in small children: many of them are symptomatic of hamartomas of the hypothalamus.

Dreifuss: Thinks that there are two different kinds of gelastic seizures: one is the pathological laughter of epileptic type, without mirth. The other one is a pathological laughter with inappropriate mirth. Dreifuss describes the case of a patient who had an epileptic laughter at his mother's funeral, just before his own funeral, when a vascular malformation ruptured in his third ventricle.

Reference

Bossi, L., Munari, C., Stoffles, C., Bonis, A., Bacia, T., Talairach, J., Bancaud, J. (1982): Somatomotor manifestations in temporal lobe seizures. In *Advances in epileptology* ed. Akimoto, Kazamatsuri, Seino, Ward, pp.29-32. Raven Press: New York.

Epileptic syndromes in infancy, child-hood and adolescence. J. Roger, C. Dravet, M. Bureau, F.E. Dreifuss and P. Wolf. John Libbey Eurotext Ltd ©1985.

Chapter 33
Progressive Myoclonic Epilepsy in Childhood and Adolescence

Joseph ROGER

Centre Saint-Paul, 300 Boulevard de Sainte-Marguerite, 13009, Marseille, France

Summary

The majority of disorders which produce during their evolution a syndrome of progressive myoclonic epilepsy (PME) with an evolution to dementia show clinical, EEG and biological characteristics which allow early recognition before the complete syndromic picture is realized (Gaucher's disease, ceroid lipofuscinosis and Lafora's disease . . .). In dyssynergia cerebellaris myoclonica with epilepsy and cherry-red spot myoclonus syndrome, the epilepsy does not generally have a progressive evolution and dementia is either delayed or absent.

For these reasons it does not seem necessary ultimately to preserve a widened PME syndrome. The inclusion of these disorders in PME syndrome are therefore no longer justified. Nevertheless it is recommended the concept of PME be retained because of the existence of cases of undetermined etiology and of which the anatomical or biochemical basis has not been defined.

Introduction

Does progressive myoclonic epilepsy (PME) merit consideration as an individual entity?

Since the first descriptions of Unverricht (1891) and Lundborg (1903-1913), this syndrome appears to have been well characterized. Its existence has been subsequently confirmed (van Bogaert, 1968; Diebold, 1973). In his work on what he proposes to call 'the genetic myoclonic epileptic dementia syndromes', Diebold proposed division of PME into two groups: one which merits characterization as a specific syndrome, which he proposes to call, 'Erbliche Myoclonisch-Epileptisch-Dementielle Kernsyndrome', where the characteristics of the syndrome are found in all of the patients suffering from certain diseases (PME, dyssynergia cerebellaris myoclonica (DCM), myoclonic variant of ceroid lipofuscinosis) and the other one, 'Erbliche Myoclonisch-Epileptisch-Dementielle Rand-Syndrome', where the syndrome develops only in a certain proportion of the patients suffering from various diseases (Leucodystrophy, Hallervorden-Spatz's disease, Wilson's disease, and Huntington's disease).

The PME syndrome is characterized clinically by the association of:
- a myoclonic syndrome associating generalized myoclonus and arrhythmic, asynchronous and asymmetrical, partial or segmental, myoclonus;
- an epileptic syndrome in which the seizures are of various types, the most frequent being generalized tonic-clonic seizures, myoclonic attacks and tonic seizures;
- a progressive mental deterioration leading to dementia;
- a neurological syndrome generally associating cerebellar, pyramidal and eventually extrapyramidal signs.

On the EEG, there exists a progressive deterioration of background rhythm, a progressive alteration in the organization of sleep patterns, paroxysmal abnormalities (association of spikes, spike-waves or generalized polyspike-wave activity, either slow or rapid and with multifocal abnormalities).

In fact few disorders that are normally classed as PME show an association of these four types of symptoms. These are the only ones which merit grouping under the heading of PME — Group I of our study.

In other disorders, there is a slow evolution with myoclonus but the epilepsy is generally less severe and dementia is delayed or even absent. These constitute Group II.

Group I

Four disorders can be characterized by their neurological and epileptic appearance.

(1) The juvenile form of Gaucher's disease (subacute juvenile neuronopathic type or type III)
The neuropsychiatric manifestations appear around 6-8 years. They consist either of neurological problems, including a cerebellar syndrome rapidly followed by pyramidal signs, or mental deterioration, or epileptic seizures of various types (generalized clonic seizures, partial motor seizures). These are often associated with myoclonus without any related EEG manifestations (Herrlin and Hillborg, 1962; Claes and Carpenter, 1967).

The EEG abnormalities appear early and can even precede the clinical signs. There is a progressive deterioration of background activity, an abnormal response to intermittent photic stimulation (IPS), some diffuse paroxysmal abnormalities and multifocal abnormalities with a clear posterior predominance (Nishimura *et al.,* 1980).

The duration of the illness is variable and death generally occurs 3 to 10 years after the onset.

(2) The juvenile form of ceroid lipofuscinosis, Spielmeyer-Vogt-Sjögren.
The age of onset of this illness is variable, but in two-thirds of cases it is between 6 and 8 years.

The initial clinical signs are practically always represented by a decrease in visual acuity, followed by a slowing of psychomotor development and by the appearance of cerebellar and extrapyramidal signs. The epilepsy generally appears 1 to 4 years after the onset of the illness. The seizures are of a generalized convulsive type sometimes associated with absences, rapidly followed by myoclonic manifestations of fragmental, segmental and massive myoclonus (Sjögren, 1931; Zeman *et al.,* 1970).

On the EEG, there are high amplitude, 1-2 c/s slow wave and slow spike-wave bursts of variable duration. There is no abnormal response to IPS. The visual evoked potentials are of low amplitude and could even disappear (Pampiglione and Harden, 1977).

The evolution is slow — the average period of survival is in the order of 10 years.

(3) *Lafora's disease*

This is a recessive hereditary disease.

The onset is between 6-19 years (mean 11.5 yrs). In 80 per cent of cases it presents with seizures. These seizures are predominantly clonic, tonic-clonic and myoclonic attacks. The frequent association of partial seizures, mainly with visual manifestations must be stressed (Roger *et al.,* 1983). The myoclonic syndrome is constant with fragmentary and segmental myoclonus and rarely massive myoclonus. The myoclonus is worsened by movement or the intention of movement.

Mental deterioration begins quickly, but may not be evident in the first few years of the disease.

Pyramidal, cerebellar and extrapyramidal manifestations appear after a variable delay (van Heycop Ten Ham and de Jager, 1963).

The EEG, at the start of the illness, can have a well-organized and reactive background activity. One observes some discharges of the polyspike and rapid polyspike-wave type which are often provoked by IPS, but whose frequency does not increase during sleep. The polygraphic examination provides evidence of erratic myoclonus without any correlation with EEG paroxysms. The EEG at this stage would be very compatible with a diagnosis of primary generalized epilepsy which is very often made, but it may already be distinguished by the existence of segmental myoclonus and the lack of activation of spike-wave discharges during sleep (Tassinari *et al.,* 1978).

After a period of variable duration (from a few months to 2-3 years), the EEG picture changes (Fig. 1): the background rhythm deteriorates, the physiological elements of sleep disappear and the different phases of sleep are not identifiable except for REM sleep. Multifocal, particularly posterior, abnormalities appear, in addition to generalized paroxysmal bursts; a major photosensitivity persists. In the terminal phase, the EEG is totally disorganized.

Death occurs an average of 5.5 years following onset. The diagnosis during life can be confirmed by cutaneous, muscular and hepatic biopsies that show the characteristic (Carpenter and Karpati, 1981; Roger *et al.,* 1983) inclusion bodies.

(4) *The so-called degenerative progressive myoclonic epilepsy*

In the literature a significant number of observations described as Unverricht-Lundborg syndrome include the association of epilepsy, myoclonus and intellectual deterioration. The neuropathological studies show non specific degenerative lesions and lack of Lafora bodies. These cases are quite heterogeneous in terms of age of onset, or rapidity of evolution and, whenever familial, of their mode of transmission. Except for some rare cases, the evolution is much slower than in Lafora's disease.

The only significant group which has been well studied, in around 100 cases, is the Finnish type of myoclonic epilepsy described by Koskiniemi *et al.* (1974 *b*). It is a recessive illness in 90 per cent of cases, starting between 8 and 13 years, most often with myoclonic jerks, but sometimes also with generalized seizures. The myoclonus is segmental, fragmentary and massive; it can appear spontaneously but is exaggerated by various stimuli and in particular by movement. The seizures are most often massive myoclonus and tonic-clonic seizures. Rare at the beginning, they increase in frequency and often occur in series. Neurologically, the first symptom, which often remains isolated, is cerebellar ataxia. Only in 30 per cent of cases are there pyramidal manifestations.

Mental deterioration is slowly progressive, since in the cases with long evolution Koskiniemi indicates that the IQ lowered by 10 points within 10 years. As far as can be judged according to the late neurological deterioration, no patient becomes completely

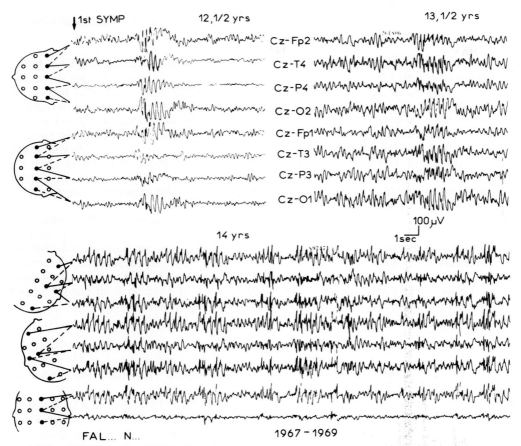

1st SYMP   12,1/2 yrs   13,1/2 yrs

Cz-Fp2
Cz-T4
Cz-P4
Cz-O2
Cz-Fp1
Cz-T3
Cz-P3
Cz-O1

14 yrs   100 μV 1 sec

FAL... N...   1967 – 1969

Fig. 1. Evolution of the EEG during Lafora's disease: *top left* — EEG carried out 6 months after the first seizures. Basal activity at 8 c/s, generalized spike-wave discharges; *top right* — 1.5 years after onset of the illness: a slowing of background activity and irregular spike-wave discharges *bottom* — 2 years after the onset of the illness: global deterioration of background activity, very frequent discharges of spikes, polyspikes, isolated or in brief bursts.

demented (Koskiniemi, 1974).

There is a progressive worsening of the myoclonus and of the cerebellar syndrome. Walking alone remains possible up to 5 to 8 years after onset, but the patients become generally bedridden 5 to 10 years after onset. According to early statistics, death occurs after a mean duration of 15 years, as a result of intercurrent complications.

The survival has improved, due to the currently available anticonvulsive treatment and a better standard of care.

On the EEG, at the beginning of the illness, there is a reduction in the alpha activity and the appearance of theta rhythm which becomes more and more prominent. In a certain number of cases one can see slower, delta wave bursts associated with rapid activity. The paroxysmal abnormalities are represented by generalized spike-waves of 3-5 c/s, predominating in the frontal region, often associated with polyspike-waves and sometimes with myoclonic jerks. Focal abnormalities do not exist. IPS is always very positive, producing generalized spike-wave and polyspike-wave discharges. The terminal phase of the EEG is very disorganized, showing theta-delta waves, some ex-

305

tremely frequent spike-wave and polyspike-wave discharges with persisting photosensitivity (Koskiniemi et al., 1974a).

Recently, in 15 families living in USA and without Finnish ascendants, Eldridge et al. (1983) observed 27 cases of PME in whom the diagnosis of Lafora disease was eliminated through pathological examinations. They thought that the clinical picture of their cases is the same than the picture seen in Finland and they proposed to name it 'Baltic myoclonus epilepsy'. They noticed that a number of patients living in Estonia, previously described by Unverricht (1895) and of patients living in south-west Sweden described by Lundborg (1903, 1913) had a similar course of disease. They thought that, in the more recent cases, this clinical picture has been modified in that the prognosis has been worsened by phenytoïn therapy, rendering the distinction from Lafora disease difficult. These authors conclude that the Baltic type can be seen outside Finland, and it is four times commoner than the Lafora type.

We believe that it is too early to include the majority of degenerative PME observed outside Finland in the disease described by Koskiniemi et al. (1974b). Firstly, despite the fact that Scandinavian neurologists are well informed about Koskiniemi disease, no other case has been reported from Scandinavia, except Finland; secondly, necropsy cases are too rare (two cases) in the report of Eldridge et al. (1983) to know if the anatomical observations are identical; thirdly, some cases of PME without Lafora bodies can have a rapid fatal evolution in the absence of any phenytoïn treatment.

Group II

(1) *Dyssynergia cerebellaris myoclonica (DCM) with epilepsy (Ramsay-Hunt syndrome)* (Hunt, 1921)

The DCM described in 1921 by Ramsay-Hunt is considered by many authors as a syndrome resulting from various pathological processes. Indeed the published cases are heterogeneous, both with respect to the age of onset, the genetic origin, the duration, the eventual association with other neurological symptoms, in particular spino-cerebellar symptoms, and the disparity of anatomical lesions observed in the rare cases which have been verified (presence or absence of atrophy of the dentate system and of associated spinal lesions). Certain cases appear to be neuropathologically quite similar to Friedriech's ataxia and to olivo-pontocerebellar atrophy. We believe however, in spite of the scarcity of anatomical verifications, that there exists a definite disorder that we shall describe according to our personal observations (Roger et al., 1968; Tassinari et al., 1974; Roger et al., 1982a).

It is a recessive disorder which starts between 6 and 20 years (mean 11.5 yrs) with a myoclonic syndrome or epileptic seizures. The myoclonic syndrome is characterized above all by a typical intention and action myoclonus, but often there also exists partial myoclonus which is evidenced by the polygraphic recording. The epilepsy is constant. It is characterized by myoclonic and, more rarely, by generalized tonic-clonic seizures. The seizures, generally sensitive to therapy, have a tendency to diminish in frequency or even to disappear in the course of their evolution. The neurological manifestations are variable and, apart from a predominantly axial cerebellar syndrome, the other neurological symptoms (signs of spino-cerebellar degeneration) are often absent. The absence of mental impairment is classical but an intellectual deterioration is observed frequently.

The evolution is very slow and characterized mainly by the accentuation of intention and action myoclonus.

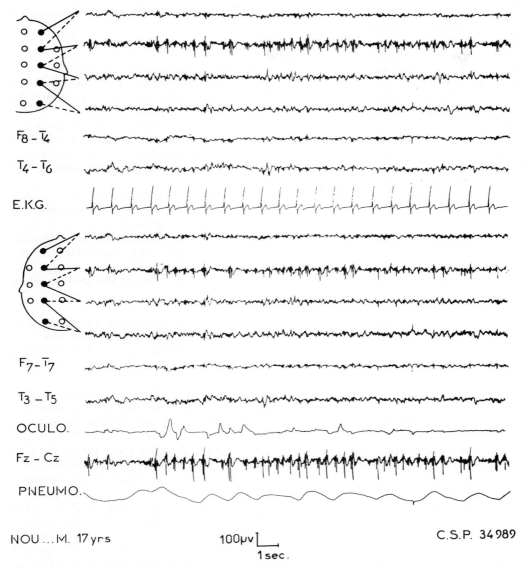

F₈ – T₄

T₄ – T₆

E.K.G.

F₇ – T₇

T₃ – T₅

OCULO.

Fz – Cz

PNEUMO.

NOU...M. 17 yrs   100μv | C.S.P. 34 989
                              1 sec.

Fig. 2. Appearance, during the course of REM sleep, of rapid polyspikes in the central and vertex regions.

On the EEG, except for transient episodes generally related to therapeutic overdosage, the background rhythm remains normal and sleep patterns are well organized. There exist generalized paroxysmal abnormalities of spikes, spike-waves and polyspike-waves precipitated by IPS, but not increased during slow wave sleep. During rapid eye movement (REM) sleep, there appear characteristic abnormalities constitued by rapid polyspikes localized in the central and vertex regions (Fig 2). The generalized paroxysmal discharges tend to diminish during the evolution (Tassinari *et al.,* 1974).

There exist typical modifications of somato-sensitive evoked potential (SEP)

(Mauguiere *et al.,* 1981) which are of a very exaggerated amplitude (often multiplied by 10 or more) — 'giant response' — .

(2) *'Cherry-red spot myoclonus syndrome'*

It is a sialidosis with an isolated deficit in neuraminidase (Rapin *et al.,* 1978).
The age of onset is variable, but it is most often in adolescence. The first manifestations are either a reduction of visual acuity, or a cerebellar syndrome, or in half the cases a myoclonus or epilepsy.

The neurological picture, when the disease is established, is very similar to that of the Ramsay-Hunt syndrome: intention and action myoclonus, photosensitivity, cerebellar syndrome, absence of mental deterioration. The only distinctive features are the nearly constant existence of amblyopia and the discovery of a cherry-red spot on funduscopic examination.

The EEG and polygraphic picture is only described in sufficient detail in a small number of cases. It resembles that of DCM, however with the following peculiarities: the massive myoclonus corresponding to the generalized polyspike-waves are much more frequent, the polyspike-wave discharges always correspond to a massive myoclonus; the discharges and the jerks are not provoked by IPS; abnormal SEPs also exist (Engel *et al.,* 1977).

The functional evolution is most often unfavourable because of the severity of the myoclonus and of its resistance to therapy.

Mention must be made of cases that are rare but which appear to be increasing in the literature, characterized by a clinical and EEG profile similar to that of Ramsay-Hunt syndrome, associated with mitochondrial myopathy (Fukhuara *et al.,* 1980; Fitzimons *et al.,* 1981; Roger *et al.,* 1982 *b).*

It appears from this survey that in fact the clinical and EEG picture and, in particular, the early manifestations of each one of the diseases that we have described are variable, and thus for each of them the differential diagnosis at onset has to be elaborately considered.

On the other hand, in a large number of cases, there are signs which permit the diagnosis of the illness before the complete picture of PME is realized: visceral signs, funduscopic abnormalities, EEG tracings, biochemical and morphological study results of lymphocyte, muscular and hepatic biopsies.

Under these conditions one can ask whether retaining the concept of PME is anything other than an old habit that should be abandoned. We feel that ultimately it should. However the problem is more complex than indicated in this review. There are still many unclassifiable observations for which the clinical presentation is extremely varied. There exist in the literature some cases of myoclonic epilepsies which are slowly progressive and associated with diverse neurological symptoms (dystonia, retinitis pigmentosa) sometimes of dominant and sometimes of recessive transmission and which do not correspond to the description of Koskiniemi PME (van Bogaert, 1968: Takahata and Suzuki, 1980)

On the other hand, there are rare observations where the clinical picture is very near to that of Lafora's disease but for which the anatomical studies only show non-specific degenerative lesions (Matthews *et al.,* 1969; Haltia *et al.,* 1969).

In anticipation of a better classification of these cases and the discovery of errors of metabolism which support them, it appears justified to retain a group that we propose to call Progressive Myoclonic Epilepsies of unknown etiology.

References

Carpenter, S., Karpati, G. (1981): Sweat gland duct cells in Lafora disease: diagnosis by skin biopsy. *Neurology* **31,** 1564-1568.

Claes, C., Carpenter, G. (1967): Sur la forme juvénile de la maladie de Gaucher. *J. Neurol. Sci.* **4,** 571-582.

Diebold, K. (1973): *Die erblichen myoklonisch-epileptisch dementiellen Kern syndrome.* Springer: Berlin.

Eldridge, R., Iivanainen, M., Stern, R., Koerber, I., Wilder, B.J., (1983): "Baltic" Myoclonus Epilepsy: hereditary disorder of childhood made worse by phenytoin. *Lancet* **2,** 838-842.

Engel, J., Rapin, I., Giblin, D.R. (1977): Electrophysiological studies in two patients with cherry red spot-myoclonus syndrome. *Epilepsia* **18,** 73-87.

Fitzimons, R.B., Clifton-Bligh, P., Wolfenden, W.H. (1981): Mitochondrial myopathy and lactic acidemia with myoclonic epilepsy, ataxia and hypothalamic infertility. A variant of Ramsay-Hunt syndrome. *J. Neurol. Neurosurg. Psychiat.* **44,** 79-81.

Fukuhara, N., Tokiguchi, S., Shirakawa, K., Tsubaki, T. (1980): Myoclonus epilepsy associated with ragged-red fibers (Mitochondrial abnormalities) disease entity or a syndrome? Light and electron microscopic studies in two cases and review of literature. *J. Neurol. Sci.* **47,** 117-133.

Haltia, M., Kristenson, K., Sourander, P. (1969): Neuropathological studies in three scandinavian cases of progressive myoclonus epilepsy. *Acta Neurol. Scand.* **45,** 63-77.

Herrlin, K.M., Hillborg, P.O. (1962): Neurological signs in a juvenile form of Gaucher's disε ;. *Acta Paediatr.* **51,** 137-157.

Hunt. J.R. (1921): Dyssynergia cerebellaris myoclonica. Primary atrophy of the Dentate system. A contribution to the pathology and symptomatology of the cerebellum. *Brain* **44,** 490-538.

Koskiniemi, M. (1974): Psychological findings in progressive myoclonus epilepsy without Lafora bodies. *Epilepsia,* **15,** 537-545.

Koskiniemi, M., Toivakka, E., Donner, M. (1974*a*): Progressive myoclonus epilepsy. Electroencephalographical findings. *Acta Neurol. Scand.* **50,** 333-359.

Koskiniemi, M., Donner, M., Majuri, H., Haltia, M., Norio, R. (1974*b*): Progressive myoclonus epilepsy. A clinical and histopatological study. *Acta Neurol. Scand.* **50,** 307-332.

Lundborg, H. (1903): *Die progressive Myoklonus epilepsie.* Almquist and Wiksell: Upsala.

Lundborg, H. (1913): *Medizinisch-biologische Familienforschung.* Fischer: Jena.

Matthews, W.B., Howell, D.A., Stevens, D.L. (1969): Progressive myoclonus epilepsy without Lafora bodies. *J. Neurol. Neurosurg. Psychiatr.* **32,** 116-122.

Mauguiere, F., Bard, J., Courjon, J. (1981): Les potentiels évoqués somesthésiques précoces dans la dyssynergie cérébelleuse myoclonique progressive. *Rev. EEG. Neurophysiol.* **11,** 174-182.

Nishimura, R., Omos-Lau, N., Ajmone-Marsan, C., Baranger, J.A. (1980): Electroencephalographic findings in Gaucher Disease. *Neurology* **30,** 152-159.

Pampiglione, G., Harden, A. (1977): So-called neuronal ceroïd lipofuscinosis. Neurophysiological studies in 60 children. *J. Neurol. Neurosurg. Psychiatr.* **40,** 323-330.

Rapin, I., Goldfischer, S., Katzman, R., Engel, J., O'Brien, J.S. (1978): The cherry-red spot — myoclonus syndrome. *Ann. Neurol.* **3,** 234-242.

Roger, J., Soulayrol, R., Hassoun, J. (1968): La dyssynergie cérébelleuse myoclonique (syndrome de Ramsay-Hunt). *Rev. Neurol.* **119,** 85-106.

Roger, J., Bureau, M., Gobbi, G. (1982*a*): L'épilepsie dans les maladies par erreur innée du métabolisme chez le grand enfant et l'adolescent. *Bol. Lega It. Epil.* **39,** 137-142.

Roger, J., Pellissier, J.F., Dravet, C., Bureau-Paillas, M., Arnoux, M., Larrieu, J.L. (1982*b*): Dégénérescence spinocérébelleuse. Atrophie optique-Epilepsie-Myoclonus-Myopathie mitochondriale. *Rev. Neurol.* **138,** 187-200.

Roger, J., Pellissier, J.F. Bureau, M., Dravet, C., Revol, M., Tinuper, P. (1983): Le diagnostic précoce de la maladie de Lafora. Importance des manifestations paroxystiques visuelles et intérêt de la biopsie cutanée. *Rev. Neurol.* **139,** 115-124.

Sjögren, T. (1931): Die Juvenile amaurotische idiotie-Klinische und Erblichkeits medizinische u:..ersuchungen. *Hereditas (Lund)* **14,** 197-426.

Takahata, N., Suzuki, H. (1980): Neuropathological studies on hereditary ataxia with variable involuntary movements. In I. Sobue, *Spinocerebellar degenerations,* pp. 209-222. University of Tokio Press.

Tassinari, C.A., Bureau-Paillas, M., Dalla Bernardina, B., Grasso, E., Roger, J. (1974): Etude électroencéphalographique de la dyssynergie cérébelleuse myoclonique avec épilepsie (syndrome de Ramsay-Hunt). *Rev. EEG Neurophysiol.* **4,** 407-428.

Tassinari, C.A., Bureau-Paillas, M., Dalla Bernardina, B., Picornell-Darder, I., Mouren, M.C., Dravet, C., Roger, J. (1978): La maladie de Lafora. *Rev. EEG Neurophysiol.* **8,** 107-122.

Unverricht, H. (1891): *Die Myoclonie.* Franz Deuticke: Leipzig.

Van Bogaert, L. (1968): L'épilepsie-myoclonie progressive d'Unverricht-Lundborg et le problème des encéphalopathies progressives associant épilepsie et myoclonies. *Rev. Neurol.* **119,** 47-57.

Van Heycop Ten Ham, M.W., De Jaeger, H. (1963): Progressive myoclonus epilepsy with Lafora- bodies. Clinical pathological features. *Epilepsia* **4,** 95-119.

Zeman, W., Donahue, S., Dyken, P., Green, J. (1970): The neuronal ceroïd-lipofuscinoses (Batten-Vogt syndrome). In *Handbook of clinical neurology,* Vol. 10, pp. 588-679, ed P.S. Vinken, G.W. Bruyn. North-Holland: Amsterdam.

*　　　　*　　　　*

Discussion
Summarized by Joseph ROGER

Aicardi considers that in the majority of cases the problem of diagnosis has to be faced before the complete PME syndrome has developed and that therefore the nosological concept of PME should not be retained. Perhaps the problem persists with respect to a heterogeneous syndrome such as DCM where various modes of transmission exist.

Roger points out that it is difficult for any observer to have an overall view of this problem since the prevalence of these different disorders varies greatly from country to country. In the north of Europe there are probably many more so-called myoclonic degenerative epilepsies of uncertain etiology than there are in Mediterranean countries.

Henriksen adds that the disorder described by Koskiniemi apparently only exists in Finland and he does not believe that cases are seen in Norway or Sweden.

Dreifuss explains that in the USA there is a not negligible number of cases of PME with a fairly slow evolution which are certainly not of the Lafora type. He has personally observed cases in three families without Finnish origin.

Lerman has also observed a certain number of cases of this type in Israel.

We therefore conclude that this syndromic concept of PME ought only to be retained for disorders of unknown etiology and of imprecise nosological diagnosis.

Epileptic syndromes in infancy, childhood and adolescence. J. Roger, C. Dravet, M. Bureau, F.E. Dreifuss and P. Wolf. John Libbey Eurotext Ltd ©1985.

Afterword
The International Classification of Epilepsies and the Marseille Workshop

Peter WOLF

Chairman of the Commission on Classification and Terminology of the International League against Epilepsy

The need for an internationally accepted classification of epileptic syndromes and epilepsies is being increasingly felt, and the process of its development is fully under way. The Commission on Classification and Terminology of the International League against Epilepsy (members: Drs Dreifuss, Martinez-Lage, Roger, Seino and Wolf) is busy with the preparation of a new proposal.

The reviews and discussions from the Marseille workshop give a lively insight into one stage of the development of this classification, as well as into many of the problems involved.

More problems were raised at this meeting than could possibly be solved and, clearly, the different syndromatic concepts have reached various stages of development. Some entities, like the major syndromes of generalized idiopathic epilepsy, are well established, and there was general agreement about their fundamental definitions. In other respects, divergent views were put forward. Some discussants searched for broad concepts of syndromes that may cover various disorders considered as subvarieties. Other participants favoured a classification which distinguishes many separate syndromes, some of which may differ only slightly from one another. In one specific instance, the conflicting views could not be resolved, and the opposing viewpoints about the nosological place of myoclonic-astatic epilepsy are, therefore, set forth side by side in this volume. Finally, the discussion of some disorders, such as epilepsy with continuous spike-waves in slow sleep, is at a very early stage and the question of the possible relationship of this disorder to the syndrome of acquired epileptic aphasia has only been touched upon fleetingly.

The nomenclature used during the workshop was all but uniform, and the editors have left it at that (except when editing some of the discussions). The attentive reader will note that the International Classification of Epileptic Seizures in its latest version has not always been respected by all authors. Within its pages, this volume thus demonstrates clearly the urgent necessity of reaching its own goal, that is the classification of syndromes as a logical complement to the classification of seizures, so that exact and unequivocal nomenclature becomes possible on both levels.

The Marseille meeting has been an important aid to the work of the Commission, and its proceedings will doubtless be reflected in the syndromic classification which will be proposed by the Commission in the coming year.

Epileptic syndromes in infancy, childhood and adolescence. J. Roger, C. Dravet, M. Bureau, F.E. Dreifuss and P. Wolf. John Libbey Eurotext Ltd ©1985.

A Proposal for a Definition of Epileptic Syndromes in Infancy, Childhood and Adolescence

On the last day of the meeting, every reviewer proposed a detailed definition of the syndrome that he had to present. This definition was discussed by all the participants.

The reviewers judged that it was not possible, in our present state of knowledge, to define accurately any syndrome of the epilepsies in inborn errors of metabolism in infants and children, photosensitive epilepsies, epilepsy with unilateral seizures and lesional partial epilepsies out of the Kojewnikow syndrome.

The definitions adopted for the other syndromes do not imply a complete and unanimous agreement but only a general consensus based on a compromise.

They are listed in the following pages.

Benign Neonatal Convulsions
Perrine Plouin

Very frequently repeated convulsions, occurring around the 5th day of life, at present without known aetiology.

In most cases interictal EEG abnormalities are 'théta pointu alternant'.

There is no recurrence of convulsions or epileptic seizures.

The psychomotor development is normal.

Benign Neonatal Familial Convulsions
Perrine Plouin

Rare syndrome, with a dominant inheritance.

Characterized by repeated convulsions occurring mostly on 2nd and 3rd days of life.

There are no EEG criteria.

In a low percentage of cases recurrent seizures can occur in childhood or later in life.

Early Myoclonic Encephalopathy

Jean Aicardi

The principal characteristics of this syndrome are:

Onset before 3 months
Fragmentary myoclonus from onset
Partial seizures (erratic)
Massive myoclonias and/or tonic spasms
EEG: suppression-burst activity
Evolving into atypical hypsarrhythmia
Severe course. Complete lack of psychomotor development. Frequently death
  before 1 year
Frequent familial cases, suggesting the possibility of one or several congenital
  metabolism errors, but this familiarity is not constant

This Early Myoclonic Encephalopathy is probably different from the Early Infantile
Epileptic Encephalopathy (EIEE) described by Ohtahara, which comprises only tonic
spasms and suppression-burst activity.

Febrile Convulsions

Niall O'Donohoe

Syndrome of late infancy and early childhood
Age-dependent: 6 months to 5 years
Incidence: 3% of population at risk
Important genetic predisposition
A response to a sudden, rapid temperature rise
Close association with virus infections
Seizures: brief, generalized, but lateralizing or focal features are common even in brief seizures.

Duration of FC: of paramount importance — if longer than 15-30 min. potentially damaging to brain. Greater risk of prolonged FC in females younger than 18 months
— majority of FCs are brief, 'simple'
— prolonged FCs are usually first attacks
— prolonged FCs, i.e. 'complicated', may give transient or permanent neurological sequelae.

Complicated seizures can occur in two circumstances:
(a) normal child, strong genetic predisposition, acute viral illness
(b) child who is neurologically and mentally suspect, due to pre- or perinatal insult, develops an acute febrile illness
Is (b) a different syndrome?

EEG: doubtful value in prognosis

Overall prognosis: excellent (less hopeful before 1 year)
Spontaneous remission is the rule
Less than 4% overall later develop epilepsy.

West Syndrome

Peter M. Jeavons

I — *Typical West syndrome*
  Spasms
  Mental retardation (or mental deterioration)
  Hypsarrhythmia
Onset before age 1 year, with a peak between 3 and 7 months.
Two types:
  (a) primary, idiopathic, cryptogenic
  (b) secondary, symptomatic.

II — May be *included* in West syndrome, as *atypical West syndromes:*
  - spasms and mental retardation without hypsarrhythmia, but with paroxysmal EEG abnormalities
  - spasms and hypsarrhythmia without mental retardation
  - mental retardation and hypsarrhythmia without spasms
  - mental retardation and hypsarrhythmia with 'staring seizures' (tonic seizures on polygraphic records). This type is probably an early Lennox-Gastaut syndrome, but borderlines are imprecise.
  - onset before 3 months
  - Aicardi syndrome.

III — Must be *excluded:*
  - benign myoclonus of early infancy (Lombroso and Fejerman)
  - early myoclonic-astatic fits
  - Early Infantile Epileptic Encephalopathy (Ohtahara)
  - onset after 4 months with two normal EEGs, including sleep
  - onset after 1 year

Infantile Myoclonic Epilepsy with Favourable Outcome or Benign Myoclonic Epilepsy in Infancy

Charlotte Dravet

Generalized *myoclonic fits,* several a day, in normal infants, without antecedents but simple febrile convulsions or family history, occurring between 6 months and 3 years

EEG — ictal: fast, generalized spike-waves and multiple spike-waves
— interictal: normal background activity, rare spike-waves,
— always spike-waves during sleep

Easily controlled by treatment
No other type of seizure
Normal psychomotor development

Severe Myoclonic Epilepsy in Infancy

Charlotte Dravet

Generalized and/or unilateral *clonic seizures,* febrile and/or afebrile, in normal infants, without antecedents but frequent family history, occurring in the first year
Later appearance of associated *myoclonic fits,* between 8 months and 4 years

EEG: normal at the initial stage, then showing fast, generalized spike-waves and focal abnormalities, not modified by sleep. ILS: early positive.

Occurrence of partial seizures and atypical absences

Inefficacy of treatment

Psychomotor development: normal in the first stage, slowing down after 2 years

Neurological signs: variable ataxia and myoclonus.

Myoclonic Astatic Epilepsy (Cortico Reticular Epilepsy with Minor Seizures (and Grand Mal) of Early Childhood)

Hermann Doose

Incidence: 1-2% of all epilepsies up to age 9
Age of onset: 7 months to 6 years, mostly between 2 and 5 years
Sex ratio: boys/girls: 2 : 1, except if onset in the first year
Individual history: mostly normal until onset, except in 12% of the cases
Genetics: 37% affected families
   prevalence in siblings: 16%
   prevalence in parents: 6%
   polygenically determined disposition.

Symptomatology:
   myoclonic fits, astatic fits, myoclonic astatic fits, absences with myoclonias and/or atonia, tonic-clonic seizures, febrile or afebrile
   frequent status (36%)
   tonic seizures only in the late course of unfavourable cases.

EEG:
   initially often only 4-7 c/s rhythms
   irregular fast spike-waves and polyspike-waves
   2-3 c/s spike-waves during status, often very irregular
   only *rarely* focal abnormalities.

Course: variable
   onset with grand mal, followed by myoclonic and/or astatic fits (and absences)
   onset with minor seizures (myoclonic and/or astatic) followed by grand mal
   only minor seizures (myoclonic and/or astatic)

Prognosis: Unfavourable in 50 % with development of dementia, persisting grand mal and tonic seizures during night. On the other hand, favourable course with good response to valproate/ethosuximid (and phenobarbital).

Differential diagnosis:
- West syndrome
- Lennox-Gastaut syndrome: mostly normal development before onset, no daytime tonic seizures, rarely typical focal seizures, no complex partial seizures, no atypical absences, no multifocal EEG abnormalities, as a rule no neurological deficits (only in the late course)

Lennox-Gastaut Syndrome

Anne Beaumanoir

Symptomatic triad

1. *Epileptic seizures* — The typical ones are:

    axial tonic seizures
    atypical absences
    atonic seizures

Other types of seizures are frequently associated: myoclonias, generalized tonic-clonic seizures, partial seizures.
All these seizures are very frequent and difficult to control from the onset.
Status epilepticus are common: stupor status with myoclonias, tonic and atonic seizures.

2. *EEG abnormalities*

- awake: abnormal background activity
           slow spike-waves, less than 3 c/s, diffuse, anteriorly accentuated
           multifocal abnormalities frequently associated
- sleep: bursts of fast rhythms, around 10 c/s.

3. *Slowing in mental development* with personality disorders

Age of onset from 1 to 8 years, rarely afterward.
Unfavourable outcome.

III — EPILEPTIC SYNDROMES IN CHILDHOOD

Childhood Absence Epilepsy

Pierre Loiseau

A form of primary generalized epilepsy occurring in normal children (peak: 6-7 years), mostly in girls
Strong genetic predisposition
Beginning with absence seizures
Very frequent absences of any kind, apart from myoclonic absences.

EEG: bilateral, synchronous, symmetrical 3 c/s spike-waves (sometimes less regular); normal background activity.

Evolution:
    1 — remission
    2 — rare persistence of absences only
    3 — tonic-clonic seizures during adolescence or later.

Epilepsy with Myoclonic Absences

Carlo Alberto Tassinari

Seizures: clonic jerks, diffuse, rhythmically repeated (in relation with 3 c/s spike-waves) and frequent association of *tonic* contraction.
    Frequency: daily.

Ictal EEG: generalized 3 c/s spike-waves, as in typical absences.
Interictal EEG: usually normal background activity and isolated generalized spike-waves

Onset around 7 years
Male preponderance
Neurological condition before MA: usually normal
Associated seizures: rare tonic-clonic seizures (20 %).

Prognosis: poor, because of:
- resistance to treatment
- mental deterioration
- evolution in other epilepsy with poor prognosis.

Benign Partial Epilepsies

Bernardo Dalla Bernardina

The following criteria concern the epilepsies of childhood with partial seizures and focal EEG abnormalities, which are age-dependent, without demonstrable anatomical lesions and which recover spontaneously.

Clinical criteria:
- no neurological deficit
- no intellectual deficit
- family history of benign epilepsy
- onset after 18 months
- seizures usually brief and rare, sometimes frequent at the onset, but only for a short period and not increasing in frequency after, responding well to treatment
- seizures variable in symptomatology but not polymorphous in the same child (neither tonic nor atonic)
- no post-ictal prolonged deficit
- no impairment of neurological and psychological development.

EEG criteria:
- normal background activity
- focal abnormalities with 'rolandic spikes-like' morphology
- possible multifocal similar independent abnormalities
- possible brief bursts of generalized spike-waves discharges, not increasing during slow sleep
- normal sleep organization
- increase of focal abnormalities during sleep, but without morphological changes, without fast polyspikes, without EEG depression following spikes, without bilateralization evoking continuous generalized spike-waves.

A number of these criteria may be lacking in certain cases of benign partial epilepsy. For example a child with a neurological deficit can have a benign partial epilepsy, or an increase of generalized spikes can occur during sleep. But, the greater the number of these criteria are fulfilled in a patient, the more probable is the diagnosis of benign partial epilepsy.

Benign Partial Epilepsy with Centro-Temporal Spikes of Childhood

Pinchas Lerman

The most frequent and the best known of the benign partial epilepsies.

Genetic predisposition
Male predominance
Onset between 3 and 13 years (peak: 9-10 years)
Recovery before 15-16 years

Seizures: brief, hemifacial motor, with frequent associated somato-sensory symptoms, usually nocturnal, sometimes tending to become generalized in this case

EEG: blunt, high voltage centro-temporal spikes, often followed by slow-waves, activated by sleep and tending to spread and/or to shift from side to side.

Benign Partial Epilepsy of Childhood with Occipital Paroxysms

Henri Gastaut

This epilepsy is characterized by:

(1) interictally, paroxysms of high amplitude spike-waves or sharp waves, recurring more or less rhythmically on the occipital and postero-temporal areas of one or both hemispheres, and occurring only when the eyes are closed.

(2) ictally, initial visual symptoms (amaurosis, phosphens, visual illusions or hallucinations), often followed by a hemiclonic seizure or by automatisms when the occipital discharge spreads to central or temporal regions.

(3) immediately after the fits, in a quarter of the cases, the appearance of migrainous cephalalgia.

The other features are those of benign partial epilepsies in general.

Other forms of Benign Partial Epilepsy

Two other forms of benign partial epilepsy have been described but their individualization is not yet evident.

I — *Benign partial epilepsy with affective symptoms during the attacks*
The ictal symptomatology is mainly constituted by a terror feeling and autonomic signs, without evident loss of consciousness. EEG abnormalities are variable, situated in frontal and mid-temporal areas.

II — *Benign partial epilepsy with extreme somato-sensory evoked potentials*
In children presenting with an extreme somato-sensory potential evoked by heel tapping, later appearance of spontaneous EEG abnormalities, located in the parietal area, and later on partial motor seizures with adversion, spontaneously recovering.

Landau-Kleffner Syndrome

Anne Beaumanoir

Language disorders: regression of previously acquired language skills, often associated with auditory agnosia and behaviour disorders, without intellectual deterioration.

EEG abnormalities:
- normal basal rhythm
- profuse and nearly always bilateral spikes or spike-waves, variable in time and space but most often temporal, and subcontinuous during slow sleep

In 2/3 of the patients *one or a few seizures* of variable types and appearing especially during sleep.

Evolution: disappearance of seizures and of EEG abnormalities before adolescence. Improvement of language in the majority of cases.

N.B. Must cases without seizures be excluded from the definition of an epileptic syndrome?

Epilepsy with Continuous Spike-Waves During Slow Sleep Otherwise Described as ESES (Epilepsy with Status Epilepticus during Slow Sleep)

Carlo Alberto Tassinari

This syndrome represents a situation resulting from the association of:

(1) various epileptic conditions, usually characterized by atypical absences with diffuse spike-waves, and rare nocturnal, partial or generalized, motor seizures, but *never tonic* seizures, and

(2) from the EEG point of view, continuous, diffuse spike-waves during slow sleep. This pattern occurs after the onset of seizures and its duration is variable, from some months to some years.

This syndrome is a self-limited, age-related condition of childhood.

Prognosis: frequently reserved because of the appearance of behavioural and various neuropsychological disturbances, despite the usually benign evolution of seizures.

IV — EPILEPTIC SYNDROMES IN CHILDHOOD AND ADOLESCENCE

Juvenile Absence Epilepsy

Peter Wolf

Primary generalized epilepsy of age-related onset, with absences that do not differ from those of childhood
Onset is around puberty
Seizure frequency is low (less than one/day), and repetition sporadic
Sex distribution is equal
If there are generalized tonic-clonic seizures they mostly occur on awakening
The EEG mostly shows rapid (> 3 c/s) spikes and waves.

Juvenile Myoclonic Epilepsy

Peter Wolf

Primary generalized epilepsy with age-related onset (pre- to post-puberty), characterized by seizures with bilateral, single or repetitive, arrhythmic, irregular myoclonic jerks, predominantly in the arms. A minority of patients may suddenly fall. No disturbance of consciousness can be noticed.
The aetiology is not known
In some of the cases the disorder is inherited
Often there are additional generalized tonic-clonic seizures
All seizures occur predominantly shortly after awakening and are often precipitated by sleep withdrawal
The ictal EEG shows rapid (> 3 c/s) generalized, often irregular spike-waves and polyspike-waves, that are also found interictally
There is no close phase correlation between EEG spikes and jerks.
Frequently the patients are photosensitive.

Epilepsy with Generalized Tonic-Clonic Seizures on Awakening

Peter Wolf

Primary generalized epilepsy with generalized tonic-clonic seizures, manifesting exclusively or predominantly (over 90%) shortly after awakening (not considering the time of day). There may be a second peak in the evening
Onset is mostly in the second decade
The aetiology is usually unknown.
If there are other seizures those are mostly absences or myoclonic seizures, like in Benign Juvenile Myoclonic Epilepsy
Seizures may be precipitated by sleep withdrawal
The EEG shows one of the patterns of generalized primary epilepsies.

Benign Partial Seizures of Adolescents

Pierre Loiseau

Onset: 10-20 years. Peak: 13-14 years
Sex: male predominance
No family or personal history of epileptic predisposition
Normal neurological and mental status
Seizures: various types, mainly with motor and/or sensory symptoms. In 2/3 of cases, secondary generalization
One seizure, or a cluster of 2-5 seizures in less than 24 hours
Normal EEG or mild abnormalities.

Kojewnikow's Syndrome

Jean Bancaud

Two types of Kojewnikow's Syndrome are now recognized but only one of these two types has to be included among the epileptic syndromes of childhood because the other one is not specifically related to this age.

The first type represents a particular form of rolandic partial epilepsy, in both adults and children, related to a variable lesion of the motor cortex. Its principal features are:
- motor partial seizures, always well localized
- often late appearance of myoclonias in the same site where there are somato-motor seizures
- EEG: normal background activity and focal paroxysmal abnormalities (spikes and slow waves)
- occurrence at any age in childhood and adulthood
- frequently demonstrable aetiology (tumoral, vascular....)
- no progressive evolution of the syndrome (neither clinical, neither electroencephalographic, nor psychological) except the evolutive character of the causal lesion.

The second type is peculiar to child and adolescent:
- onset between 2 and 10 years (peak at 6 years)
- unknown aetiology
- seizures are motor partial seizures but often associated with other types of seizures
- myoclonias early appear in the course of the illness (before the seizures or simultaneously), are initally localized then become erratic and diffuse, and persist during sleep
- a progressive motor deficit occurs and other neurological signs can be associated with it
- a mental deterioration is observed
- EEG: abnormal background activity, which is asymmetric and slow, diffuse delta slow waves, numerous ictal and interictal discharges not strictly limited to the rolandic area
- the anatomical lesion, demonstrated by neuroradiological investigation, is diffuse and progressive.

The electro-clinical picture is that of a malignant progressive disease of which a viral aetiology is strongly suspected.

Progressive Myoclonic Epilepsy of Unknown Aetiology

Joseph Roger

Progressive myoclonic epilepsy is *clinically* characterized by:
(1) a myoclonic symptomatology, including combined fragmentary and segmentary, arrhythmic, asynchronous, asymmetric myoclonias and massive myoclonias
(2) an epileptic symptomatology, with seizures of various types, mostly generalized tonic-clonic, myoclonic and tonic
(3) a progressive mental deterioration leading to dementia
(4) a progressive neurological symptomatology with cerebellar, pyramidal and extra-pyramidal signs.

Concerning the EEG there is:
 - a deterioration of the background rhythms
 - a progressive alteration of the sleep organization
 - paroxysmal abnormalities such as generalized, fast or slow spikes and spike-waves and multifocal abnormalities.

Specific diseases which can realize this electro-clinical picture are usually recognizable and their early diagnosis is possible (ceroid-lipofuscinosis, Lafora disease...).
But other specific diseases have a different course and never give exactly this type of picture (cherry-red spot myoclonus, dyssynergia cerebellaris myoclonica).

Index

Encephalitis, 297
Encephalopathy
    early infantile epileptic, 20, 27-28, 47
    early myoclonic, 12-21, 46, 315
    non progressive, 68-72
Epilepsy
    benign myoclonic in infants, 46, 51-57, 65, 318
    benign partial, 95, 137-149, 322
    benign partial with affective seizures, 137-149, 171-175, 324
    benign partial with centro-temporal spikes, 116-117, 137-149, 150-158, 179, 201, 211, 282, 323
    benign partial with extreme somato-sensory evoked potentials, 176-180, 324
    benign partial with occipital paroxysms, 137-149, 159-170, 323
    childhood absence, 106-120, 321
    idiopathic generalized, 242-246, 247-258, 259-270, 320, 326, 327
    — see also primary generalized epilepsy
    intermediate generalized, 116, 128, 272
    juvenile absence, 242-246, 326
    juvenile myoclonic, 128, 247-258, 326
    lesional with partial seizures, 95, 115, 161-162, 173-174, 217-220, 278-285
    myoclonic astatic, 46, 66, 78-88, 95-96, 319
    myoclonic in non progressive encephalopathy, 68-72
    myoclonic with mitochondrial myopathy, 76, 308
    partialis continua, 286-298, 328
    photosensitive, 232-236, 237-241
    primary generalized, 34, 56, 78-79, 117, 130-136, 220
    — see also idiopathic generalized epilepsy
    progressive myoclonic, 256-257, 302-310, 329
    secondary generalized, 65-66, 96, 128
    severe myoclonic, 55-56, 58-67, 318
    with centro-temporal spikes — see benign partial
    with continuous spike-waves during slow sleep, 194-204, 205-212, 325
    with generalized convulsive seizures in childhood, 130-136
    with generalized tonic-clonic seizures on awakening, 259-270, 327
    with myoclonic absences, 121-129, 321
    with occipital paroxysms — see benign partial epilepsy
    with unilateral seizures, 216-221, 222-227
Ethosuximide, 7, 240
Evoked potentials
    somato-sensory, 176-180, 324
    visual, 75-76

F
Febrile convulsions, 34-41, 59, 65, 79, 80, 316
Fever — see febrile convulsions

G
Gaucher's disease, 303
Genetics, 7-8, 18-19, 34-35, 43, 51-52, 59, 73-77, 79-80, 90, 108-109, 122, 138, 155, 215, 243, 248-249, 261, 302-310

Grand mal — see generalized tonic-clonic seizures

H
Hematoma (intracerebral), 26
HHE (Hemiconvulsion-Hemiplegia-Epilepsy syndrome), 36, 39, 41, 216, 221, 226, 280
Hyperglycinaemia (non ketotic), 19, 23, 74
Hypsarrhythmia, 15, 44

I
Inborn errors of metabolism, 19-20, 73-77, 302-310
Infantile spasms, 42-50, 73, 86
Infarct (cerebral), 26, 279
IPS — see photosensitivity

J
Jansky-Bielschowsky disease, 75-76

K
Kojewnikow syndrome, 286-298, 328

L
Lafora disease, 304
Landau-Kleffner syndrome, 142, 181-191, 192-193, 202, 214, 324
Lennox-Gastaut syndrome, 42, 44, 47, 55, 65, 75, 86, 89-99, 100-104, 127, 183, 202, 205-212, 217-220, 320
    myoclonic variant, 71, 94

M
Malformations (cerebral), 19-20, 23, 28-29, 45, 47, 266-268
Mental impairment, 65, 82-86, 93-94, 115, 127, 156-157, 182, 199-200, 214, 249, 263-264, 289, 296-297, 302-306
Migraine, 162, 213
Mucolipidosis type 1, 75-76
Myoclonus
    benign of early infancy, 46, 55
    epileptic, 14-17, 51-57, 59, 74-76, 234-235, 287-295, 302-310
    physiological, 257
Myopathy (mitochondrial), 76, 308

N
Neonatal convulsions, 2-11, 12-22, 23-31
    benign, 2-11, 314
    familial benign, 7-8, 314
    idiopathic (5th day), 4-6, 314
Neuropathology, 19, 266-268

P
Pavor nocturnus, 173
Petit mal, 106-108, see also childhood absence epilepsy
    impulsive — see juvenile myoclonic epilepsy

intermediate — see intermediate generalized epilepsy
myoclonic — see juvenile myoclonic epilepsy and benign myoclonic epilepsy in infancy
myoclonic-astatic, 46, 56, 78-88, 95-96
Phenobarbital, 156, 173, 179, 256, 269
Phenytoin, 156, 179, 269, 306
Photosensitivity, 53, 60, 76, 82, 232-236, 237-241, 245, 250-254, 265, 303-308
Poliodystrophy, 19
Prognosis, 6, 7, 10-11, 28, 36-37, 46, 55, 64-65, 71, 82-86, 96, 113-115, 127, 136, 156, 161, 173-174, 196, 245, 256, 268-269, 275, 283-284
Prophylaxis, 37
Psychic symptoms — see mental impairment
Pyknolepsy, 107-108, 242
    — see also childhood absence epilepsy
Pyridoxine-dependency, 26, 73-74

R
Ramsay-Hunt syndrome, 306-308
Rhythms
    10 c/s, fast, 93, 123
    theta 4-7 c/s, 60, 82, 86
    delta posterior, 112-113, 114

S
Sandhoff disease, 74-75
Santavuori-Haltia-Hagberg disease, 74
Seizures
    atonic or astatic, 81, 92, 101
    benign partial s. of adolescence, 274-277, 327
    clonic, 3, 4, 7, 24, 59, 64, 69, 82, 92
    complex partial, 160, 162, 172, 217, 275, 280
    generalized tonic-clonic, 82, 114, 127, 130-136, 196, 244, 249, 262
    grand mal — see generalized tonic-clonic s.
    hemiclonic — see unilateral s.
    inborn errors of metabolism (in), 73-77,
    jacksonian — see motor partial s.
    motor partial, 152-153, 195, 208-209, 288-296
    myoclonic, 52-53, 59-64, 80, 92, 249, 262
    myoclonic atonic or myoclonic astatic, 81, 92
    nocturnal, 82, 86, 90-91, 151-153, 172-173, 195-196
    partial, 14, 59-60, 139
    partial with affective symptoms, 172
    psychomotor — see complex partial s.
    self-induced, 64, 235, 238
    simple partial, 152-153, 160, 178, 195, 209, 275, 280
    tonic, 64, 82, 90-91, 127, 209
    unilateral, 59, 160, 216-221, 222-227
    visual partial, 160, 304
Sialidoses, 75-76, 308
Sleep — see nocturnal seizures and sleep EEG
Spasms, 14-15
    — see also infantile spasms

334

Spielmeyer-Vogt-Sjögren disease, 76, 303
Spike-waves (continuous during slow sleep) — see electrical status during slow sleep
Status epilepticus, 59, 73, 81, 85, 93, 127, 178, 216-221, 297
      electrical during slow sleep, 141, 183, 194-204, 205-212, 325
      myoclonic, 69-70
      neonatal, 4-6, 24-27
Sturge-Weber disease, 279
Suppression-burst, 15-17, 20, 27-28, 44, 74

T
Tay-Sachs disease, 74
Théta pointu alternant, 3-7
Treatment, 37, 45-46, 49, 55, 113-114, 117, 127-128, 156, 245, 256, 268-269
      overdose, 95
Tumor (intracranial), 279

U
Unverricht-Lundborg syndrome, 256, 302, 304-306

V
Valproate (sodium valproate, valproic acid), 39-40, 55, 85, 127, 200, 234, 240, 256
Vanishing EEG, 74

W
West syndrome, 24, 42-50, 55, 90, 317

Z
Zinc deficiency, 6